Dental Implant Prosthetics

Dental Implant Prosthetics

Editor: Victor Martinez

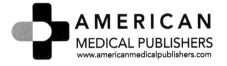

AMERICAN
MEDICAL PUBLISHERS
www.americanmedicalpublishers.com

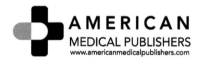
AMERICAN
MEDICAL PUBLISHERS
www.americanmedicalpublishers.com

Cataloging-in-Publication Data

Dental implant prosthetics / edited by Victor Martinez.
   p. cm.
Includes bibliographical references and index.
ISBN 978-1-63927-652-3
1. Dental implants. 2. Prosthodontics. 3. Dentistry. 4. Mouth--Surgery.
5. Mouth--Diseases--Treatment. I. Martinez, Victor.
RK667.I45 D46 2023
617.693--dc23

American Medical Publishers,
41 Flatbush Avenue,
1st Floor, New York,
NY 11217, USA

ISBN 978-1-63927-652-3 (Hardback)

Contents

Preface

Dental implant is a procedure in which an intraoral prosthesis made from titanium screws is implanted into the jawbone to correct defects, like missing teeth, or missing hard or soft structures of the jaw. The principal dental implant prostheses include dental crown, dental bridge, dentures, palatal obturator and orthodontic appliance. The main objective of dental implant prosthetics is to enhance aesthetics, improve mastication and support speech. Fixed prosthodontics or removable dentures can be used for treatment, depending on the health condition of the patient. The angle and position of adjacent teeth determines the position where implants will be fixed. The position is assessed by utilizing computed tomography with CAM simulations, lab simulations and through surgical stents. This book covers in detail some existent and innovative concepts revolving around dental implant prosthetics. It presents researches and studies performed by experts across the globe. This book will prove to be immensely beneficial to students and researchers in this field.

This book is a result of research of several months to collate the most relevant data in the field.

When I was approached with the idea of this book and the proposal to edit it, I was overwhelmed. It gave me an opportunity to reach out to all those who share a common interest with me in this field. I had 3 main parameters for editing this text:

1. Accuracy – The data and information provided in this book should be up-to-date and valuable to the readers.

2. Structure – The data must be presented in a structured format for easy understanding and better grasping of the readers.

3. Universal Approach – This book not only targets students but also experts and innovators in the field, thus my aim was to present topics which are of use to all.

Thus, it took me a couple of months to finish the editing of this book.

I would like to make a special mention of my publisher who considered me worthy of this opportunity and also supported me throughout the editing process. I would also like to thank the editing team at the back-end who extended their help whenever required.

Editor

Development of a New Drill Design to Improve the Temperature Control during the Osteotomy for Dental Implants: A Comparative In Vitro Analysis

Sergio Alexandre Gehrke [1,2,*], Raphaél Bettach [3,4], Benoit Cayron [5], Gilles Boukhris [6], Berenice Anina Dedavid [7] and Juan Carlos Prados Frutos [8]

1 Biotecnos Research Center, Montevideo 11100, Uruguay
2 Department of Biotechnology, Catholic University of Murcia, 30107 Murcia, Spain
3 Department of Cariology and Comprehensive Care, New York University, New York, NY 10010, USA; rbettach@gmail.com
4 Private practice, 77220 Gretz-Armainvilliers, France
5 Private practice, 37000 Tours, France; cayron.benoit@gmail.com
6 Private practice, 75012 Paris, France; boukhrisgilles@gmail.com
7 Department of Materials Engineering, Pontifical Catholic University of Rio Grande do Sul, Porto Alegre 90619-900, Brazil; berenice@pucrs.br
8 Department of Medicine and Surgery, Faculty of Health Sciences, Rey Juan Carlos University, 28933 Madrid, Spain; juancarlos.prados@urjc.es
* Correspondence: sergio.gehrke@hotmail.com

Abstract: The present in vitro study evaluated a new drill design to improve the temperature control during the osteotomies for dental implant installation, comparing with two drill designs that use conventional external irrigation. Three blocks of synthetic cortical bone were used for osteotomy procedures. Three groups were created: control group 1 (Con1), where a conical multiple drill system with a conventional external irrigation system was used; control group 2 (Con2), where a single bur with a conventional external irrigation system was used; and, test group (Test), where the new single bur (turbo drill) with a new irrigation system was used. Twenty osteotomies were made without irrigation and with intense irrigation, for each group. A thermocouple was used to measure the temperature produced during the osteotomies. The measured temperature were: 28.9 ± 1.68 °C for group Con1; 27.5 ± 1.32 °C for group Con2; 26.3 ± 1.28 °C for group Test. Whereas, the measured temperatures with irrigation were: 23.1 ± 1.27 °C for group Con1; 21.7 ± 1.36 °C for group Con2; 19.4 ± 1.29 °C for group Test. The single drill with a new design for improving the irrigation and temperature control, in comparison with the drill designs with conventional external irrigation.

Keywords: dental implants; drill design; irrigation system; osteotomy; thermocouple

1. Introduction

The osteotomy protocols, regardless of the system used, determine that it should be performed with a low-temperature variation, never exceeding 47 °C, as it could denature bone tissue proteins and generate necrosis in that area [1]. Several studies have been developed with different irrigation systems and with different drill designs to improve and decrease trauma during the osteotomy procedure for installing implants and, consequently, reducing inflammatory reactions [2–4].

Recently, Salles and Collaborators (2015) [5], reported through an experimental study using an immunohistochemical analysis for the inflammatory factor NFkB (nuclear factor kappa-light-chain-enhancer of activated B cells), that irrigation plays an important role in controlling this endonuclease and, obviously, in controlling the intensity of the inflammatory process. In this sense, other histological studies have also shown that the healing response of bone tissue around implants can be improved when using drilling systems designed to reduce the trauma caused during osteotomy procedures [6–8].

Regarding the instruments and techniques used to perform osteotomies for the installation of implants, different factors must be considered and analyzed, such as irrigation method (external or internal), drill design, drilling speed, the number of drills (single or multiples), drill material, drilling movement (continuous or intermittent), equipment used (rotary or oscillatory), force applied, among others. For these findings, the methods of evaluating the efficiency of the systems proposed for performing osteotomies, the most used is the evaluation of temperature control during the procedure. To perform these experiments, thermosensors installed near the location where the drilling or infrared sensors can be used, both of which have similar results, but may vary in practicality to the operator during the tests [2,4,9]. In addition, several substrates are used to perform this type of in vitro test, mainly, bone of animal origin and synthetic bone [10].

However, there is no consensus on the ideal system for osteotomy, both in terms of the number of drills, and in terms of their ideal design. In this sense, a device was developed and coupled to the drill shank, creating a new drill design, which has the function of boosting and directing the flow of the irrigating liquid into the bone tissue, thus increasing the effectiveness of refrigeration during the osteotomy procedure. Then, the present in vitro study evaluated this new drill design to improve the temperature control during the osteotomies, comparing with two drill designs (single and multiple sequence) that use conventional external irrigation.

2. Materials and Methods

In this study, two groups of drill systems with conventional external irrigation were used as control and, compared with the new drill design (TURBOdrill®, Implants Diffusion International, Montreuil, France) that features a device attached to its stem to boost and direct the flow of the liquid used for irrigation. This device featured a titanium cylinder with an inverted propeller that received the liquid and, with the rotation of the drill, worked as a turbine. Then, the liquid was driven by the blades down into the socket. In addition, the device served as a stopper to control the exact drilling depth. Figure 1 presents the main characteristics of this new drill design.

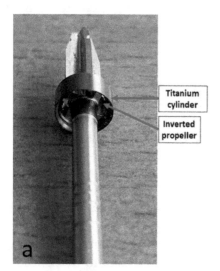 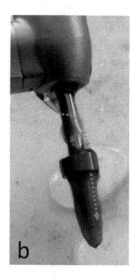 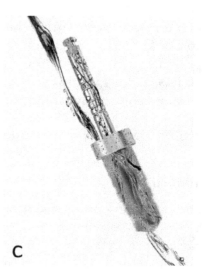

Figure 1. Representative image of the details of new drill design (**a**), that present an accoupled cylinder with an inverted propeller to improve the irrigation. (**b**) The blue arrows indicate the liquid is driven by the propeller down into the blades. (**c**) Schematic image of the path taken by the irrigating liquid.

Thus, three experimental groups were formed, as described below:

Control group 1 (Con1): Multiple drill sequence for a conical implant of 10 mm in length and 4.1 mm in diameter, Straumann (Basel, Switzerland): drill diameters were 2.2 mm (used at 800 rpm), 2.8 mm (600 rpm) and 3.5 mm (500 rpm) [11].

Control group 2 (Con2): One single drill for a conical implant of 10 mm in length and 4.2 mm in diameter for conical IDAll implant, Implants Diffusion International (Montreuil, France). The speed recommended and used was 1500 rpm.

Test group (Test): One single drill (TURBOdrill®) for a conical implant of 10 mm in length and 4.2 mm in diameter for conical IDAll implant, Implants Diffusion International (Montreuil, France). The speed recommended and used was 1500 rpm. Figure 2 shows an image of the drills used for each group.

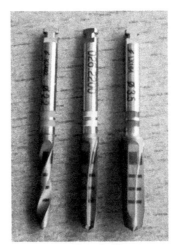

Con1

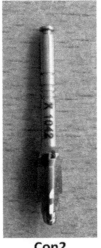

Con2

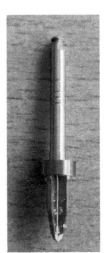

Test

Figure 2. Image of the drill systems used for the osteotomies in the 3 groups.

Three synthetic cortical bone blocks manufactured in polyurethane foam with a density of 40 pounds per cubic foot (PCF), corresponding to 0.62 g/cm^3 (Nacional Ossos, Jaú, Brazil), were used (one per group). The blocks presented the following dimensions: width of 9.7 cm, height of 5 cm and length of 10 cm. Initially, a perforation to install the sensor was performed with a conical carbide bur at 1 mm in diameter and 3 mm in depth, at a distance previously calculated so that after the osteotomy completed with the proposed system for each group, the final distance between the two perforations was 1 mm. Figure 3 shows these details.

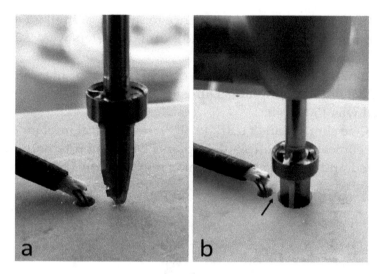

Figure 3. The thermocouple type k positioned in the perforation and the drill positioned before starting the osteotomy (**a**) and after the osteotomy finished (**b**), where the arrow indicates the distance of 1 mm to the sensor.

A type K thermocouple device (Mod. TP-01, Lutron Electronics Co., Inc., Coopersburg, PA, USA) was used for measuring the temperature during the osteotomies, which was coupled to a digital thermometer (Lutron Electronics Co., Inc.) with a resolution of 0.1 °C. Whenever one osteotomy was completed, the next was only started after the temperature returned to the initial level of 18 ± 1 °C (baseline temperature).

For drilling, a drilling machine controlled by an automated system was used, which was used in other previous studies [4,12]. The device controls the milling speed, the load applied during the osteotomy, irrigation volume and intermittent movements. All osteotomies were performed by applying a load of 2 kg, intermittent movements (4 mm, 8 mm and, finishing at 10 mm) and with intense irrigation of 50 mL/min (in condition 2). Irrigation was carried out with distilled water. Then, within these described conditions, twenty osteotomies were performed without irrigation and another 20 with irrigation for each group.

The range of temperature variation was calculated using the maximum temperature value measured and the baseline temperature (ΔT). The data were compared statistically using the ANOVA One-Way test to verify differences between the 3 groups in the two proposed conditions (without and with irrigation). Additionally, Bonferroni's multiple comparison test was used to determine the individual difference between the 3 groups. All cases where $p < 0.05$ were considered statistically significant. All data were analyzed using GraphPad Prism version 5.01 for Windows (GraphPad Software, San Diego, CA, USA).

3. Results

The measured data of the temperature generated during the osteotomies were collected in an electronic sheet, and the differences between the initial and maximum temperatures were calculated. A normal distribution result was detected of the groups after applied the normality test.

Significant differences for the measured temperatures during the osteotomies without and with irrigation were detected, in both cases with $p < 0.0001$. Considering absolute values, the Con2 group and Test group (both using one single drill) yielded similar results (not significantly different) in the condition 1 (without irrigation). However, in the Con1 group, significantly higher temperatures were recorded concerning the other 2 groups in both conditions (without and with irrigation). The Box Plot graphs shown in Figure 4 presented the medians, quartiles and ranges of the 3 groups analyzed in both conditions (without and with irrigation) and the statistical comparison between the groups.

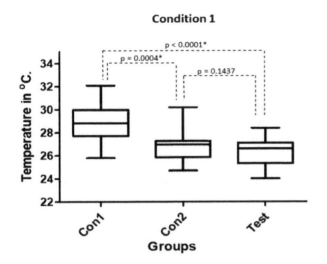
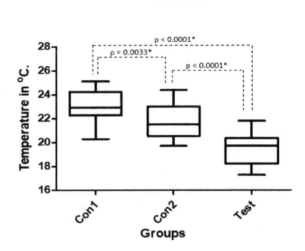

Figure 4. Box Plot graphs presenting the medians, quartiles and ranges of the 3 groups analyzed in both conditions tested (without and with irrigation, respectively) and the statistical comparison between the groups. * shows that they are statistically different.

The mean, standard deviation (SD), median and range values of the maximum temperature measured for each group in the 2 conditions proposed are summarized in Table 1.

Table 1. Mean, standard deviation (SD), median and range values of the maximum temperature measured for each group in the 2 conditions proposed. Values in centigrade degrees (°C).

Variables	Condition 1			Condition 2		
Groups	Mean and SD	Median	Range Values	Mean and SD	Median	Range Values
Con1	28.9 ± 1.68	28.8	25.8 to 32.1	23.1 ± 1.27	22.9	20.3 to 25.1
Con2	26.9 ± 1.31	27.0	24.7 to 30.2	21.7 ± 1.36	21.5	19.7 to 24.4
Test	26.3 ± 1.28	26.6	24.0 to 28.4	19.4 ± 1.29	19.7	17.3 to 21.8

The one single drill used in the Con2 and Test groups produced a smaller variation of temperature in comparison with the multiple sequence drills used in the Con1 group, as demonstrated follow the means ± standard deviations concerning baseline values (ΔT). Firstly, the calculated variation of temperature data in the osteotomies without irrigation were: 10.40 ± 1.85 °C for Con1 group; 8.34 ± 1.23 °C for Con2 group; 7.77 ± 1.26 °C for Test group. Whereas, in the osteotomies with irrigation, the calculated values were: 4.54 ± 1.39 °C for Con1 group; 3.14 ± 1.34 °C for Con2 group; 0.93 ± 1.47 °C for Test group. A significant difference was recorded for ΔT between the groups in both conditions ($p < 0.0001$). However, when the groups were compared against each other, only in condition 1 did the Con2 and Test group shows no statistical differences. The calculated values of the temperature variation as well as the statistical comparison between the groups are shown graphically in Figure 5.

Regarding the time required for osteotomy in each group, the average was ~10 s for the Con2 and Test groups, and ~80 s for the Con1 group (including three consecutive drilling sequence plus the time for substitution the drills). The time needed to return to baseline temperature after each implant site preparation procedure was a mean of 10 ± 2 min.

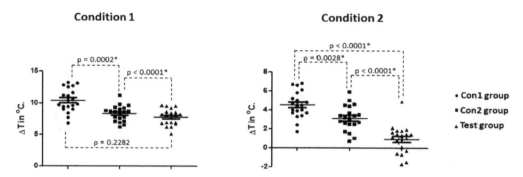

Figure 5. Points graph of the calculated temperature variation (ΔT) between the initial temperature and maximums temperature for each group in both conditions tested and the statistical difference between the groups. * shows that they are statistically different.

4. Discussion

The control of trauma during the handling of peri-implant tissues in surgical procedures for the installation of implants is of fundamental importance to obtain satisfactory results and free of complications. Among the maneuvers performed during surgery to install implants, an osteotomy can be considered the most traumatic step, then this topic has been the subject of several studies and the development of new technologies to minimize the effects of this procedure. In this sense, a new drill design was developed featuring a titanium tube with an internal helix on its stem, which aims to direct the flow of irrigating liquid into the drill blades, improving the cooling of bone tissue during the drilling for osteotomy. Then, our objective was to compare this new drill design with two other drill systems, measuring and comparing the temperature during the drilling procedure performed in a block of synthetic bone. The results showed that the new drill design was more effective in the control of heat production during the osteotomies performed, in comparison with the other two drill systems used as control groups.

This new drill design uses the concept of a single cutter to perform an osteotomy, which, according to previous publications, when compared to conventional drill systems that use a multiple drill sequence, showed a better performance in controlling the temperature [12], and similar healing of bone tissue around the implants installed in prepared beds using a single drill [7,12,13]. In addition to these results from in vitro and preclinical studies in rabbits, a study in humans was presented demonstrating a high success rate (98% of implant survival) with the use of a single drill to install the implants, in which 350 implants were evaluated [14]. Conversely, as described by Li et al. [15], there is a great concern for the risk of heat generation during milling with a single cutter, mainly in higher density bone tissue and for the accumulation of bone chips inside the drill. This accumulation of residues inside the cutting part of the drill and its contact with the side of the drilling will result in additional heat generation [15]. In this sense, the device coupled to the stem of the new drill design, which works as a propeller turbine for the cooling liquid, in addition to increasing the temperature control of the drill blades, can eliminate the bone residues inside of the drill. Still, the intermittent movements applied during the performance of the osteotomy help this elimination of bone residues and are important in controlling the temperature [4].

Other authors have reported that the drilling procedures for osteotomy should be minimally traumatic, which would be highly recommended to preserve the bone tissue by preventing damage to its healing potential [16]. In addition, the drilling to perform the surgical bed (osteotomy) for the installation of endosseous implants, produces a large local inflammatory reaction, which can be controlled and/or reduced by the use of adequate irrigation technique [5]. The results obtained in the present study showed a lower temperature rise in the groups where a single drill was used to perform the osteotomy (Con2 group and Test group), in comparison with the group where a drilling system with multiple drills (Con1 group) was used. Comparing the data with irrigation, that is a more similar condition with a clinical scenario, the Test group was 16% < Con1 group and 11% < Con2, whereas the Con2 was 6% < Con1 group.

The manufacture of cutters and their performance is directly related to engineering factors and mechanical functioning. For example, drills with double-positive cutters reduce the cutting pressure, consume less power and create less heat [17]. Then, the test carried out without irrigation (condition 1) serves, mainly, to analyze the efficiency of the different types of cutters. From the results obtained in the present study, when the samples were tested without irrigation, it was demonstrated that the 3 drill systems tested present high quality in their designs and excellent performance since the variation in general average from the initial temperature to final temperature was relatively low. Moreover, the heat generated in the drilling operation is also roughly proportional to the undeformed chip thickness and cutting forces [18].

Other authors have described that mechanical factors (drill and blade design, cutting precision, drill diameter) and technical factors (drilling protocol, speed and force applied, drill angulation, irrigation system and torque applied), are important in determining the physical stress generated [19,20]. Then, as the mechanical factors are determined by the manufacturer of the drilling system, it is the technical factors that may vary during its execution, as clinically this will depend directly on the operator. However, in our study, automated equipment was used so that there were no variations and/or errors during the execution of predetermined technical factors for each drilling systems tested. Regards to the technique applied for the groups, only the drill speed was different between them, which followed the recommendation of each manufacturer. In this sense, a variety of propositions were described in the literature [10], however, the drill design (project) must determine the ideal speed for each drilling system.

Another important factor to note is the characteristics of bone density used in our experiment. The cortical bone presented the mayor density and, as described by Sener et al. (2009) [21], that most heat changes are generated in the most superficial part of this compact bone. Then, the sensor was installed at a depth of 3 mm, although the bone block used had the same density throughout its structure. Still, regarding the drilling time, several authors have described that the drilling time can influence the temperature variation values during osteotomy [19]. In this point, the measured time for drilling in the Con1 group (multiple sequences), obviously was superior due to the need to replace the drills, because it is a sequence of 3 cutters, compared to the groups Con2 and Test that use only one drill. This possibility of performing osteotomy with a low-temperature variation using only one drill may prove beneficial to tissues reducing the local damage as well as the patients' discomfort.

Some limitations and clinical care of this in vitro study must be considered, such as the fact that an all-cortical bone model and automated equipment were used to perform osteotomies, as this does not reflect the clinical reality. On the other hand, when analyzing from the point of view of the proposed and tested techniques, the use of a single cutter for the preparation of the implant bed does not allow for direction corrections after its execution, unlike the use of multiple cutters, where it is possible correct any direction error during the passage from one to the other drill sequence. Thus, we can say that the use of a single cutter requires greater precision during its use. Another important observation is that the initial temperature of the specimens in this study was ~18 °C, while in the patient we have an initial temperature of ~37 °C, which gives us a variation limit of ~10 °C. Then, when we calculate the temperature variation values with the corporal temperature, in the Con1 group in the condition 1 (without irrigation), the temperature could exceed the critical limit and be causing bone necrosis (~37 °C + 10.4 °C = ~47.4 °C). This scenario could occur due to a failure of the irrigation during the surgical procedure. However, in the other two groups a with an average temperature variation of 8.1 °C, even without irrigation, the value was below the critical point (~37 °C + 8.1 °C = ~45.1 °C). Still, in all groups when the osteotomies were performed using irrigation the values were far removed from the critical value.

5. Conclusions

Within the limitations of the present in vitro study, we can conclude that the single drill with the new design for improving the irrigation and temperature control, demonstrated that the new device coupled to the drills (TURBOdrill®) increases and directs the flow of the irrigation liquid and results in better temperature control during the osteotomy, in comparison with the drill designs that use conventional external irrigation.

Author Contributions: Conceptualization, J.C.P.F. and G.B.; Data curation, S.A.G. and B.A.D.; Formal analysis, S.A.G. and B.C.; Investigation, S.A.G., R.B. and B.A.D.; Methodology, S.A.G., J.C.P.F. and G.B.; Resources, G.B.; Software, R.B.; Supervision, R.B.; Validation, J.C.P.F.; Writing—original draft, S.A.G. and B.C.; Writing—review & editing, J.C.P.F. and B.A.D. All authors have read and agreed to the published version of the manuscript.

References

1. Eriksson, A.R.; Albrektsson, T. Temperature threshold levels for heat-induced bone tissue injury: A vital-microscopic study in the rabbit. *J. Prosthet. Dent.* **1983**, *50*, 101–107. [CrossRef]
2. Sannino, G.; Capparé, P.; Gherlone, E.F.; Barlattani, A. Influence of the implant drill design and sequence on temperature changes during site preparation. *Int. J. Oral Maxillofac. Implants* **2015**, *30*, 351–358. [CrossRef] [PubMed]
3. Bernabeu-Mira, J.C.; Pellicer-Chover, H.; Peñarrocha-Diago, M.; Peñarrocha-Oltra, D. In Vitro Study on Bone Heating during Drilling of the Implant Site: Material, Design and Wear of the Surgical Drill. *Materials* **2020**, *19*, 1921. [CrossRef] [PubMed]
4. Gehrke, S.A.; Loffredo Neto, H.; Mardegan, F.E. Investigation of the effect of movement and irrigation systems on temperature in the conventional drilling of cortical bone. *Br. J. Oral Maxillofac. Surg.* **2013**, *51*, 953–957. [CrossRef] [PubMed]
5. Salles, M.B.; Gehrke, S.A.; Shibli, J.A.; Allegrini, S., Jr.; Yoshimoto, M.; König, B., Jr. Evaluating Nuclear Factor NF-κB Activation Following Bone Trauma: A Pilot Study in a Wistar Rats Model. *PLoS ONE* **2015**, *14*, e0140630. [CrossRef] [PubMed]
6. Gehrke, S.A. Evaluation of the Cortical Bone Reaction around of Implants Using a Single-Use Final Drill: A Histologic Study. *J. Craniofac. Surg.* **2015**, *26*, 1482–1486. [CrossRef] [PubMed]
7. Gehrke, S.A.; Bettach, R.; Aramburú Júnior, J.S.; Prados-Frutos, J.C.; Del Fabbro, M.; Shibli, J.A. Peri-Implant Bone Behavior after Single Drill Versus Multiple Sequence for Osteotomy Drill. *Biomed. Res. Int.* **2018**, *11*, 9756043. [CrossRef] [PubMed]
8. Trisi, P.; Falco, A.; Berardini, M. Single-drill implant induces bone corticalization during submerged healing: An in vivo pilot study. *Int. J. Implant Dent.* **2020**, *15*, 2. [CrossRef] [PubMed]
9. Scarano, A.; Lorusso, F.; Noumbissi, S. Infrared Thermographic Evaluation of Temperature Modifications Induced during Implant Site Preparation with Steel vs. Zirconia Implant Drill. *J. Clin. Med.* **2020**, *5*, 148. [CrossRef] [PubMed]
10. Mishra, S.K.; Chowdhary, R. Heat Generated by Dental Implant Drills During Osteotomy-A Review: Heat Generated by Dental Implant Drills. *J. Indian Prosthodont. Soc.* **2014**, *14*, 131–143. [CrossRef] [PubMed]
11. Available online: https://www.straumann.com/content/dam/media-center/straumann/en/documents/brochure/technical-information/490.038-en_low.pdf (accessed on 23 May 2020).
12. Gehrke, S.A.; Bettach, R.; Taschieri, S.; Boukhris, G.; Corbella, S.; Del Fabbro, M. Temperature Changes in Cortical Bone after Implant Site Preparation Using a Single Bur versus Multiple Drilling Steps: An in Vitro Investigation. *Clin. Implant Dent. Relat. Res.* **2015**, *17*, 700–707. [CrossRef] [PubMed]
13. Jimbo, R.; Giro, G.; Marin, C.; Granato, R.; Suzuki, M.; Tovar, N.; Lilin, T.; Janal, M.; Coelho, P.G. Simplified drilling technique does not decrease dental implant osseointegration: A preliminary report. *J. Periodontol.* **2013**, *84*, 1599–1605. [CrossRef] [PubMed]
14. Bettach, R.; Taschieri, S.; Boukhris, G.; Del Fabbro, M. Implant Survival after Preparation of the Implant Site Using a Single Bur: A Case Series. *Clin. Implant Dent. Relat. Res.* **2015**, *17*, 13–21. [CrossRef] [PubMed]
15. Li, L.; Zhu, Z.; Li, L. Letter to the editor. Re: Simplified drilling technique does not decrease dental implant osseointegration: A preliminary report. *J. Periodontol.* **2014**, *85*, 512–513. [CrossRef] [PubMed]

16.   Romeo, U.; Del Vecchio, A.; Palaia, G.; Tenore, G.; Visca, P.; Maggiore, C. Bone Damage Induced by Different Cutting Instruments—An in Vitro Study. *Braz. Dent. J.* **2009**, *20*, 162–168. [CrossRef] [PubMed]

17.   Stephenson, D.A.; Agapiou, J.S. Cutting Tools Metal. In *Cutting Theory and Practice*, 3rd ed.; Front Cover; CRC Press: Boca Raton, FL, USA, 2016.

18.   Cubberly, W.; Bakerjian, R. *Tool and Manufacturing Engineers Handbook*; Desk Edition; (v. 1–5): Books; Society of Manufacturing Engineers: Dearborn, MI, USA, 1989.

19.   Sumer, M.; Misir, A.F.; Telcioglu, N.T.; Guler, A.U.; Yenisey, M. Comparison of heat generation during implant drilling using stainless steel and ceramic drills. *J. Oral Maxillofac. Surg.* **2011**, *69*, 1350–1354. [CrossRef] [PubMed]

20.   Augustin, G.; Zigman, T.; Davila, S.; Udilljak, T.; Staroveski, T.; Brezak, D.; Babic, S. Cortical bone drilling and thermal osteonecrosis. *Clin. Biomech.* **2012**, *27*, 313–325. [CrossRef] [PubMed]

21.   Sener, B.C.; Dergin, G.; Gursoy, B.; Kelesoglu, E.; Slih, I. Effects of irrigation temperature on heat control in vitro at different drilling depths. *Clin. Oral Implants Res.* **2009**, *20*, 294–298. [CrossRef] [PubMed]

2

Treatment of Full and Partial Arches with Internal-Conical-Connection Dental Implants: Clinical Results after 5 Years of Follow-Up

Diego Lops [1,*]**, Riccardo Guazzo** [2]**, Alessandro Rossi** [1]**, Antonino Palazzolo** [1]**, Vittorio Favero** [3]🆔**,
Mattia Manfredini** [4]🆔**, Luca Sbricoli** [2]🆔 **and Eugenio Romeo** [1]

[1]   Department of Prosthodontics, School of Dentistry, University of Milan, 20142 Milan, Italy;
     alessandroluigirossi@gmail.com (A.R.); antonino.palazzolo@unimi.it (A.P.); eugenio.romeo@unimi.it (E.R.)
[2]   Department of Neurosciences, University of Padua, 35121 Padua, Italy; riccardo.guazzo@unipd.it (R.G.);
     luca.sbricoli@unipd.it (L.S.)
[3]   Section of Dentistry and Maxillofacial Surgery, Department of Surgery, University of Verona,
     37134 Verona, Italy; vittorio_favero@yahoo.it
[4]   Department of Oral Surgery, Fondazione Policlinico Ca' Granda, 20141 Milan, Italy;
     mattia.manfredini@unimi.it
*   Correspondence: diego.lops@unimi.it

Abstract: The aim of the present investigation is to evaluate the implant therapy outcomes over a period of 5 years and to analyze several patient risk factors influencing the stability of the peri-implant tissues. Seventy-eight patients were consecutively treated between 2009 and 2017 and restored with implant-supported fixed prostheses. The following inclusion criteria were considered: partial or complete edentulism; residual bone volume of at least 3.3 mm in diameter and 8 mm in length; a favorable relationship between maxilla and mandible; at least a minimum 5 year follow-up for each implant included in the statistical analysis. Intraoral radiographs were taken at implant loading and every 12 months during the follow-up visits. They were subsequently stored on a personal computer and analyzed to determine the changes in bone level. Seventy-eight patients receiving 209 implants completed a minimum follow-up period of 5 years. One-hundred dental implants were inserted in the maxilla while 109 were placed in the mandible. Eleven (14.1%) out of 78 treated patients who received 29 (13.9%) dental implants were considered as drop-outs. On the whole, peri-implantitis was diagnosed in three implants. The average final pocket probing depth at implant level was 2.5 ± 1.2 mm. The average final bone loss after 5 years was 0.3 ± 0.4 mm, both at the mesial and distal aspect of the implant. The effects of the prosthesis type, sex and implant site did not statistically influence the marginal bone loss; on the contrary, a statistically significant difference regarding marginal bone loss was detected between smoker and non-smoker patients ($p = 0.021$). Implants with internal-conical abutment connection showed stable peri-implant bone levels at the medium-term follow-up. Nevertheless, further prospective long-term clinical studies are necessary to confirm these data.

Keywords: internal-conical-connection; partial fixed dentures; marginal bone level

1. Introduction

Nowadays, partially and completely edentulous patients can be treated with implant-supported prosthesis as a reliable and predictable treatment option [1,2]. A pivotal contribution in reaching this goal was provided by the continuous improvement in quality of prosthetic components. As far as esthetics and function are concerned, several implant-supported prosthetic solutions can satisfy patient expectations [3,4]. To this purpose, Romeo et al., in their prospective longitudinal study on partial edentulism [5], reported high prognostic rates: success ranged from 89% to 95.3% while cumulative survival ranged from 93.6% to 96.7%, after 3 to 7 years of loading, respectively.

Precisely, the most frequent long-term complications associated with dental implants are mucositis and peri-implantitis [6]. As a matter of fact, peri-implantitis is highly prevalent and may affect 7.8–43.3% of all implants studied and reported in dental literature [6–10].

On the whole, an initial peri-implant bone loss of 2–3% has been reported that is followed by a further 2–3% loss over a period of 5 years regarding implants supporting fixed partial dentures (FPDs) [11]. On the other hand, concerning fixed prosthesis longevity, a 5 year survival rate of 96.5% for single tooth replacement, 95.4% for partial implant-supported fixed prosthesis and 90.1% for implant-tooth reconstruction were shown in several systematic reviews [12–14].

Hence, due to the high success and survival rates available in the literature concerning dental implants, "classical" Albrektsson success criteria [15] underwent an evolution; nowadays, clinicians and researchers all over the world are mainly paying attention to the marginal bone level changes over the years [16,17].

Nevertheless, it has to be highlighted that higher survival and lower complication rates also depend on a positive learning curve in implant dentistry, as reported in recent clinical studies [18]. Related to this, it is widely reported that an internal-conical-connection between the abutment and the implant may contribute to the stability of peri-implant hard tissues, if compared to flat-to-flat interfaces [19–22]. However, recent outcomes from a systematic review and meta-analysis comparing the conical internal connection (IC) with the external hexagonal connection (EH) on the occurrence of marginal bone loss (ΔMBL) disagreed with this statement [23]. In fact, no statistically significant differences were found for ΔMBL one, three and five at one, three and five years after loading between implant connections ($p < 0.05$), and statistically significant differences were found for PD between EH and IC implants (1 year follow-up) −0.53 (95%CI −0.82 to −0.24, $p = 0.0004$). On the contrary, the role of platform switching in implant abutment is still unclear [24,25].

The present prospective longitudinal study aimed at evaluating the radiographical and peri-implant clinical outcomes of dental implants characterized by internal-conical-connection and platform switching after an observation period of 5 years.

Moreover, several potential patient-related risk factors influencing the peri-implant tissues and implant failures were analyzed.

2. Material and Methods

Seventy-eight patients were consecutively treated between 2009 and 2017 at the Dental Clinic, Department of Medicine and Surgery, University of Milan, Italy. The fundamental principles of the Declaration of Helsinki were followed in the conduction of the study. Before participating in the study, all patients signed a specifically designed consent form. No ethical committee document was provided as the reported treatments and the follow-up procedures only consisted of standard treatments and control visits.

Inclusion criteria were as follows: partial or complete edentulism; residual ridge volume of at least 3.3 mm in diameter and 8 mm in length as evaluated both clinically and radiographically; a favorable relationship with respect to the opposing dental arches; each dental implant included in the measurements needed a minimum 5 year follow-up. Only one type of implant-supported restoration for each patient was included in the present study. There was a yearly follow-up visit, in which oral hygiene control was carefully checked.

The following exclusion criteria were considered: active periodontal disease, heart disease, coagulation or leukocyte diseases, metabolic disorders, radiotherapy in the head and neck area, parafunctions such as clenching or bruxism, a smoking habit (more than 10 cigarettes per day), alcohol or drug abuse.

Patients were restored with implants with an internal-conical-connection (Astra Tech, Mölndal, Sweden), which supported fixed prostheses.

Peri-implant tissues were evaluated for concerns regarding probing pocket depth, bleeding on probing (bleeding index score of 0 to 3), and plaque index scores (on a scale of 0 to 3) [5].

Intraoral radiographs were taken using the paralleling technique to control projection geometry, with exposure parameters of 65 to 90 kV, 7.5 to 10 mA, and 0.22 to 0.25 seconds [5]. They were subsequently stored on a personal computer and analyzed using the program ImageJ (US National Institute of Mental Health, Bethesda, MD, USA) to determine bone level changes. Peri-implant bone resorption was assessed both mesially and distally, taking the implant head as a reference point. Radiographs were taken at baseline (loading time) and at the 5 year follow-up visit, which were analyzed and compared to verify any change in the peri-implant marginal bone level (Figure 1). A radiographic control was performed during the yearly follow-up visits as well.

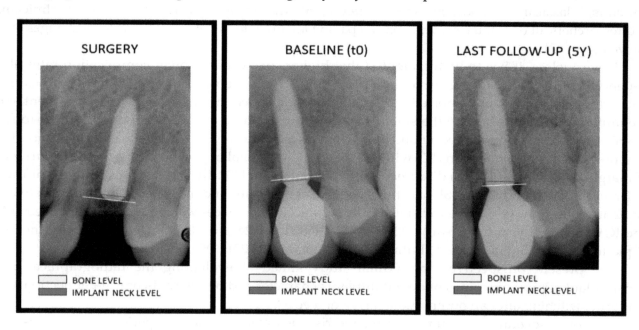

Figure 1. Radiographs performed after implant placement, at baseline (time of loading) and at the 5 year follow-up visit.

Several reference measurements were also considered: (i) implant neck diameter; (ii) implant length as the distance between the implant neck and the most apical point of each implant, along an ideal line running parallel to the implant axis. All measurements were performed by a single calibrated operator (A.P.). Calibration consisted of three-time measurements at three different time points by assessing fifteen radiographs with another author (D.L.) acting as reference examiner. Subsequently, intra-examiner and inter-examiner reliability were calculated (k = 0.90 and k = 0.85, respectively).

After a 3 month submerged healing, transmucosal healing abutments were connected at surgical re-entry. Hence, pre-prosthetic evaluation was performed 3 months after implant placement. Two weeks after surgical re-entry, an implant impression was taken, and a provisional restoration was screwed into position. Therefore, after maturation of the peri-implant soft tissues (2–3 months after provisional delivery), a second implant impression was taken for the final implant-supported restoration. Definitive abutments were screwed into position using 35 Ncm of torque. For all the fixed prostheses, a platform switching connection between fixture and abutment was provided. Cemented prostheses were fixed with zinc oxyphosphate cement or zinc-eugenol oxide cement, while screw-retained prostheses were secured by applying a 15 Ncm torque to the abutment framework screw using a manual torque driver.

Statistical Analysis

Mean values, standard deviations (SDs) and cumulative frequencies were calculated for the above-mentioned implant-related biometric parameters. The efficacy variable was the change in the peri-implant bone-level. Clinical data were considered as descriptors. The peri-implant bone level data were analyzed at implant and patient level. Bivariate analysis was performed either considering dental implant or patient as statistical unit. Analysis of variance and post hoc analysis with Bonferroni correction when indicated were formulated in order to evaluate marginal bone level in the different time intervals, while a multilevel analysis was used to evaluate the influence of different factors affecting bone loss at implant level. A p-value less than 0.05 was considered as statistically significant. A specifically designed software (SPSS 21.0; SPSS, Inc., Chicago, IL, USA) was used for all the statistical analyses.

3. Results

Seventy-eight patients receiving 209 implants were enrolled in the present clinical investigation. Forty-three patients were male (55.1%) and thirty-five patients were female (44.9%). Patients' mean age at time of surgery was 55.4 ± 10.7 years (range 26–84 years). Sixteen patients (20.5%) were smokers and sixty-two (79.5%) were non-smokers as reported in Table 1.

Table 1. Patients' features.

Gender (male/female)	43/35
Smokers/Non-smokers	16/62
Age (years)	55.4 (10.7)

One-hundred implants were placed in the maxilla (21 in the anterior and 79 in the posterior segment) and 109 in the mandible (25 in the anterior and 84 in the posterior segment), respectively (Table 2).

Table 2. Implant sites.

	Anterior	Posterior	Total
Maxilla	21	79	100
Mandible	26	83	109

Implants length was 8 (two implants), 9 (32), 11 (105), 13 (65) 15 (5) mm, respectively. All implants features are reported in Table 3.

Table 3. Implant features.

Implant Length (mm)	Maxilla	Mandible	Total
8	2	0	2
9	7	25	32
11	48	57	105
13	43	22	65
15	0	5	5
Total	100	109	

Out of 78 treated patients, 11 (14.1%) with 29 (13.9%) dental implants dropped out and were not considered in the statistical analysis (Table 4). One patient dropped out after 1 year of follow up. Six patients were lost after two years. Four patients who received two implants each were lost after 3 years.

Table 4. Drop-outs' features.

Patient ID	Gender	Age	Smoke	Number of Implants	Last Follow-Up (years)
21	M	57	No	4	2
22	F	55	No	5	3
23	F	60	No	2	2
29	F	60	No	2	2
31	F	84	No	2	3
45	F	37	Yes	1	3
50	F	74	No	1	4
61	M	51	Yes	2	1
64	M	63	No	2	2
67	F	59	No	2	2
78	M	42	Yes	6	2

No implants were lost during the osseointegration period. One implant affected by peri-implantitis was removed four years post-insertion. No specific anatomical condition was detected as promoting an inflammatory status of peri-implant hard and soft tissues. On the contrary, peri-implantitis was successfully treated in two different patients (one implant each). In all cases, the patients were smokers.

The average final pocket probing depth at implant level was 2.5 ± 1.2 mm. Probing depths at mesial, distal, buccal, and lingual sites of 3 mm or less were observed at 89.4%, 89.9%, 90.4%, 90.9% of all implants, respectively. An overall success rate of 90.1% was calculated after 5 years of follow-up.

Standardized periapical radiographs were used to measure bone loss. The average final bone loss after 5 years of evaluation was 0.3 ± 0.4 mm, both at the mesial and distal aspect of the implant.

The effects of multiple implants in the same patient were analyzed and were not statistically significant ($p = 0.605$).

The effects of the prosthesis type on marginal bone loss were analyzed, even if no statistical difference was noticed ($p = 0.092$). Three different sub-groups were considered for the statistical analysis: single tooth (79 prostheses), partial (98) and full (32) prostheses, respectively. Similarly, no statistical difference was calculated for each sub-group ($p = 0.103$, 0.098 and 0.127, respectively).

Moreover, sex was not correlated to peri-implant marginal bone loss ($p = 0.125$). Prosthesis type and distribution are reported in Table 5.

Table 5. Prosthesis type and distribution.

Type of Prosthesis	n.
Single tooth	77
Single tooth with distal cantilever	2
Partial	30
Toronto	5
Full fixed prostheses	27
Splint	48
Partial with mesial cantilever	15
Partial with distal cantilever	5

Furthermore, smoking and its potential effect on implant peri-implant bone stability was analyzed. To this purpose, an average marginal bone loss of 0.3 ± 0.3 mm was calculated for implants placed in non-smoker patients while implants placed in smoker patients showed an average marginal bone loss of 0.5 ± 0.5 mm. Such difference was statistically significant ($p = 0.021$).

Data on different parameters and the respective effect on marginal bone loss are reported in Table 6.

Table 6. Clinical parameters and the respective effect on marginal bone loss.

Parameters	p-Value	Significant (YES/NO)
Prosthesis sub-group single tooth	0.103	No
Prosthesis sub-group partial dentures	0.098	No
Prosthesis sub-group full dentures	0.127	No
Sex	0.125	No
Smoking habit	0,021	Yes

Moreover, the site of implant placement and the respective effect on the bone loss was considered. In the anterior maxilla, an average bone remodeling of 0.3 ± 0.3 mm was found while an average bone remodeling of 0.4 ± 0.6 mm was found in the posterior maxilla. Similarly, in anterior and posterior mandibula, a mean bone remodeling of 0.5 ± 0.4 and 0.3 ± 0.4 mm were calculated, respectively. All these comparisons were not statistically significant ($p > 0.05$).

Average bone loss cumulative frequency distribution at implant level is presented in Figure 2 while cumulative frequency distribution of average bone loss at patient level is reported in Figure 3. After five years of loading, 12.2% of implants showed a mean 1 mm of marginal bone loss; at the same time, 30% of implants showed 0.5 mm of radiographic bone loss, while 8% of implants showed a marginal bone gaining.

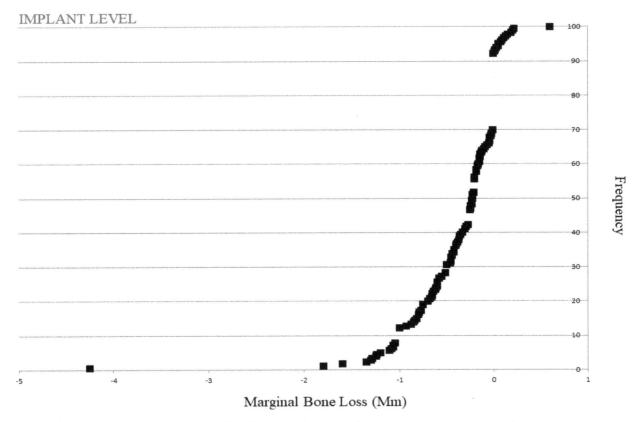

Figure 2. Cumulative frequency distribution of average bone loss at implant level (every square is an implant. The x axis is a mm scale and in the y axis we have the cumulative frequencies).

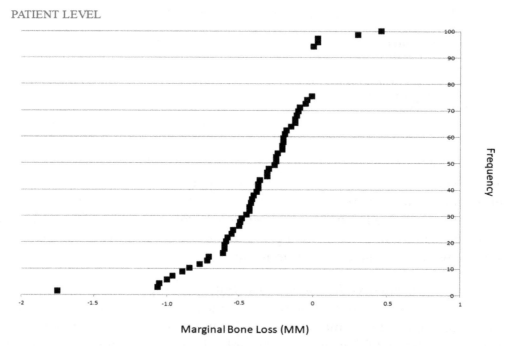

Figure 3. Cumulative frequency distribution of average bone loss at patient level (every square is a patient. The x axis is a mm scale and in the y axis we have the cumulative frequencies).

The 5 year marginal bone loss (MBL) changes from the implant loading are shown in Figure 4.

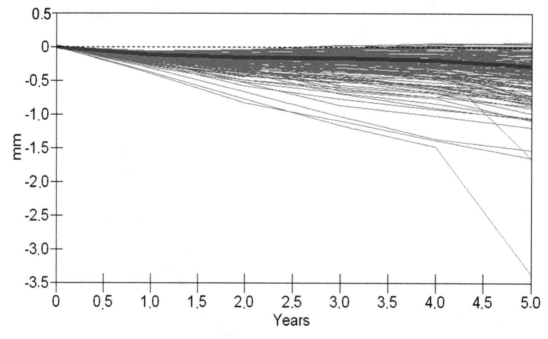

Figure 4. The 5 year marginal bone loss changes from the implant loading are shown in Figure 4. Every line is an implant, and the red line is the mean value of marginal bone loss.

4. Discussion

The present retrospective longitudinal study aimed to evaluate the outcome of implant-supported restorations after 5 years of function. Regarding the present study outcomes, the marginal bone level stability measurements could be addressed to the implant to abutment stability. This is directly influenced by the type of connection, even if platform switching may help achieve ridge dimension preservation and enhance the stability of peri-implant soft tissues [26]. In fact, the role of platform switching on the stability of the peri-implant hard tissue is still unclear [24,25,27,28], and controversy on hard tissue preservation with the platform switching technique remains unsolved [29]. Nevertheless, bone-level implants have been created with many connection configurations. Locking-taper conical connection implants have proven superior to buttress joint implants at achieving a tight seal and eliminating the micro-gap at the implant-to-abutment junction and have demonstrated improvements in crestal bone maintenance. According to these findings, the internal-conical-connection of the implants included in the present report seemed to positively influence the peri-implant bone stability [19–22].

Several potential risk factors that might influence peri-implant tissues and implant failures were also evaluated. Other studies by Wennström et al. [26] reported a similar 5 year failure rate, specifically a failure rate of 5.3% at the PFD (partial fixed dentures) level and 2.7% at implant level were calculated and a good medium-term prognosis of implant-supported rehabilitations was confirmed.

Only a smoking habit, even related to smokers that smoke up to 10 cigarettes per day, was found to be statistically significant as far as bone loss is concerned. Indeed, 0.5 ± 0.5 mm of bone loss was suffered by implants placed in smoker patients while non-smoker patients experienced an average marginal bone loss of 0.3 ± 0.3 mm. It could be assumed that patients reporting to be light smokers stated facts that were not entirely true. Similarly, a systematic review conducted by Moraschini et al. in 2016 [30] agreed with such outcomes, reporting a statistically significant difference of marginal bone loss when considering smokers versus non-smokers. To be more precise, a range of bone loss between 0.07 and 0.9 mm with a mean value of 0.5 mm was reported. Nevertheless, the clinical significance of 0.2 mm of bone loss might be questioned. Since smoking was the only statistically significant risk factor, no multilevel analysis was performed to compare other variables. In the end, average bone loss around implants might not be affected by factors such as sex, insertion site and prosthesis type. In this respect, the same parameters were evaluated in a prospective study accounting for 630 patients and 1569 implants, which was conducted by Rammelsberg et al. [31] in 2017. The authors reported that incidence of implant-related complications was not significantly influenced by implant location, age, sex, or implant placement associated with GBR procedures.

In the present study, Figure 3 on 5 year bone loss changes could be superimposed to the outcomes of Fransson and Tomasi [16]. In such a scenario, the authors analyzed the bone loss pattern of peri-implantitis-associated bone loss on 419 implants with up to 23 years of observation. To summarize, a tendency of 0.15 mm peri-implant bone loss per year was predicted by the authors. In the present analysis, a similar trend is displayed.

Finally, implant-supported restorations showed a high success rate and a tendency of implant loss similar to previous studies considering at least 5 years of function [1–5]. Smoking was the only variable showing statistical significance with respect to bone loss. Nevertheless, it should be highlighted that this finding might not be correlated to a poorer prognosis from a clinician's point of view.

5. Conclusions

Within the limits of the present clinical study, dental implants with internal-conical-connection showed stable peri-implant bone levels at the medium-term follow-up (5 years). Nevertheless, further clinical studies with adequate methodology and sample size and with a more consistent observation period are warranted to confirm the trends and results found in the present report.

Author Contributions: D.L. study coordinator; R.G. statistics; A.R. surgical procedures; A.P. surgical procedures; V.F. data análisis; M.M. measurements; L.S. paper writing; E.R. study coordinator; All authors have read and agreed to the published version of the manuscript.

Acknowledgments: We would like to thank Chiara Burgio who reviewed the manuscript and helped throughout the submission.

References

1. Jung, R.; Zembic, A.; Pjetursson, B.E.; Zwahlen, M.; Thoma, D.S. Systematic review of the survival rate and the incidence of biological, technical, and aesthetic complications of single crowns on implants reported in longitudinal studies with a mean follow-up of 5 years. *Clin. Oral Implant. Res.* **2012**, *23*, 2–21. [CrossRef]

2. Pjetursson, B.E.; Thoma, D.; Jung, R.; Zwahlen, M.; Zembic, A. A systematic review of the survival and complication rates of implant-supported fixed dental prostheses (FDPs) after a mean observation period of at least 5 years. *Clin. Oral Implant. Res.* **2012**, *23*, 22–38. [CrossRef]

3. Laurell, L.; Lundgren, D. Marginal Bone Level Changes at Dental Implants after 5 Years in Function: A Meta-Analysis. *Clin. Implant. Dent. Relat. Res.* **2011**, *13*, 19–28. [CrossRef]

4. Ravald, N.; Dahlgren, S.; Teiwik, A.; Gröndahl, K. Long-term evaluation of Astra Tech and Brånemark implants in patients treated with full-arch bridges. Results after 12–15 years. *Clin. Oral Implant. Res.* **2013**, *24*, 1144–1151. [CrossRef] [PubMed]

5. Romeo, E.; Lops, D.; Margutti, E.; Ghisolfi, M.; Chiapasco, M.; Vogel, G. Long-term survival and success of oral implants in the treatment of full and partial arches: A 7-year prospective study with the ITI dental implant system. *Int. J. Oral Maxillofac. Implant.* **2004**, *19*, 247–259.

6. Berglundh, T.; Persson, L.; Klinge, B. A systematic review of the incidence of biological and technical complications in implant dentistry reported in prospective longitudinal studies of at least 5 years. *J. Clin. Periodontol.* **2002**, *29*, 197–212. [CrossRef] [PubMed]

7. Zitzmann, N.U.; Berglundh, T. Definition and prevalence of peri-implant diseases. *J. Clin. Periodontol.* **2008**, *35*, 286–291. [CrossRef]

8. Ferreira, S.D.; Silva, G.L.M.; Cortelli, J.R.; Costa, J.E.; Costa, F.O. Prevalence and risk variables for peri-implant disease in Brazilian subjects. *J. Clin. Periodontol.* **2006**, *33*, 929–935. [CrossRef]

9. Roos-Jansaker, A.-M.; Lindahl, C.; Renvert, H.; Renvert, S. Nine- to fourteen-year follow-up of implant treatment. Part II: Presence of peri-implant lesions. *J. Clin. Periodontol.* **2006**, *33*, 290–295. [CrossRef]

10. Koldsland, O.C.; Scheie, A.A.; Aass, A.M. Prevalence of Peri-Implantitis Related to Severity of the Disease with Different Degrees of Bone Loss. *J. Periodontol.* **2010**, *81*, 231–238. [CrossRef]

11. Holm-Pedersen, P.; Lang, N.P.; Müller, F. What are the longevities of teeth and oral implants? *Clin. Oral Implant. Res.* **2007**, *18*, 15–19. [CrossRef] [PubMed]

12. Lang, N.P.; Pjetursson, B.E.; Tan, K.; Bragger, U.; Egger, M.; Zwahlen, M. A systematic review of the survival and complication rates of fixed partial dentures (FPDs) after an observation period of at least 5 years. II. Combined tooth-implant-supported FPDs. *Clin. Oral Implant. Res.* **2004**, *15*, 643–653. [CrossRef] [PubMed]

13. Bragger, U.; Karoussis, I.; Persson, R.; Pjetursson, B.; Salvi, G.; Lang, N.P. Technical and biological complications/failures with single crowns and fixed partial dentures on implants: A 10-year prospective cohort study. *Clin. Oral Implant. Res.* **2005**, *16*, 326–334. [CrossRef]

14. Jung, R.E.; Pjetursson, B.E.; Glauser, R.; Zembic, A.; Zwahlen, M.; Lang, N.P. A systematic review of the 5-year survival and complication rates of implant-supported single crowns. *Clin. Oral Implant. Res.* **2008**, *19*, 119–130. [CrossRef] [PubMed]

15. Albrektsson, T. On long-term maintenance of the osseointegrated response. *Aust. Prosthodont. J.* **1993**, *7*, 15–24.

16. Fransson, C.; Tomasi, C.; Pikner, S.S.; Grondahl, K.; Wennstrom, J.L.; Leyland, A.H. Severity and pattern of peri-implantitis-associated bone loss. *J. Clin. Periodontol.* **2010**, *37*, 442–448. [CrossRef]

17. Cecchinato, D.; Parpaiola, A.; Lindhe, J. A cross-sectional study on the prevalence of marginal bone loss among implant patients. *Clin. Oral Implant. Res.* **2012**, *24*, 87–90. [CrossRef]

18. Pjetursson, B.E.; Asgeirsson, A.G.; Zwahlen, M.; Sailer, I. Improvements in Implant Dentistry over the Last Decade: Comparison of Survival and Complication Rates in Older and Newer Publications. *Int. J. Oral Maxillofac. Implant.* **2014**, *29*, 308–324. [CrossRef]

19. Hurson, S. Implant/Abutment Biomechanics and Material Selection for Predictable Results. *Compend. Contin. Educ. Dent.* **2018**, *39*, 440.

20. Lops, D.; Meneghello, R.; Sbricoli, L.; Savio, G.; Bressan, E.; Stellini, E. Precision of the Connection Between Implant and Standard or Computer-Aided Design/Computer-Aided Manufacturing Abutments: A Novel Evaluation Method. *Int. J. Oral Maxillofac. Implant.* **2018**, *33*, 23–30. [CrossRef]

21. Zipprich, H.; Weigl, P.; Ratka, C.; Lange, B.; Lauer, H.-C. The micromechanical behavior of implant-abutment connections under a dynamic load protocol. *Clin. Implant. Dent. Relat. Res.* **2018**, *20*, 814–823. [CrossRef] [PubMed]

22. Bressan, E.; Stocchero, M.; Jimbo, R.; Rosati, C.; Fanti, E.; Tomasi, C.; Lops, D. Microbial Leakage at Morse Taper Conometric Prosthetic Connection: An In Vitro Investigation. *Implant Dent.* **2017**, *26*, 756–761. [CrossRef] [PubMed]

23. Rosa, E.C.; Deliberador, T.M.; Nascimento, T.C.D.L.D.; Kintopp, C.C.D.A.; Orsi, J.S.R.; Wambier, L.M.; Khajotia, S.S.; Florez, F.L.E.; Storrer, C.L.M. Does the implant-abutment interface interfere on marginal bone loss? A systematic review and meta-analysis. *Braz. Oral Res.* **2019**, *33*, e068. [CrossRef] [PubMed]

24. Canullo, L.; Goglia, G.; Iurlaro, G.; Iannello, G. Short-term bone level observations associated with platform switching in immediately placed and restored single maxillary implants: A preliminary report. *Int. J. Prosthodont.* **2009**, *22*, 277–282.

25. Saito, H.; Chu, S.; Zamzok, J.; Brown, M.; Smith, R.; Sarnachiaro, G.; Hochman, M.; Fletcher, P.; Reynolds, M.; Tarnow, D. Flapless Postextraction Socket Implant Placement: The Effects of a Platform Switch–Designed Implant on Peri-implant Soft Tissue Thickness—A Prospective Study. *Int. J. Periodontics Restor. Dent.* **2018**, *38*, s9–s15. [CrossRef]

26. Wennström, J.L.; Ekestubbe, A.; Gröndahl, K.; Karlsson, S.; Lindhe, J. Oral rehabilitation with implant-supported fixed partial dentures in periodontitis-susceptible subjects. A 5-year prospective study. *J. Clin. Periodontol.* **2004**, *31*, 713–724. [CrossRef]

27. Calvo-Guirado, J.L.; Ortiz-Ruiz, A.J.; López-Marí, L.; Delgado-Ruiz, R.; Maté-Sánchez, J.; Bravo Gonzalez, L.A. Immediate maxillary restoration of single-tooth implants using platform switching for crestal bone preservation: A 12-month study. *Int. J. Oral Maxillofac. Implant.* **2009**, *24*, 275–281.

28. Crespi, R.; Capparè, P.; Gherlone, E. Radiographic evaluation of marginal bone levels around platform-switched and non-platform-switched implants used in an immediate loading protocol. *Int. J. Oral Maxillofac. Implant.* **2009**, *24*, 920–926.

29. Lang, N.P.; Pun, L.; Lau, K.Y.; Li, K.Y.; Wong, M.C. A systematic review on survival and success rates of implants placed immediately into fresh extraction sockets after at least 1 year. *Clin. Oral Implant. Res.* **2011**, *23*, 39–66. [CrossRef]

30. Moraschini, V.; Velloso, G.; Luz, D.; Cavalcante, D.M.; Barboza, E.D.S.P. Fixed Rehabilitation of Edentulous Mandibles Using 2 to 4 Implants. *Implant. Dent.* **2016**, *25*, 435–444. [CrossRef]

31. Rammelsberg, P.; Kappel, S.; Bermejo, J.L. Effect of prosthetic restoration on implant survival and success. *Clin. Oral Implant. Res.* **2016**, *28*, 1296–1302. [CrossRef] [PubMed]

3

Osseointegration of Maxillary Dental Implants in Diabetes Mellitus Patients: A Randomized Clinical Trial Human Histomorphometric Study

Lyly Sam [1], Siriporn Chattipakorn [2] and Pathawee Khongkhunthian [1,*]

[1]   Center of Excellence for Dental Implantology, Faculty of Dentistry, Chiang Mai University, Chiang Mai 50200, Thailand; lyly_sam@cmu.ac.th

[2]   Department of Oral Biology and Diagnostic Sciences, Faculty of Dentistry, Chiang Mai University, Chiang Mai 50200, Thailand; siriporn.c@cmu.ac.th

*   Correspondence: pathawee.k@cmu.ac.th

Abstract: *Background*: Survival of dental implants in well-controlled Type 2 diabetes (T2DM) was found to be comparable to that in healthy patients. However, to our best knowledge, there have been no studies of the bone histomorphometry of osseointegration in patients with Type 2 diabetes. *Purpose*: To compare bone-implant-contact (BIC) and new bone formation between well-controlled Type 2 diabetes with HbA1c of less than 8% and healthy controls. *Methods*: 10 diabetic (T2DM) patients and 10 healthy controls were selected. Each patient received a 2.5 mm × 5 mm micro-implant in the maxilla, in either the premolar or first molar area. After 8 weeks of healing, the micro-implant was retrieved using a trephine bur and sent for bone histomorphometric analysis. A commercial titanium implant was immediately placed as the conventional treatment. *Results*: The mean BIC (30.73%) in T2DM patients was significantly lower than in the healthy patients (41.75%) ($p = 0.01$). New bone formation around the implant surface was reduced in T2DM patients (36.25%) compared to that in the control group (44.14%) ($p = 0.028$). The Pearson correlation coefficient revealed a strong correlation between increased HbA1c and decreased BIC ($p < 0.05$) and decreased new bone formation ($p < 0.05$). *Conclusions*: Within the limitation of this study, bone-to-implant contact and bone healing around dental implants in T2DM patients were significantly lower than in healthy patients.

Keywords: dental implants; type 2 diabetes; osseointegration; obesity; bone histomorphometry

1. Introduction

The connections between success of dental implantation and various systemic conditions have been started to be investigated and published during the past decade [1–3]. It is well known that any conditions that interfere with normal homeostasis of bone might have detrimental effects on the survival of dental implants [4]. Understanding the medically-compromised conditions that might affect dental implants, for example diabetes mellitus or osteoporosis, helps reduce failures and complications following the treatment [3]. Diabetes mellitus impairs bone healing, therefore, this systemic condition has to be taken into the consideration for dental implant treatment.

Four hundred and twenty-two million people worldwide were diagnosed with diabetes mellitus (DM) in 2014 and the number of affected people is estimated to be on the rise [5]. The increasing number of DM cases is due to increasing prevalence of obesity, since these two disorders are metabolically associated [6]. Increasing sugar intake, physical inactivity and sedentary life are the key factors for developing these two disorders, commonly found among people in developed countries [7,8].

The most common forms of DM are type 1 and type 2. Type 1 (T1DM), or insulin-dependent diabetes mellitus is the result of failure of the pancreas to produce insulin. Type 2 (T2DM), or non–insulin-dependent diabetes, results from deficiency in insulin production, or its mechanism of action, or both. Unlike T1DM, T2DM is linked to obesity, which is the predominant form in the adult population, contributing about 90% to 95% of diabetes cases [9]. This form of diabetes is characterized by insulin resistance, hyperglycemia and dysfunction of the pancreas to produce sufficient insulin. All of these disorders can be seen in the late stage of T2DM [10]. In addition, obesity and T2DM contribute to metabolic syndrome, which is associated with abdominal obesity, blood lipid disorders, inflammation, insulin resistance or full-blown diabetes, and increased risk of developing cardiovascular disease [11]. T2DM is associated with various systemic complications, including microvascular and macrovascular complications, such as retinopathy, nephropathy, neuropathy, cerebrovascular disease and cardiovascular disease [12]. Furthermore, DM has been found to be associated with increased prevalence of periodontitis and tooth loss [13], impaired wound healing, and increased susceptibility to infection [14].

Glycemic control is important for long term maintenance of DM to prevent associated major complications, such as cardiovascular diseases [15]. Glycosylated hemoglobin percentage (HbA1c) is considered a more reliable indicator for glycemic level in the previous six to eight weeks than fasting plasma glucose (FPG) [16]. The quality of glycemic control was found, in some studies [17–20], to affect the survival of dental implants and the healing of their supporting bone whereas, in others studies no differences were found [21–23]. "Well-controlled: "better-controlled," "moderately-controlled," and "poorly-controlled" DM are among the common terms to describe the quality of diabetic condition by different researchers in their respective studies. To determine the cut-off point for HbA1c to differentiate between well- and poorly-controlled DM is unclear, although many authors consider HbA1c of more than 8% as poorly-controlled [24]. This is possibly the reason why the results of bone healing around dental implants in T2DM were inconsistent due to different methods to define the glycemic status of the patients.

The long-term clinical performance of dental implants in diabetic patients is less than in healthy individuals [25–27]. Moreover, many clinical studies have investigated the effect of T2DM on soft and hard tissue healing following dental implant treatment [18–20,28]. In a recent systematic review, it was concluded that dental implant treatment is safe and predictable for diabetic patients; patients with well-controlled DM were able to achieve similar implant survival compared to healthy controls [29]. However, in poor-controlled DM, many studies reported impaired osseointegration [17,21], higher risk of peri-implantitis [18] and higher level of implant failure [27]. Clinically, the osseointegration in well-controlled DM has not been investigated.

A number of animal studies have evaluated bone healing around implants in patients with DM to understand its effects on osseointegration [30–33]. The results from these studies were convincing that DM adversely affects bone healing around implants by decreasing intrafibrillar collagen mineralization [30], trabecular bone formation [31], bone removal torque [32], bone mineralization and bone-implant contact significantly [33].

Various kinds of animal models have been used as testing steps with dental implants before clinical applications in human. The most commonly-used animals for evaluation of bone implant interaction are the dog, sheep, goat, pig and rabbit [34]. Among many characteristics to be considered when choosing a specific animal for an experiment, bone macrostructure, microstructure, composition and remodeling are the most important factors for consideration. The pig is considered a good likeness to human; however, size and ease of handling may limit its use for research [34]. There are a number of studies evaluating bone-implant contact (BIC) in humans [35–39]. For ethical reasons, dental implants placed in humans jaw bone and later retrieved for histologic evaluation are mostly used as transitional implants to support provisional dentures during the healing period.

Several studies conducted in animals show the adverse effect of DM such as peri-implantitis and disintegration on survival and healing of dental implants [30–33]; however, the similarity of bone healing around biocompatible materials still varies between animals and humans.

Therefore, the clinical study on humans is more appropriate for evaluating the effect of DM on bone healing and bone-implant contact. The purpose of this study was to compare bone-implant contact (BIC) and new bone formation at the bone implant connection in maxilla between healthy subjects and those with T2DM. The null hypothesis is no significant difference in bone implant contact and new bone formation between healthy and T2DM patients.

2. Materials and Methods

According to the WMA Declaration of Helsinki-Ethical Principles for Medical Research Involving Human Subjects, this study was approved by the Human Experimentation Committee of the Faculty of Dentistry, Chiang Mai University (No. 33/2561) and Thai Clinical Trials Registry (TCTR20190103004). All patients involving in the study have signed the inform consents. This prospective clinical study was designed (following the consort guideline) to compare BIC between well-controlled T2DM and healthy group. Ten T2DM and 10 healthy volunteers participated in this study. Patients who needed an implant in upper premolar and molar region were included in the study. All participants were well informed regarding to the whole procedure and an informed consent form was signed. For the T2DM patients, only those with well-controlled condition (HbA1c ≤ 8%) were admitted.

General inclusion criteria were physically healthy (ASA I or II), emotionally and psychologically stable and local inclusion criteria were tooth loss at premolar and molar area (at least 6months extraction), and sufficient keratinized tissue (>4 mm). Exclusion criteria were cardiovascular complications, history of bone fracture during the last 6 months, HIV, smoking and any type of cancers. List of all inclusion and exclusion criteria were presented in Figure 1. After intra-oral examination, patients were sent for dental cone-beam computed tomography to determine the bone width and height, which is the final criteria required for participating in this project.

Under local anesthesia, both groups had a micro-implants with 2.5 mm in diameter and 5 mm in length placed in their right or left maxilla in the premolar and first molar edentulous area. After eight weeks of healing, another surgery was performed to retrieve the micro-implant using trephine bur, and the retrieved micro-implant was sent for bone histomorphometric analysis to evaluate BIC and new bone formation. Upon removal of the micro implant, the bone bed was prepared for conventional implant placement. Either 4.2 mm or 5 mm diameter of conventional implant was used depends on the width of alveolar bone and location of implant placed. Dental prosthesis was delivered after 12 weeks of uneventful healing. Height, weight, and waist circumference were recorded and blood was taken at the baseline and two months after healing of micro-implants to evaluate FPG, HbA1c, cholesterol, triglycerides, HDL-C and LDL-C. A summary of the research protocol is shown in Figure 2.

Inclusion criteria

General

1. Physically healthy (ASA I or II classification)
2. Psychological and emotional stable
3. No history of bone fracture during the last 12 months
4. No smoking
5. Be compliant with dental appointment and instruction
6. Understand the overall procedure and sign the informed consent.

Local

1. Tooth loss at upper premolar or molar area (at least 6 months removal) & seeking dental implant placement
2. Properly healed edentulous area (no infection, no pus, no swelling, no bleeding)
3. Sufficient keratinized gingival at least 4 mm.
4. Alveolar bone width of at least 6 mm and height of 12 mm (by CBCT)
5. No bone augmentation procedure needed before and during implant placement
6. Stable dental occlusion

Exclusion criteria

1. HbA1c level above 8% for test group
2. Pregnant or lactating females
3. Use of anti-inflammatory and immunosuppressive drugs
4. HIV
5. Current smoking or ex-smoker
6. Patients with major complications of diabetes (cardiovascular and peripheral vascular disease, neuropathy and nephropathy)
7. History of chemotherapy or radiotherapy around head and neck area
8. Third molar and anterior edentulous area
9. Antiosteoporotic drugs & other medications (e.g., hormonal contraceptives, corticosteroids, aromatase inhibitors).
10. Osteoporosis

Discontinuation criteria

1. Uncooperative
2. Not compliant with the proposed procedure and
3. Request for treatment termination.

Figure 1. Criteria for participating in this study.

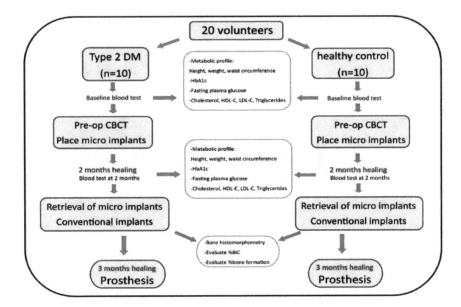

Figure 2. Summary of research protocol.

2.1. Micro-Implant Design and Characteristics

All micro-implants (Novem, PW plus Company, Nakorn Pathom, Thailand) were made from commercially available pure (CP) titanium grade 4.

The implants have minimal surface roughness by sandblast acid etch technique the same as a commercial dental implant. The implant has 2.5 mm of diameter and 5 mm of length with characteristics of four outer rings and three chambers similar to the implants used in another study [40] (Figure 3).

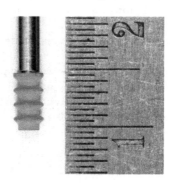

Figure 3. Micro-implant design with outer diameters of 2.5 mm and length 5 mm. the implant is designed with 3 bone chambers and 4 outer rings.

2.1.1. Surgical Procedure

Micro-Implant Placement

Edentulous area in the maxillary premolar and first molar region both right and left side were included in the experiment protocol with bone diameter of at least 6 mm in order to accommodate the future conventional implant of between 4.2 mm to 5 mm and bone length of at least 10 mm to 12 mm. All of patients in control and test groups first underwent surgical placement of a 2.5 mm × 5 mm micro-implant (Figure 4c). Local anesthesia was administered using articaine 4% with epinephrine 1:100,000 concentration (Septanest SP, Septodont, Saint-Maur-des-Fosses, France) and mid-crestal incision was made using number 15c carbon steel blade (Swann-Morton, Sheffield, England) and full thickness flap was raised using periosteal elevator. Implant bed was made using a cylindrical carbide bur drilled in the middle of the crestal bone and the micro-implant was placed by press-fit technique using percussion manually until all the threads completely embedded in the alveolar bone. The mucoperiosteal flap was then repositioned and 4-0 nylon suture (Sofilon, Novamedic, Samut Prakan, Thailand) was used to close the surgical site. Analgesic (paracetamol 500 mg, GPO, Bangkok, Thailand) and antibiotics (either amoxycillin 500 mg (GPO) or clindamycin 150 mg (GPO) were prescribed for all patients for 3 days and 7 days respectively. Sutures were removed after 7 days post-operation, and wound healing was monitored at 1 week, 4 weeks and 8 weeks after implant placement before retrieval and placement of conventional implants.

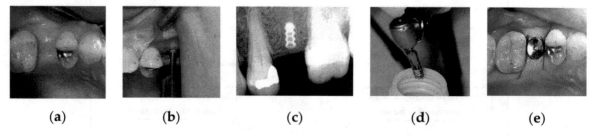

| (a) | (b) | (c) | (d) | (e) |

Figure 4. Surgical placement of micro-implant. (**a**). Initial situation with one missing tooth on maxillary second pre-molar area; (**b**). Full thickness flap raised and micro implant was inserted; (**c**). Periapical radiograph immediately after the surgery; (**d**). Trephine bur was used to retrieve the implant after 8 weeks of healing; (**e**). Conventional implant was placed immediately after removal of the micro-implant and healing abutment was used.

Conventional Implant Placement

After 8 weeks healing of micro-implants, all patients were appointed for another surgery to retrieve the integrated micro-implant. A conventional dental implant (Novem, PW plus) was placed in the existing socket as part of a missing tooth replacement with implant supported prosthesis. The surgical procedure began with local anesthesia administration with articaine 4% with epinephrine 1:100,000 concentration (Septanest SP, Septodont, Saint-Maur-des-Fossés, France). A 15c scalpel blade (Swann-Morton, Sheffield, England) was used to make mid-crestal incision before full thickness flap was raised with periosteal elevator. Upon the exposure of micro-implant head, trephine bur was used to remove the implant along with intact bone surrounding (Figure 4d). The specimen was then placed in 10% buffered formalin solution and sent to the laboratory for histomorphometric evaluation. In the same surgical site, implant bed was further prepared by implant shaping and final drills following the implant manufacturer's instruction of drilling protocol. Implant of 4.2 mm or 5 mm diameter and 10 mm or 12 mm in length was then placed (Figure 4e) followed by insertion torque and resonance frequency analysis (RFA) to measure implant stability as part of conventional implant surgery procedure. Transmucosal healing abutment was tightened on top of the conventional implant fixture and the soft tissue was repositioned with 4-0 nylon sutures (Sofilon, Novamedic, Samut Prakan, Thailand). Patients were appointed for 1 week follow up and suture removal. After 12 weeks of uneventful healing, dental impression was made and sent to dental laboratory for prosthesis fabrication.

2.2. Blood Test

All participants were required to fast for at least 10 h before blood withdrawal to evaluate HbA1c, FPG, cholesterol, HDL-C, LDL-C and triglycerides at baseline and 8 weeks after micro-implant placement. Ten milliliters of blood was collected from median cubital vein and separated into 3 different tubes for different parameters. Whole blood in EDTA tube was for testing HbA1c and sodium fluoride tube was for fasting plasma glucose. Another tube (red tube) with no anticoagulant or preservative was used for testing of cholesterol, HDL-C, LDL-C and triglycerides. All data was analyzed and correlated with the value of BIC and new bone formation.

2.3. Histological Preparation and Histomorphometric Analysis

Sample processing included fixation, dehydration, infiltration and embedding following the method described by Donath et al. [41]. The final thickness after grinding the sample was about 8–10 μm. After staining with toluidine blue, image processing was captured by Carl Zeiss microscope and analyzed by AxioVision SE64 Rel. 4.9.1 Software (Carl Zeiss, Jena, Germany). The total length of implant surface and the length of the surface where the bone tissue directly contacted the implant were measured to calculate bone contact with the implant surface. For the new bone formation, the total area of implant chamber and the area of new bone growth were measured to calculate the percentage of bone formation. Two separated evaluators analyzed and calculated the samples and inter-calibration between the examiners was done before statistical analysis.

2.4. Statistical Analysis

Sample size calculation was based on a previous study which could provide an α error of 5 and 90% power of test [33]. Shapiro-Wilk test was used to test the normality between test and control groups. All variances were compared using independent t-test. The Pearson correlation coefficient was performed to find any correlation between the parameters. $p < 0.05$ was considered significantly different.

3. Results

Ten T2DM (5 males and 5 females) and ten healthy (3 males and 7 females) participants were included in this study (No drop-outs of patients). T2DM patients were significantly older than the control group (50.3 years ± 3.1 years vs. 60.5 years ± 1.2 years, $p = 0.01$). Anthropometric measurement showed no significant difference of body mass index (BMI) (T2DM 24.1 ± 1.0; controls 24.6 ± 1.2) and waist circumference (T2DM 33.4 ± 1.3 inches; control 33.6 ± 1.2 inches) ($p > 0.05$) (Table 1).

Table 1. Comparison of anthropometry (BMI and waist circumference) between T2DM group and control group.

		Participant	Gender		Age	BMI	Waist Circumference (WC)
		n	Male	Female	Mean ± SE	Mean ± SE	Mean ± SE
Group	Control	10	3	7	50.3 ± 3.1 (years)	24.6 ± 1.2	33.6 ± 1.2 (inches)
	T2DM	10	5	5	60.5 ± 1.2 (years)	24.1 ± 1.0	33.4 ± 1.3 (inches)
Total number		20					
Significance					$p = 0.01$	$p = 0.844$	$p = 0.796$

Results from blood test of metabolic parameters and lipid profile at both baseline and at 8 weeks are shown in Table 2. FPG (122.6 mg/dL vs. 77 mg/dL, $p < 0.05$) and HbA1c in T2DM (6.47% vs. 5.16%, $p < 0.05$) at 8 weeks were significantly higher than in controls as expected although the other lipid profile parameters (cholesterol, HDL-C, LDL-C and triglycerides) were not significantly different (Table 2).

Table 2. Comparison of lipid profile of control and T2DM groups. Only fasting plasma glucose (FPG) and HbA1c showed significant difference ($p < 0.05$).

	Control ($n = 10$)	T2DM ($n = 10$)
FPG at baseline	80.4 ± 8.9 (mg/dL)	117.1 ± 20.5 (mg/dL) *
FPG at 8 weeks	77 ± 6.4 (mg/dL)	122.6 ± 26.1 (mg/dL) *
HbA1c at baseline	5.3 ± 0.2 (%)	6.43 ± 0.6 (%)
HbA1c at 8 weeks	5.1 ± 0.1 (%)	6.47 ± 0.6 (%) *
Cholesterol at baseline	222.1 ± 43.7 (mg/dL)	164.3 ± 48.9 (mg/dL)
Cholesterol at 8 weeks	213.1 ± 51.8 (mg/dL)	164.9 ± 44.6 (mg/dL)
HDL-C at baseline	61 ± 16.1 (mg/dL)	53.7 ±17 (mg/dL)
HDL-C at 8 weeks	60.7 ± 17.8 (mg/dL)	55.2 ± 17.3 (mg/dL)
LDL-C at baseline	136.3 ± 42 (mg/dL)	90.5 ± 35.1 (mg/dL)
LDL-C at 8 weeks	134.2 ± 46.8 (mg/dL)	87.1 ± 37.3 (mg/dL)
Triglycerides at baseline	124 ± 96.6 (mg/dL)	101 ± 49.9 (mg/dL)
Triglycerides at 8 weeks	91.4 ± 40.5 (mg/dL)	112.8 ± 80.7 (mg/dL)

* significant difference between the groups ($p < 0.05$).

Data from bone histomorphometric analysis demonstrated that the collected data from both groups were normally distributed by using Kolmogorov-Smirnov and Shapiro-Wilk test. After 8 weeks of placement, all micro-implants placed in both groups showed no sign of failure from both clinical evaluation and periapical radiograph; therefore, osseointegration occurred (Figure 5).

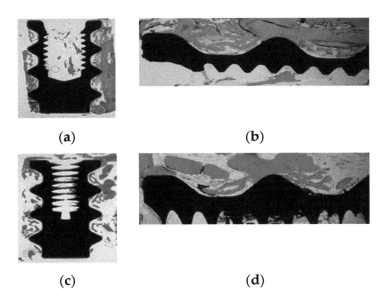

(a)   (b)

(c)   (d)

Figure 5. Histomorphometric examination of micro-implant of control (**a,b**) and T2DM group (**c,d**). T2DM group showed less bone implant contact (BIC) and new bone formation inside the implant thread.

The calculation of BIC from both groups showed that T2DM had significantly lower BIC (30.73%) than its control counterpart (41.75%) ($p = 0.01$). Similarly, new bone formation in the implant chamber was reduced in the tested group (36.25%) compared to the healthy group (44.14%) ($p = 0.028$). The Pearson correlation indicated that higher FPG was closely related to higher HbA1c. Moreover, higher HbAc1 was adversely related to lowered BIC and new bone formation on titanium implants surface indicating that the higher HbA1c, the lower bone formation around implants (Figures 6 and 7). However, other parameters including cholesterol, HDL-C, LDL-C and triglycerides did not show any correlation with BIC and new bone formation.

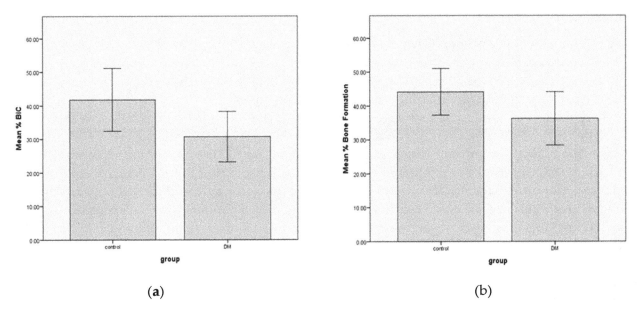

(a)   (b)

Figure 6. Comparison of %BIC and % bone formation between T2DM and controls. %BIC and % bone formation in T2DM group were significantly lower than their counterpart. ((**a**) % BIC) ((**b**) % Bone formation).

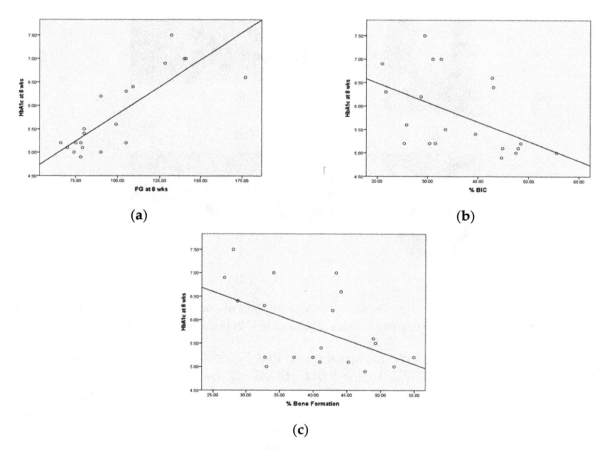

Figure 7. Correlation between fasting glucose (FG) and HbA1c (**a**), HbA1c and %BIC (**b**), HbA1c and % bone formation (**c**). There was a strong correlation between increased HbA1c and decreased BIC ($p < 0.05$) and decreased new bone formation ($p < 0.05$).

4. Discussion

T2DM is the most common form of all DM and the number of affected patients were on the rise. T2DM was linked to being overweight and obese [6]. BMI and waist circumference are the most common measurements for obesity. In this study, both T2DM and healthy had normal range of BMI and WC demonstrating that none of the participants were obese.

There were studies about the success and survival of dental implants in T2DM patients in recent systematic reviews [29,42]. Good glycemic control seemed to be closely associated with the higher survival rate and fewer complications of dental implants in T2DM patients. FPG and HbA1c are the most commonly used parameters to determine glycemic status for T2DM; however, HbA1c is considered more reliable since it indicates the average glycemic status of T2DM patients in the last 3 months due to the life cycle of red blood cells [16]. Only T2DM patients with well-controlled glycemic status having HbA1c below 8% were included in this study. Clinically and histologically, all implants were successfully integrated to the alveolar bone.

Only patients with a missing tooth on the maxilla in the premolar and molar region were included in this study. Peri-implant bone healing in the posterior maxilla is more rapid than in other areas of the jaw bones. Posterior maxilla consists of almost all trabecular bone; therefor, bone regeneration and remodeling are far quicker than in cortical bone. In addition, osteoconduction and de-novo bone formation only occur in peri-implant healing in trabecular bone [43]. Therefore, premolar and molar of maxilla were chosen for this study.

Bone histomorphometry is crucial for understanding osseointegration of dental implant. Osseointegration has been defined as a direct and functional connection between bone and an artificial implant. Both macroscopic and microscopic characteristics of dental implants could influence the success of these procedures. There were animal studies regarding to bone healing around implants in diabetic models [30–32]. In hyperglycemia condition, it was found that early bone mineralization was interrupted [30], trabecular bone, signaling molecules of fibronectin and Integrin α5β1 were reduced [31], BIC and implant removal torque were lower comparing to controls [32]. However, there are a few downsides of using animals for experiments. In case of DM, the diabetic animals might not accurately represent the pathologic condition of the T2DM in human as animals were either drug-induced or genetically modified to create the diabetic condition. In addition, bone healing and turnover rates of these animals such as rats and rabbits are not comparable to human [33,34]. All of these might interfere with the interpretation of the data received. Interesting, our study showed similar result of negative effects of hyperglycemia or DM on BIC and new bone formation in the implant thread indicating that bone healing capacity of T2DM patients was significantly lower than in those healthy group. Moreover, In genetically modified and drug-induced diabetic rats, it was found that new trabecular bone around implant surfaces was reduced compared to those rats treated with insulin [31,32] and thus presented lower removal torque values [32]. Most of our T2DM patients were using anti-diabetic medications to control their blood glucose to a well-controlled state. However, that was not effective in increasing BIC and new bone formation around dental implants in our findings which is contradicted with what was found in the animal experiments.

Another significant finding was the strong correlation between HbA1c and BIC and new bone formation. The higher HbA1c, the lower bone formation around implants (Figure 7b,c) and this finding might explain the result from the studies regarding to the lower resonance frequency analysis (RFA) of dental implants in clinical situation [17,21]. Clinically, it is impractical to retrieve implant for histomorphometric analysis even though it is a more reliable method to observe the osseointegration phenomenon. Thus, a less invasive method to reflect the healing process of dental implant is to measure implant stability by RFA. Oates and colleges [17,21] found that the implant stability of T2DM with higher HbA1c was significantly lower than those with lower HbA1c and required longer time to return to baseline stability indicating that the healing capacity of hyperglycemic condition in T2DM was adversely affected. These findings supported the result of our study of the association between higher HbA1c and lower BIC and new bone formation which in turn demonstrated lower implant stability clinically.

Previous studies showed that success of dental implants in diabetic patient ranged from 92% [44] to 97.2% [23], which was comparable to their healthy counterparts. Long-term clinical comparison was reported in a prospective study up to 12 years which showed no significant difference between T2DM and controls for simple dental implants placement as well as more complicated cases such as sinus lift and bone augmentation [23]. However, other studies demonstrated the adverse effect of DM on dental implants in terms of success rate [25–27], osseointegration by resonance frequency test [17,21], and peri-implant tissue such as increased bleeding on probing (BOP) [19] and peri-implantitis [28]. For these inconsistent reports of the clinical outcome of DM on dental implants, a few factors should be considered. Firstly, the study of success of dental implant in diabetic patients were conducted in different manners such as retrospective, prospective and cross-sectional studies as shown in recent literature reviews; therefore, a meta-analysis was not possible [29,45]. Secondly, not all the studies stated the type of their diabetic patients whether they are type 1 or type 2. In addition, the status of their glycemic control was not clearly defined; for instance, most authors considered HbA1c below 8% well-controlled while some others accepted less than 8%, used other parameter such as fasting plasma glucose, or did not even report the glycemic status of the participants. To our best knowledge, this study is the first clinical study that compared histologically osseointegration between healthy and T2DM patients. From the results of our study, dental implants in T2DM patients had lower osseointegration although all implants show 100% success clinically within our study period; therefore, long-term follow-up is required.

5. Conclusions

Within the limitations of this study, it can be concluded that bone healing around dental implants of T2DM patients was significantly lower than healthy patients. Long term follow-up for the clinical results of dental implant treatment in patients with DM is required.

Author Contributions: L.S.: conception, design, data collection, data interpretation, manuscript. S.C.: conception, design, data interpretation, manuscript revision. P.K.: conception, design, data analysis and interpretation, critical revision of the manuscript, final approval of manuscript. All authors have read and agreed to the published version of the manuscript.

References

1.   Alsaadi, G.; Quirynen, M.; Komarek, A.; van Steenberghe, D. Impact of local and systemic factors on the incidence of oral implant failures, up to abutment connection. *J. Clin. Periodontol.* **2007**, *34*, 610–617. [CrossRef]

2.   Mombelli, A.; Cionca, N. Systemic diseases affecting osseointegration therapy. *Clin. Oral Implant. Res.* **2006**, *17*, 97–103. [CrossRef] [PubMed]

3.   Diz, P.; Scully, C.; Sanz, M. Dental implants in the medically compromised patient. *J. Dent.* **2013**, *41*, 195–206. [CrossRef] [PubMed]

4.   Marx, R.E.; Garg, A.K. Bone structure, metabolism, and physiology: Its impact on dental implantology. *Implant. Dent.* **1998**, *7*, 267–276. [CrossRef]

5.   World Health Organization. Global Report on Diabetes 2016. Available online: http://www.who.int/diabetes/global-report/en/ (accessed on 15 April 2019).

6.   Mokdad, A.H.; Ford, E.S.; Bowman, B.A.; Dietz, W.H.; Vinicor, F.; Bales, V.S.; Marks, J.S. Prevalence of obesity, diabetes, and obesity-related health risk factors, 2001. *JAMA* **2003**, *289*, 76–79. [CrossRef] [PubMed]

7.   Zimmet, P.; Alberti, K.; Shaw, J. Global and societal implications of the diabetes epidemic. *Nature* **2001**, *414*, 782–787. [CrossRef]

8.   Hu, F.B.; Leitzmann, M.F.; Stampfer, M.J.; Colditz, G.A.; Willett, W.C.; Rimm, E.B. Physical activity and television watching in relation to risk for type 2 diabetes mellitus in men. *Arch. Intern. Med.* **2001**, *161*, 1542–1548. [CrossRef]

9.   Americal Diabetes Association. Diagnosis and classification of diabetes mellitus. *Diabetes Care* **2010**, *33*, 62–69. [CrossRef]

10.   DeFronzo, R.A. Pathogenesis of type 2 diabetes mellitus. *Med. Clin. N. Am.* **2004**, *88*, 787–835. [CrossRef]

11.   Després, J.P.; Lemieux, I. Abdominal obesity and metabolic syndrome. *Nature* **2006**, *444*, 881–887. [CrossRef]

12.   Cade, W.T. Diabetes-related microvascular and macrovascular diseases in the physical therapy setting. *Phys. Ther.* **2008**, *88*, 1322. [CrossRef] [PubMed]

13.   Khader, Y.S.; Dauod, A.S.; El-Qaderi, S.S.; Alkafajei, A.; Batayha, W.Q. Periodontal status of diabetics compared with nondiabetics: A meta-analysis. *J. Diabetes Complicat.* **2006**, *20*, 59–68. [CrossRef]

14.   Abiko, Y.; Selimovic, D. The mechanism of protracted wound healing on oral mucosa in diabetes. review. *Bosn. J. Basic Med. Sci.* **2010**, *10*, 186–191. [CrossRef] [PubMed]

15.   Ahmed, A.A. Glycemic Control in Diabetes. *Oman Med. J.* **2010**, *25*, 232–233. [CrossRef] [PubMed]

16.   Bonora, E.; Tuomilehto, J. The pros and cons of diagnosing diabetes with A1C. *Diabetes Care* **2011**, *34*, 184–190. [CrossRef] [PubMed]

17.   Oates, T.W.; Dowell, S.; Robinson, M.; McMahan, C.A. Glycemic control and implant stabilization in type 2 diabetes mellitus. *J. Dent. Res.* **2009**, *88*, 367–371. [CrossRef]

18.   Aguilar-Salvatierra, A.; Calvo-Guirado, J.L.; Gonzalez-Jaranay, M.; Moreu, G.; Delgado-Ruiz, R.A.; Gomez-Moreno, G. Peri-implant evaluation of immediately loaded implants placed in esthetic zone in patients with diabetes mellitus type 2: A two-year study. *Clin. Oral Implant. Res.* **2016**, *27*, 156–161. [CrossRef]

19.   Gomez-Moreno, G.; Aguilar-Salvatierra, A.; Roldan, J.R.; Guardia, J.; Gargallo, J.; Calvo-Guirado, J.L. Peri-implant evaluation in type 2 diabetes mellitus patients: A 3-year study. *Clin. Oral Implant. Res.* **2015**, *26*, 1031–1035. [CrossRef]

20. Ghiraldini, B.; Conte, A.; Casarin, R.C.; Casati, M.Z.; Pimentel, S.P.; Cirano, F.R.; Ribeiro, F.V. Influence of Glycemic Control on Peri-Implant Bone Healing: 12-Month Outcomes of Local Release of Bone-Related Factors and Implant Stabilization in Type 2 Diabetics. *Clin. Implant. Dent. Relat. Res.* **2016**, *18*, 801–809. [CrossRef]

21. Oates, T.W.; Galloway, P.; Alexander, P.; Green, A.V.; Huynh-Ba, G.; Feine, J.; McMahan, C.A. The effects of elevated hemoglobin A1c in patients with type 2 diabetes mellitus on dental implants. *J. Am. Dent. Assoc.* **2014**, *145*, 1218–1226. [CrossRef]

22. Dowell, S.; Oates, T.W.; Robinson, M. Implant success in people with type 2 diabetes mellitus with varying glycemic control: A pilot study. *J. Am. Dent. Assoc.* **2007**, *138*, 355–361. [CrossRef] [PubMed]

23. Tawil, G.; Younan, R.; Azar, P.; Sleilati, G. Conventional and advanced implant treatment in the type II diabetic patient: Surgical protocol and long-term clinical results. *Int. J. Oral Maxillofac. Implant.* **2008**, *23*, 744–752.

24. Americal Diabetes Association. The absence of a glycemic threshold for the development of long-term complications: The perspective of the Diabetes Control and Complications Trial. *Diabetes* **1996**, *45*, 1289–1298. [CrossRef]

25. Busenlechner, D.; Fürhauser, R.; Haas, R.; Watzek, G.; Mailath, G.; Pommer, B. Long-term implant success at the Academy for Oral Implantology: 8-year follow-up and risk factor analysis. *J. Periodontal Implant. Sci.* **2014**, *44*, 102–108. [CrossRef]

26. Morris, H.F.; Ochi, S.; Winkler, S. Implant survival in patients with type 2 diabetes: Placement to 36 months. *Ann. Periodontol.* **2000**, *5*, 157–165. [CrossRef]

27. Daubert, D.M.; Weinstein, B.F.; Bordin, S.; Leroux, B.G.; Flemmig, T.F. Prevalence and predictive factors for peri-implant disease and implant failure: A cross-sectional analysis. *J. Periodontol.* **2015**, *86*, 337–347. [CrossRef]

28. Ferreira, S.; Silva, G.; Cortelli, J.; Costa, J.; Costa, F. Prevalence and risk variables for peri-implant disease in Brazilian subjects. *J. Clin. Periodontol.* **2006**, *33*, 929–935. [CrossRef]

29. Naujokat, H.; Kunzendorf, B.; Wiltfang, J. Dental implants and diabetes mellitus—A systematic review. *Int. J. Implant. Dent.* **2016**, *2*, 5. [CrossRef]

30. Ajami, E.; Bell, S.; Liddell, R.S.; Davies, J.E. Early bone anchorage to micro- and nano-topographically complex implant surfaces in hyperglycemia. *Acta Biomater.* **2016**, *39*, 169–179. [CrossRef]

31. Liu, Z.; Zhou, W.; Tangl, S.; Liu, S.; Xu, X.; Rausch-Fan, X. Potential mechanism for osseointegration of dental implants in Zucker diabetic fatty rats. *Br. J. Oral Maxillofac. Surg.* **2015**, *53*, 748–753. [CrossRef]

32. De Molon, R.S.; Morais-Camilo, J.A.; Verzola, M.H.; Faeda, R.S.; Pepato, M.T.; Marcantonio, E., Jr. Impact of diabetes mellitus and metabolic control on bone healing around osseointegrated implants: Removal torque and histomorphometric analysis in rats. *Clin. Oral Implant. Res.* **2013**, *24*, 831–837. [CrossRef] [PubMed]

33. Von Wilmowsky, C.; Stockmann, P.; Harsch, I.; Amann, K.; Metzler, P.; Lutz, R.; Moest, T.; Neukam, F.W.; Schlegel, K.A. Diabetes mellitus negatively affects peri-implant bone formation in the diabetic domestic pig. *J. Clin. Periodontol.* **2011**, *38*, 771–779. [CrossRef] [PubMed]

34. Pearce, A.; Richards, R.; Milz, S.; Schneider, E.; Pearce, S. Animal models for implant biomaterial research in bone: A review. *Eur. Cell Mater.* **2007**, *13*, 1–10. [CrossRef] [PubMed]

35. Grassi, S.; Piattelli, A.; De Figueiredo, L.C.; Feres, M.; De Melo, L.; Iezzi, G.; Alba, R.C.; Shibli, J.A. Histologic evaluation of early human bone response to different implant surfaces. *J. Periodontol.* **2006**, *77*, 1736–1743. [CrossRef] [PubMed]

36. Wei, N.; Bin, S.; Jing, Z.; Wei, S.; Yingqiong, Z. Influence of implant surface topography on bone-regenerative potential and mechanical retention in the human maxilla and mandible. *Am. J. Dent.* **2014**, *27*, 171–176. [PubMed]

37. Shibli, J.A.; Mangano, C.; Mangano, F.; Rodrigues, J.A.; Cassoni, A.; Bechara, K.; Ferreia, J.D.B.; Dottore, A.M.; Iezzi, G.; Piattelli, A. Bone-to-Implant Contact Around Immediately Loaded Direct Laser Metal-Forming Transitional Implants in Human Posterior Maxilla. *J. Periodontol.* **2013**, *84*, 732–737. [CrossRef] [PubMed]

38. Degidi, M.; Perrotti, V.; Piattelli, A.; Iezzi, G. Mineralized bone-implant contact and implant stability quotient in 16 human implants retrieved after early healing periods: A histologic and histomorphometric evaluation. *Int. J. Oral Maxillofac. Implant.* **2010**, *25*, 45–48.

39. Mangano, C.; Shibli, J.A.; Pires, J.T.; Luongo, G.; Piattelli, A.; Iezzi, G. Early bone formation around immediately loaded transitional implants inserted in the human posterior maxilla: The effects of fixture design and surface. *BioMed Res. Int.* **2017**, *2017*, 4152506. [CrossRef]

40. Buser, D.; Broggini, N.; Wieland, M.; Schenk, R.; Denzer, A.; Cochran, D.; Hoffmann, B.; Lussi, A.; Steinemann, S. Enhanced bone apposition to a chemically modified SLA titanium surface. *J. Dent. Res.* **2004**, *83*, 529–533. [CrossRef]

41. Donath, K.; Breuner, G. A method for the study of undecalcified bones and teeth with attached soft tissues* The Säge-Schliff (sawing and grinding) Technique. *J. Oral. Patho. Med.* **1982**, *11*, 318–326. [CrossRef]

42. Shi, Q.; Xu, J.; Huo, N.; Cai, C.; Liu, H. Does a higher glycemic level lead to a higher rate of dental implant failure?: A meta-analysis. *JADA* **2016**, *147*, 875–881. [PubMed]

43. Davies, J.E. Understanding peri-implant endosseous healing. *J. Dent. Educ.* **2003**, *67*, 932–949. [PubMed]

44. Anner, R.; Grossmann, Y.; Anner, Y.; Levin, L. Smoking, diabetes mellitus, periodontitis, and supportive periodontal treatment as factors associated with dental implant survival: A long-term retrospective evaluation of patients followed for up to 10 years. *Implant. Dent.* **2010**, *19*, 57–64. [PubMed]

45. Oates, T.W.; Huynh-Ba, G.; Vargas, A.; Alexander, P.; Feine, J. A critical review of diabetes, glycemic control, and dental implant therapy. *Clin. Oral Implant. Res.* **2013**, *24*, 117–127.

4

Modeling of Dental Implant Osseointegration Progress by Three-Dimensional Finite Element Method

Iulia Roatesi [1] and Simona Roatesi [2],* (iD)

[1]   Department of Histology and Cytology, Dental Medicine Faculty, *Carol Davila* University of Medicine and Pharmacy, 050474 Bucharest, Romania; iulia.roatesi@umfcd.ro
[2]   Department of Applied Informatics, *Ferdinand I* Military Technical Academy, 050141 Bucharest, Romania
*   Correspondence: simona.roatesi@yahoo.fr or simona.roatesi@mta.ro

Abstract: As osseointegration is a time-dependent process, biomechanical assessment is thought to determine whether a fibrous encapsulation or a bone covering will develop around an implant, according to the stress in the implant and surrounding bone. This study proposes a model for stress evaluation by finite element method (FEM) during the osseointegration progress, the main factor implied in implant success or failure. The loadings due to masticatory forces generate stress concentration and consequently, an adequate risk concerning the implant stability should be assessed. An accurate FEM model is used to calculate the stress and displacement in the whole implant–bone system during the osseointegration progress. This process is simulated by taking into account the gradual increase in the damaged biomechanical properties of the cortical bone. The results reveal that as the implant osseointegration occurs gradually, the bone stiffness from the peri-implant area increases gradually, such that in the end (healing) we observed that the cortical bone begins to take over the bending loading. In addition, the displacements decrease as the osseointegration gradually occurs and the cortical bone stress reaches higher values, which are placed in the mandibular ridge. The FEM is suitable to model the osseointegration progress, offering valuable information concerning the stress concentration zones in the implant–bone system and consequently, the risk evaluation, both for pre- and post-osseointegration.

Keywords: dental implantation; dental crown; biomechanics; numerical modeling; dental implant stability

1. Introduction

Finite element method (FEM) is a helpful tool in the study of dental implantology as it allows the determination of the state of stress, strain and displacement in the implant and the surrounding bone [1–4]. A FEM analysis is very important in implants' optimal design [5–8], in assessing the factors that influence the whole process of pre- and post-osseointegration [9–11], or they are dedicated to oral rehabilitation [12,13], etc.

A very important issue in oral implantology is the study of the osseointegration process [14,15]. It is difficult to rigorously assess this process, whereas the biomechanical response differs from one patient to another [16,17] and moreover, the process itself depend on the specific factors that may relate to osseous healing around an implant.

Generally, FEM allows the study of the behavior of the implant and surrounding bone tissue after the osseointegration process termination [18]. In this context, it is considered a fixed contact between the bone tissue and implant throughout the bone–implant interface, i.e., under loading, there is no relative motion between the bone and implant, which would model complete osseointegration. In this case, the analysis carried out corresponds to a completely osseointegrated implant, and so for a time at least six months after the insertion of the implant. There are FEM analyses focusing on the investigation of the interaction between the implant and peri-implant bone tissue [19] or on the biomechanical of marginal bone resorption around osseointegrated implants [20].

Instead, if we consider an analysis of stress and displacement state during a period in the first few weeks or months after the implant insertion, when osseointegration is not fully attained, we propose an original method of an incomplete osseointegration modeling.

The numerical simulation using FEM determines the stress and displacement state both immediately after the implant insertion, as well as during the consolidation process of the bone–implant interaction phenomena until complete healing. The model under consideration in our study is that of a premolar implant on the jaw with a temporary crown for aesthetic reasons, in a lighter contact.

Therefore, the aim of this paper is to study by FEM the osseointegration process modeling since the first weeks of installing the implant to the complete osseointegration.

2. Materials and Methods

As the geometric model of the structure which is made up of the dental implant, bone and crown needs special preprocessing resources, the Solid Works program [21] was used to realize the model. The geometric model produced with this program was exported and used for calculations by the Cosmos program.

This study was dedicated to the analysis of the process of insertion of a dental implant into a section of jaw, with particular emphasis on highlighting the estimation for the various stages of osseointegration of the stress concentration zone in the bone and implant components under mastication loads. These areas represent the most vulnerable areas, in which the eventual yielding, rupture, damage of the structure may occur.

2.1. The Geometric Model of the Dental Implantation

The model of our analysis was static and elastic materials were considered.

Both the geometric and the finite element (FE) models of implant components and bone tissue were conducted with high accuracy, taking into account all the constructive and functional details (connection radii, threads, release cutting, contacts) so that the model could be as close as possible to reality.

Considering the case of a system made up of an implant [4], Rootform type, with a length of 11.5 mm, with a maximum thickness of 3.8 mm with two threaded areas (fine and large pitch) inserted in a portion of jaw extended for about 20 mm from the implant axis, as shown in Figure 1a,b.

The geometric model was made on one hand of the biological material, the jaw, composed of trabecular bone and cortical bone, and on the other hand, the implant, abutment and crown (Figure 1b). All these components were created by computer and used in the calculation by FEM. The implant was considered to be made of titanium alloy, the abutment of magnesium alloy and the crown of ceramic.

The implant is cone-shaped with two threaded zones (Figure 2).

The interior of the implant allowed the insertion with no thread of the intermediate part (abutment) (Figure 2b). At the top, it had a hexagonal reaming used to mount it in the jaw using an Allen key. The inner screw served to assemble the implant with the abutment by a titanium M2 screw (Figure 2b).

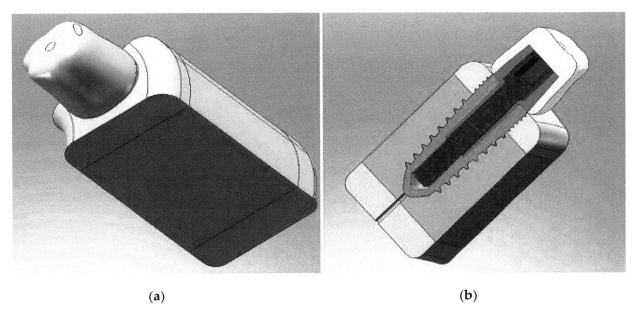

(a)   (b)

Figure 1. Geometrical model of the crown–implant–bone structure: (a) structure overview; (b) structure section.

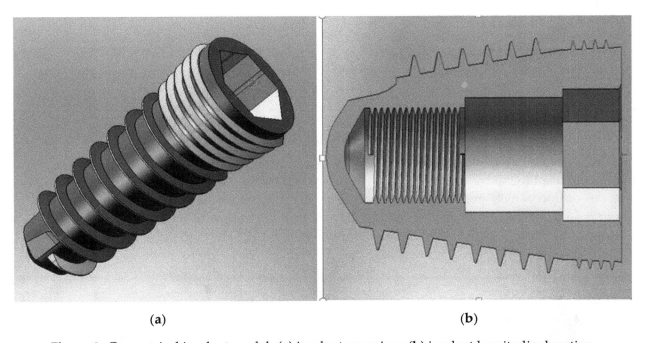

(a)   (b)

Figure 2. Geometrical implant model: (a) implant overview; (b) implant longitudinal section.

The crown geometrical model was shaped as close as to the actual shape (Figure 3a), being prepared to take into account in detail the crown characteristics, to avoid the biting force application on an almost flat surface that could affect the force transmission. The crown material was ceramic, even it was considered a provisional one. If there is no question of cost, and given that the mechanical properties of ceramics are clearly superior, this material is not outworn over time, referring to the masticatory surface (the resin from which the temporary crown is usually made easily becomes abrasive and in a short period of time), this solution can be adopted. Moreover, by using ceramics, which provide the brightness and translucency of the natural tooth, the aesthetic part is clearly superior, and if the patient, even if for a short period has maximum aesthetic requirements, it can use this solution. The supporting bone is represented by a portion of jaw around the implant on a certain distance to a boundary to which it is considered that there is no longer the influence of implant surgery.

Jaw modeling takes into account the different structure of the bone tissue (trabecular and cortical) (Figure 3b) by designating the respective zones to the corresponding material properties.

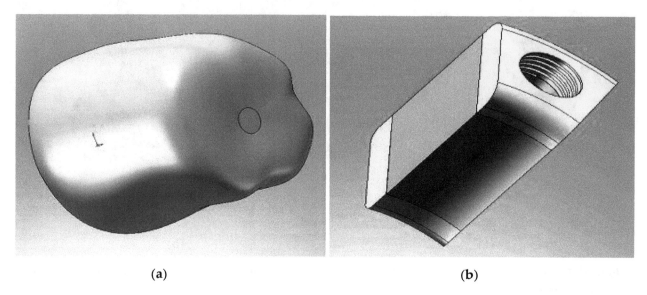

(a)   **(b)**

Figure 3. (**a**) Crown; (**b**) bone tissue with the layers of cortical bone (yellow) and trabecular bone (brown).

All components were modeled respecting in detail all the features of the actual model (threads, tapers, undercut, neck, etc.). The system is designed in such a way to transmit the masticatory force from the crown to the intermediate component and then to the upper annular part of the implant. During the transmission mechanism of mastication, force does not intervene in any threaded assembling.

2.2. Finite Element Model of the Dental Implantation

The 3D model used to study an implant in a portion of the jaw was built with the SolidWorks program and used tetraedrale elements in the implant and in the bone tissue as well [21]. The following shows one option of mesh which permits easy the observation of details under consideration. The finite element model consists of the corresponding parts of implant components, as shown in Figure 4a and the supporting bone. Figure 4b represents the finite element (FE) model of the whole system.

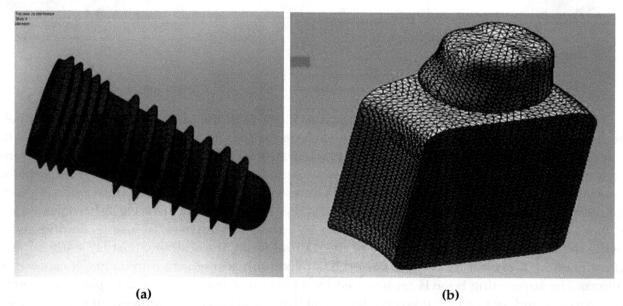

(a)   **(b)**

Figure 4. (**a**) FE model of the implant; and (**b**) FE model of the whole system.

In the FE model, there is a big number of finite elements due to the fact that there are fine structural elements, the mesh fineness appears as a necessity for a more realistic modeling of high-finesse constructive forms, such as threads and undercuts.

2.3. Contact Modeling

Osseointegration, as considered by a clinical point of view, refers more to the stability of the implant subjected to chewing loading and in close contact with the bone [22] rather than to the actual microscopic connection of bone tissue and implant surface. This connection is due to biological events which lead to the interaction of bone cells with implant surface after the surgical procedure.

The contact between the implant threads and bone is made on the thread sides. In our calculations, we considered a surface-to-surface contact (no penetration and preventing the interference between the implant and bone but allowing them to move away from each other to possibly form clearances) at the implant–one interface at the first stages of the osseointegration (lower values of E of the cortical bone), while a bonded contact, so without slipping, without friction at the final stage (the maximum E of the cortical bone). The FEM modeling was performed in order to capture the interaction between all the components of the implant and the bone, and the whole system was studied.

2.4. Material Models

In this section, the types of materials are presented, as are the main material constants for each component, i.e., bone (trabecular and cortical bone), implant and crown. These data are available from the literature [23] and from the data provided by the technical presentation of the implants used in this analysis. They are used as input data in the numerical calculations carried out in this study.

The most significant material constants used, respectively, for the implant, the abutment, the crown, trabecular bone and cortical bone are presented in Tables 1 and 2 [4] as follows:

Table 1. Material constants of the implant, its components and crown [4].

Constant name	Magnesium Alloy (Intermediate Part)		Titan Alloy (Implant and Screw)		Ceramic (Crown)	
	Value	Unit	Value	Unit	Value	Unit
Elastic modulus	4.2×10^{10}	N/m^2	1.048×10^{11}	N/m^2	2.2059×10^{11}	N/m^2
Poisson Coefficient	0.33		0.31		0.22	

Table 2. Material constants for the two types of bone [4].

Constant name	Trabecular Bone		Cortical Bone	
	Value	Unit	Value	Unit
Elastic modulus	1.8×10^8	N/m^2	$0.2 \times 10^9 – 1.8 \times 10^{10}$	N/m^2
Poisson coefficient	0.3		0.25	

2.5. Boundary Conditions

In general, in structural analysis, boundary conditions are put in displacements and/or forces in those regions of the structure where these entities are known. Zero displacement restrictions should be placed on some model boundaries to ensure equilibrium of the solution. In addition, restrictions must be set in nodes that are distant from the region of interest, which in our case, is the area surrounding the implant. It proceeds in this way to prevent the overlapping stress or strain field associated with the reaction forces, with the bone–implant interface.

In the FEM models considered in this paper, the lateral faces and bottom of the bone tissue are considered without displacement (nodes movements are fixed on those faces in all directions), (Figure 5a), considering that the influence of the loading no longer exists at that certain distance.

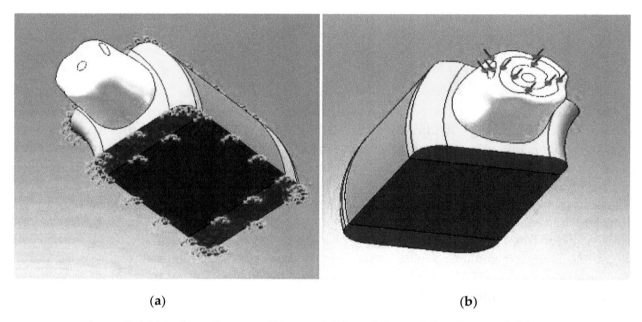

(a)   (b)

Figure 5. (a) The boundary condition; and (b) applying axial and non-axial forces.

2.6. Applying Loads

Since the purpose of this study was to analyze osseointegration in progress, we considered applying a load of very low intensity to simulate the immediate loading of an implant of a jaw premolar, with a temporary crown for aesthetic reasons, in a lighter contact.

In the actual mastication, the repetitive pattern of cyclical forces [24] transmits the loading to the peri-implant bone via the dental implant. This determines the stress around the ridge and prosthetic structure.

Since the cyclic character of mastication is difficult to simulate [25], most FE studies use axial and/or non-axial forces, and a more appropriate simulation typically uses a combination of vertical and oblique forces (axial and non-axial). Non-axial loads generate a destructive stress especially in the cortical bone ridge in peri-implant bone region and clinically disturbing for prosthesis [26].

The masticatory force size can be variable depending on age, sex, edentulous, habits and may vary from anterior to posterior in the same mouth. The loads that simulate mastication forces generate stress concentration to be assessed and therefore should be considered an appropriate risk [27].

In this study, we used a realistic simulation of mastication forces by the simultaneous application of axial and non-axial loading with a range between 20 N–30 N on sufficiently large surfaces (Figure 5b).

Before analyzing the osseointegtation progress, convergence tests were performed, keeping the mesh refined until a little change in our solution was obtained.

3. Results

The FEM analysis usually calculates von Mises stress, i.e., equivalent stress, a scalar quantity that characterizes the amount of stress and that is very important in formulating criteria of damage, plasticity, fracture, etc. In this study, this was used to evaluate the effect of loading in the dental implant, prosthesis and surrounding bone.

The following will present the results of numerical calculation by FEM by figures representing von Mises stress, displacement and safety factor. In the figures below, the most favorable areas are the minimum values of stress or displacement, while areas with the greatest damage and high risk are characterized by higher values.

The safety factor is the ratio of admissible limit values and actual FEM calculated values of stress. The admissible limit values of stress are specific to each material and adopted in specific conditions described in the literature. The figures representing the safety factor may indicate the necessity of appropriate design solutions adoption that eliminates risky zones that have a low safety factor.

In this study, we performed the calculations for different values of cortical bone Young's modulus, E. The corresponding values of Young's modulus, E lower (E = 0.2×10^8 MPa) refers to the immediate phase after the implant insertion, which simulates a weaker biomechanical implantation medium, more damaged.

Increasing values for E means that a gradual osseointegration occurs. Achieving a value of E of intact bone is considered to signify the osseointegration process's completion.

We conducted two sets of calculations and summarized the results in the following two tables: Table 3 corresponds to set no.1, when the axial force is 20 N and the oblique force is 20 N, whereas Table 4 corresponds to the set no.2, when the axial force is 30 N and the oblique force is 30 N.

Table 3. Set no.1, the axial force is 20 N, and the oblique force is 20 N.

Elasticity Modulus E	$\sigma_{max}[\frac{N}{mm^2}]$	$u_{res}[mm]$	Minimum FOS
1.8×10^{10}	7.987×10^7 (in cortical bone)	4.309×10^{-6}	5.87 (in cortical bone)
1.4×10^9	7.798×10^7 (in cortical bone)	5.25×10^{-6}	6.006 (in crown)
1.0×10^9	6.897×10^7 (in implant)	5.77×10^{-6}	6.893 (in crown)
0.6×10^9	8.044×10^7 (in implant)	7.17×10^{-6}	6.893 (in crown)
0.2×10^9	12.66×10^7 (in implant)	10.01×10^{-6}	6.893 (in crown)

Table 4. Set no.2, the axial force is 30 N, and the oblique force is 30 N.

Elasticity Modulus E	$\sigma_{max}[\frac{N}{mm^2}]$	$u_{res}[mm]$	Minimum FOS
1.8×10^{10}	1.288×10^8 (in cortical bone)	6.829×10^{-6}	3.668 (in cortical bone)
1.4×10^9	1.173×10^8 (in cortical bone)	7.853×10^{-6}	4.015 (in cortical bone)
1.0×10^9	1.033×10^8 (in implant)	9.832×10^{-6}	4.595 (in crown)
0.6×10^9	1.288×10^8 (in implant)	11.93×10^{-6}	4.595 (in crown)
0.2×10^9	1.899×10^8 (in implant)	17.51×10^{-6}	4.595 (in crown)

Tables 3 and 4 present the values of the main quantities calculated during the various stages of osseointegration as simulated in our numerical model, namely considering the damaged properties of cortical bone immediately after implant surgery, and further, as osseointegration progresses, cortical bone becomes stronger, so that in the end its mechanical properties are identical to those of intact bone. The total displacement or resulting displacement u_{res} is calculated by the formula:

$$u_{res} = \sqrt{u_x^2 + u_y^2 + u_z^2}$$

where u_x, u_y, u_z are the displacements along the axes x,y,z, while the factor of safety (FOS) is calculated by the ratio allowable stress/calculated stress. The calculated stress can be any considered stress: von Mises (the most used), Tresca and others. As a rule, the calculated stress is that corresponding to a failure criterion. We used von Mises and Tresca criterion and the differences were negligible. We present in this paper the values obtained by the von Mises criterion.

The following figures present the cases of maximum values of E (8×10^{10} Pa), corresponding to a full osseointegration and the case of minimum values of E (0.2×10^{10} Pa) corresponding to a time immediately after implant insertion, and therefore an early osseointegration as well.

Thus, Figure 6a,b represent the von Mises stress distribution for E minimum (a) and maximum (b), respectively.

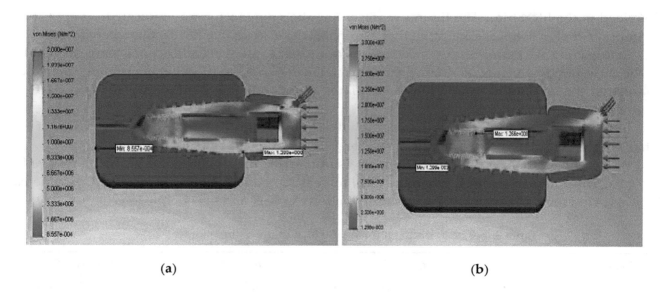

(a)

(b)

Figure 6. Distribution of the von Mises stress for the minimum E (**a**) and maximum E (**b**).

Figure 7a,b represent the displacement distribution for minimum E (a) and maximum E (b), respectively.

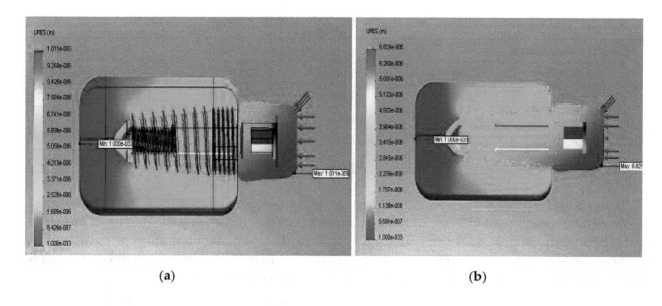

(a)

(b)

Figure 7. Displacement distribution for the minimum E (**a**) and maximum E (**b**).

Figure 8a,b represent the safety factor distribution for E minimum (a) and maximum (b), respectively.

It was observed that the rigid implant distributed the bending stress to its peak, and as the structure became stiffer, the cortical bone began to take over the bending loading. Displacements decreased as the bone–implant structure was reinforced and the most critical zone was within the upper cortical bone.

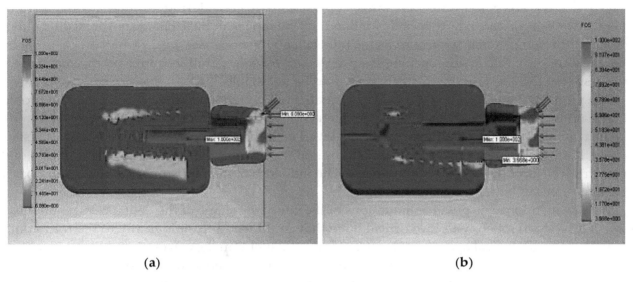

(a) (b)

Figure 8. Distribution of the safety factor for the minimum E (**a**) and maximum E (**b**).

4. Discussion

The results obtained in this study were in full compliance with the clinical practice and with the results from the literature [5,9,10,28], as it follows. As implant osseointegration develops, the rigidity of the peri-implant bone grows, so that in the end (healing) we can observe that the cortical bone is the one that provides the rigidity and stability of the implant, and the cortical bone stress reaches highest values, placed at the level of the mandibular ridge. During the period after the osseointegration process, the displacements are lower and they are placed only in the cortical bone area [1,29].

The oral implant insertion implies the incurrence of a microcraking field in the bone tissue at the implant–bone interface [30]. This leads to the mechanical properties' damage of the cortical bone and the decrease in the bone tissue stiffness around the implant. This is illustrated by the stress field aspect which is characterized by low stress values and their distribution extends along the implant [9]. It also finds that the bone–implant interface displacement has the highest values [10].

The limitations of the study were caused by several aspects, as it follows.

Osseointegration is a growth-increased change of bone structure between implant surface and bone tissue, and in the change of the osseointegration were included both the structure distribution and bone quantity to reflect the stability of the dental implant. This study partially took into account the complexity of the osseointegration progress modeling.

The results of the FEM analysis cannot be implemented directly in clinical situations, but one can design a model such that to simulate a real situation as well as possible [4]. Simplifications and method assumptions are, however, some limitations of studies using FEM.

FEM analysis should be interpreted carefully. In most cases, the numerical studies of oral implantology, e.g., using homogeneous, elastic and isotropic materials, which remain after the loading to which they are subjected, do not reflect the real situation. Taking into account these issues, it would require very laborious calculations and complicated laboratory tests to determine the material constants for a biological material, which behaves as nonlinear, heterogeneous, etc. [31].

As the cortical layer is an important structure that affects the stress distribution and stress shielding for a dental implant, the thickness of the cortical layer should be considered as a study issue, for instance. The effect of the cortical layer would be discussed as a relationship between the osseointegration progress and the biomechanical influence. On the other hand, to work with a simpler model, we adopted damaged mechanical properties for the entire cortical bone layer in the geometric model for the initial period after implant surgery, although for a more realistic approach, only a smaller area around the implant.

We used the von Mises stress as a stress representation, considering it rather a convenient one, rather than an appropriate one, especially for bone and ceramic materials that are not at all ductile as the von Mises criterion requires. Moreover, as the trabecular bone possesses weaker mechanical properties, it plays a secondary role in approaching the progress of osseointegration from a biomechanical point of view, so that the effect on the calculations would be negligible.

The problem domain could be considered small, but enough to have a correctly defined problem. The domain is chosen correctly, as long as the interaction of the neighborhood does not exist. That was proven in our model by the results and can be observed in the figures representing the stress, for instance. The fact that we obtained almost zero stress at boundaries shows the correctness of the choice of the domain, as well as of the boundary conditions. The influence of implant surgery is small and does not affect large areas of bone.

We also mentioned as possible limitations of the study the shape of the dental crown and the fact that it is directly in touch with the cortical bone that could lead physiologically to the formation of the well known biological space of at least 2–3 mm. We mention, however, that it was considered a provisional crown for a period of several months, so that the impact can be negligible.

The contact issue in the models focusing on the osseointegration progress is a delicate one. We used in our calculations a surface-to-surface contact at the interface implant–bone during the first stages of the osseointegration, and a bond contact at the final stage of it, for a maximum E of cortical bone.

On the other hand, the FEM model represents a static situation for a certain time and loading, and does not represent an actual clinical situation. Moreover, the system loading is rather dynamic and cyclical.

In addition, osseointegration is a complex process, implying both biological and mechanical factors [24], so that the FEM represents only a certain segment of the analyze.

Therefore, the results by FEM must be correlated with preclinical and clinical long-standing studies in order to obtain their validation.

The numerical model under consideration must run for as many scenarios, e.g., for different values of loads, their various plausible locations, for various values of biological material.

The numerical model requires a thorough validation, which is mandatory and it is done [32] either by the comparison of results for the same scenario using several numerical codes or standard FE programs; or comparing the results, at least qualitatively, with real clinical situations and the comparison of numerical results with the results obtained by available laboratory tests. In this study, we conducted a thorough validation of the criteria outlined previously.

Note that we made several versions of the mesh to a fineness which does not lead to errors greater than a 3.5% solution [33]. Element convergence tests were performed in order to obtain a reliable FE model to study the osseointegration progress.

5. Conclusions

In this article, an original approach using FEM calculation was used to model the osseointegration process progress. The stress and displacement in the dental implant and surrounding bone was calculated, being used to assess the biomechanical behavior of the whole assembly made up of implant system, ceramic crown and surrounding bone.

The novelty of this study included, firstly, the achievement of an accurate modeling of the bone–implant–crown system, particularly in terms of the implant (the geometrical model is an exact replica of a real implant) and secondly, the simulation in a realistic way of the osseointegration progress by taking into account the gradual increase in the damaged mechanical properties of the cortical bone. The model also includes a realistic simulation of loadings, simultaneously containing vertical and oblique forces acting on a certain surface of the crown.

The results obtained by FEM are complementary to other clinician information and they should be related to preclinical and long-term clinical trials for conclusions and right decisions.

Author Contributions: Conceptualization, I.R. and S.R.; methodology, I.R.; software, S.R.; validation, I.R. and S.R.; formal analysis, S.R.; investigation, I.R.; resources, I.R.; data curation, I.R.; writing—original draft preparation, S.R.; writing—review and editing, I.R. and S.R.; visualization, S.R.; supervision, I.R.; project administration, I.R. All authors have read and agreed to the published version of the manuscript.

Acknowledgments: We wish to thank E. Avram E. for unconditional support for the realization of the geometrical model and the FEM calculation. Both thank to V. Năstăsescu for high professionalism and expertise on FEM use.

References

1. Geng, J.P.; Tan, K.B.; Liu, G.R. Application of finite element analysis in implant dentistry: A review of the literature. *J. Prosthet. Dent.* **2001**, *85*, 585–598. [CrossRef] [PubMed]
2. Santos, M.B.F.; Silva Neto, J.P.; Consani, R.L.X.; Mesquita, M.F. Three-dimensional finite element analysis of stress distribution in peri-implant bone with relined dentures and different heights of healing caps. *J. Oral Rehabil.* **2011**, *38*, 691–696. [CrossRef] [PubMed]
3. Bahuguna, R.; Anand, B.; Kumar, D.; Aeran, H.; Anand, V.; Gulati, M. Evaluation of stress patterns in bone around dental implant for different abutment angulations under axial and oblique loading: A finite element analysis. *Natl. J. Maxillofac. Surg.* **2013**, *4*, 46–51. [PubMed]
4. Roateşi, I. Sress and strain calculation in implant and surrounding bone by FEM. *J. Stomatol.* **2014**, *60*, 227–234.
5. Winter, W.; Klein, D.; Karl, M. Effect of model parameters on finite element analysis of micromotions in implant dentistry. *J. Oral Implant.* **2013**, *39*, 23–29. [CrossRef]
6. Chu, C.M. Influences of internal tapered abutment designs on bone stresses around a dental implant: Three-dimensional finite element method with statistical evaluation. *J. Periodontol.* **2012**, *83*, 111–118. [CrossRef]
7. Li, T.; Kong, L.; Wang, Y.; Hu, K.; Song, L.; Liu, B. Selection of optimal dental implant diameter and length in type IV bone: A three-dimensional FE analysis. *Int. J. Oral Maxillofac. Surg.* **2009**, *38*, 1077–1083. [CrossRef]
8. Tang, C.B.; Liu, S.Y.; Zhou, G.X.; Yu, J.H.; Zhang, G.D.; Bao, Y.; Wang, Q.J. Nonlinear finite element analysis of three implant–abutment interface designs. *Int. J. Oral Sci.* **2012**, *4*, 101–108. [CrossRef]
9. Jimbo, R.; Janal, M.N.; Marin, C.; Giro, G.; Tovar, N.; Coelho, P.G. The effect of implant diameter on osseointegration utilizing simplified drilling protocols. *Clin. Oral Implant. Res.* **2014**, *25*, 1295–1300. [CrossRef]
10. Papavasiliou, G.; Kamposiora, P.; Bayne, S.C.; Felton, D.A. 3D-FEA of osseointegration percentages and patterns on implant-bone interfacial stresses. *J. Dent.* **1997**, *25*, 485–491. [CrossRef]
11. Zheng, L.; Yang, J.; Hu, X.; Luo, J. Three dimensional finite element analysis of a novel osteointegrated dental implant designed to reduce stress peak of cortical bone. *Acta. Bioeng. Biomech.* **2014**, *16*, 21–28. [PubMed]
12. Shigemitsu, R.; Yoda, N.; Ogawa, T.; Kawata, T.; Gunji, Y.; Yamakawa, Y. Biological-data-based finite-element stress analysis of mandibular bone with implant-supported overdenture. *Comput. Biol. Med.* **2014**, *54*, 44–52. [CrossRef] [PubMed]
13. Kasai, K.; Takayama, Y.; Yokoyama, A. Distribution of occlusal forces during occlusal adjustment of dental implant prostheses: A nonlinear finite element analysis considering the capacity for displacement of opposing teeth and implants. *Int. J. Oral Maxillofac. Implant.* **2012**, *27*, 329–335.
14. Vanegas-Acosta, J.C.; Landinez, P.N.S.; Garzón-Alvarado, D.A.; Casale, R.M.C. A finite element method approach for the mechanobiological modeling of the osseointegration of a dental implant. *Comput. Methods Programs Biomed.* **2011**, *101*, 297–314. [CrossRef] [PubMed]
15. Lee, J.S.; Cho, I.H.; Kim, Y.S.; Heo, S.J.; Kwon, H.B.; Lim, Y.J. Bone-implant interface with simulated insertion stress around an immediately loaded dental implant in the anterior maxilla: A three-dimensional finite element analysis. *Int. J. Oral Maxillofac. Implant.* **2012**, *27*, 295–302.
16. Mathieu, V.; Vayron, R.; Richard, G.; Lambert, G.; Naili, S.; Meningaud, J.P. Biomechanical determinants of the stability of dental implants: Influence of the bone-implant interface properties. *J. Biomech.* **2014**, *47*, 3–13. [CrossRef]
17. Jofre, J.; Cendoya, P.; Munoz, P. Effect of splinting mini-implants on marginal bone loss: A biomechanical model and clinical randomized study with mandibular overdentures. *Int. J. Oral Maxillofac. Implant.* **2010**, *25*, 1137–1144.
18. O'Mahony, A.; Bowles, Q.; Woolsey, G.; Robinson, S.J.; Spencer, P. Stress distribution in the single-unit osseointegrated dental implant: Finite element analyses of axial and off-axial loading. *Implant Dent.* **2000**, *9*, 207–218. [CrossRef]

19. Natali, A.N.; Pavan, P.G.; Ruggero, A.L. Analysis of bone–implant interaction phenomena by using a numerical approach. *Clin. Oral Implant. Res.* **2006**, *17*, 67–74. [CrossRef]

20. Kitamura, E.; Stegaroiu, R.; Nomura, S.; Miyakawa, O. Biomechanical aspects of marginal bone resorption around osseointegrated implants: Considerations based on a three-dimensional finite element analysis. *Clin. Oral Implant. Res.* **2004**, *15*, 401–412. [CrossRef]

21. Lombard, M. *SolidWorks 2013 Bible*; John Wiley & Sons: Indianapolis, IN, USA, 2013.

22. Brånemark, P.I.; Hansson, B.O.; Adell, R.; Breine, U.; Lindström, J.; Hallén, O. Osseointegrated implants in the treatment of the edentulous jaw. Experience from a 10-year period. *Scand. J. Plast. Reconstr. Surg. Suppl.* **1977**, *16*, 1–132. [PubMed]

23. Gultekin, B.A.; Gultekin, P.; Yalcin, S. Application of finite element analysis in implant dentistry. In *Finite Element Analysis: New Trends and Developments*; Intech: Rijeka, Croatia, 2012; pp. 21–54.

24. Misch, C.E. Bone Response to Mechanical Loads. Stress Treatment Theorem for Implant Dentistry: The Key to Implant Treatment Plans. In *Contemporary Implant Dentistry*, 3rd ed.; Mosby: St. Louis, MO, USA, 2008.

25. Kishen, A. Periapical biomechanics and the role of cyclic biting force in apical retrograde fluid movement. *Int. Endod. J.* **2005**, *38*, 597–603. [CrossRef] [PubMed]

26. Torcato, L.B.; Pellizzer, E.P.; Verri, F.R.; Falcón-Antenucci, R.M.; Júnior, J.F.S.; de Faria Almeida, D.A. Influence of parafunctional loading and prosthetic connection on stress distribution: A 3D finite element analysis. *J. Prosthet. Dent.* **2014**, *114*, 644–651. [CrossRef] [PubMed]

27. Nishigawa, K.; Suzuki, Y.; Matsuka, Y. Masticatory performance alters stress relief effect of gum chewing. *J. Prosth. Res.* **2015**, *59*, 262–267. [CrossRef] [PubMed]

28. Koka, S.; Zarb, G. On osseointegration: The healing adaptation principle in the context of osseosufficiency, osseoseparation, and dental implant failure. *Int. J. Prosthod.* **2012**, *25*, 48–52.

29. Shibata, Y.; Tanimoto, Y.; Maruyama, N.; Nagakura, M. A review of improved fixation methods for dental implants. Part II: Biomechanical integrity at bone–implant interface. *J. Prosth. Res.* **2015**, *59*, 84–95.

30. Chang, P.C.; Giannobile, W.V. Functional assessment of dental implant osseointegration. *Int. J. Periodontics Restor. Dent.* **2012**, *32*, 147–153.

31. Elias, C.N.; Meirelles, L. Improving osseointegration of dental implants. *Expert Rev. Med. Devices* **2010**, *7*, 241–256. [CrossRef]

32. Roatesi, I. Biomaterials for dental implants. *Rom. J. Mater.* **2015**, *45*, 282–289.

33. Roateşi, I.; Roateşi, S. Numerical FEM Modeling in Dental Implantology. *AIP Conf. Proc.* **2016**, *1738*. [CrossRef]

5

Vertical Bone Construction with Bone Marrow-Derived and Adipose Tissue-Derived Stem Cells

Thaiz Carrera-Arrabal [1], José Luis Calvo-Guirado [2], Fabricio Passador-Santos [1],
Carlos Eduardo Sorgi da Costa [1], Frank Róger Teles Costa [1], Antonio Carlos Aloise [1],
Marcelo Henrique Napimoga [1], Juan Manuel Aragoneses [3] and André Antonio Pelegrine [1,*]

[1] Faculdade São Leopoldo Mandic, Instituto de Pesquisas São Leopoldo Mandic, Campinas 13045-755, Brazil;
thaizarrabal@gmail.com (T.C.-A.); fabricio.passador-santos@slmandic.edu.br (F.P.-S.);
du_studio_oral@yahoo.com.br (C.E.S.d.C.); frankrogertc@gmail.com (F.R.T.C.);
aca.orto@uol.com.br (A.C.A.); marcelo.napimoga@slmandic.edu.br (M.H.N.)

[2] Department of Oral and Implant Surgery. Faculty of Health Sciences, Universidad Católica San Antonio de
Murcia (UCAM), 30002 Murcia, Spain; jlcalvo@ucam.edu

[3] Department of Dental Research in Universidad Federico Henríquez y Carvajal (UFHEC),
Santo Domingo 10107, Dominican Republic; jmaragoneses@gmail.com

* Correspondence: andre.pelegrine@slmandic.edu.br

Abstract: The purpose of this study was to conduct a histomorphometric analysis of bone marrow-derived and adipose tissue-derived stem cells, associated with a xenograft block, in vertical bone constructions in rabbit calvaria. Ten rabbits received two xenograft blocks on the calvaria, after decortication of the parietal bone. The blocks were fixed with titanium screws. The blocks were combined with the bone marrow-derived mesenchymal stem cells in the bone marrow stem cell (BMSC) group (right side of the calvaria) or with the adipose tissue-derived mesenchymal stem cells in the adipose tissue stem cell (ATSC) group (left side of the calvaria). After 8 weeks, the animals were sacrificed and their parietal bones were fixed in 10% formalin for the histomorphometric analysis. The following parameters were evaluated—newly formed bone (NFB), xenogeneic residual particles (XRP), and non-mineralized tissue (NMT). The histomorphometric analysis revealed $11.9 \pm 7.5\%$ and $7.6 \pm 5.6\%$ for NFB, $22.14 \pm 8.5\%$ and $21.6 \pm 8.5\%$ for XRP, and $65.8 \pm 10.4\%$ and $70.8 \pm 7.4\%$ for NMT in groups BMSC and ATSC, respectively, with statistically significant differences in the NFB and the NMT between the groups, but no differences in the XRP. Therefore, it can be concluded that the bone marrow-derived stem cells seem to have more potential for the bone formation than do the adipose tissue-derived stem cells when used in combination with the xenogenous blocks in the vertical bone construction.

Keywords: bone marrow cells; grafts; adipose tissue-derived stem cells

1. Introduction

Large bone constructions represent a challenge for the implant therapy team. In these situations, a bone graft is commonly considered the biological gold standard, once it has osteogenic, osteoinductive, and osteoconductive potentials [1]. However, autografts have a few disadvantages, such as prolonged surgical time and the need for an additional surgery to harvest tissue from the patient at the donor site, which can result in higher morbidity [2,3]. Thus, the study of different types of cell therapy is justified as they present minimal donor site morbidity and a lower risk of autoimmune rejection and disease transmission [4].

Concerning the usage of cell therapy in dentistry, there are many studies on the potential of stem cells for the regeneration of some tissues, such as periodontal tissues [5,6], bone [7,8], and the dentin–pulp complex [9,10]. Most of these studies focused on the use of stem cells from different sources (e.g., bone marrow, adipose tissue, periodontal ligament, and pulp). However, there are a limited number of studies comparing the results of tissue regeneration with stem cells from different sources.

Most bone substitute biomaterials have only osteoconductive potential due to the lack of proteins and of a cellular component [11]. However, the adjunctive use of stem cells with the possibility of osteoblastic differentiation could theoretically result in a composite graft (i.e., stem cell scaffold construct) with osteoconductive, osteoinductive, and osteogenic potential, as demonstrated by Victorelli et al. [12]. Autologous stem cells are adult stem cells that are considered undifferentiated cells found in specialized postnatal tissues and organs. Autologous mesenchymal stem cells have the capacity to differentiate into specialized cells of at least one mesenchymal lineage such as bone, cartilage, fat, or muscle [13], and they can be found in some types of postnatal tissues, such as bone marrow [14], adipose tissue [15], dental tissue [16], and gingival tissue [17].

Therefore, studies comparing the capacity of mesenchymal stem cells from different sources are of major importance in bone tissue engineering, especially in critical situations such as vertical bone constructions. In this study, as in a previous study by our group [7], we compared two of the most frequent types of tissue used in cell therapy—adipose tissue and bone marrow. However, as the delivery vehicle is important to the performance of mesenchymal stem cells [18,19], in the present study, we used a scaffold in block form, which is a common clinical strategy when treating bone defects that require appositional reconstructions.

2. Materials and Methods

This study was analyzed and approved by the Research Ethics Committee of the São Leopoldo Mandic Dental School, Campinas, SP, Brazil (process 0191/14).

2.1. Bone Marrow Harvest by Aspiration

Autologous bone marrow was obtained by aspiration after anesthesia in all 10 animals. Anesthesia was induced with ketamine (40 mg/kg), midazolam (2 mg/kg), and fentanyl citrate (0.8 μg/kg), and maintained with isoflurane/nitrous oxide (1:1.5%) and oxygen (2/3:1/3) with a pediatric facemask. In addition, a local anesthesia was provided via 1 mL of 2% lidocaine HCl and epinephrine 1:100,000 diluted in 1 mL of physiological saline solution.

Two-milliliters of bone marrow aspirates were obtained from each tibia of the ten rabbits using disposable 40 × 10 needles (1.10 mm × 38 mm) and 20-mL disposable syringes previously heparinized to prevent blood clotting.

2.2. Culture of Adult Bone Marrow-Derived Mesenchymal Stem Cells

The procedure to obtain the BMSCs followed the standard guidelines and was completely described in a previous publication of our group (Coelho de Faria et al.) [7].

The BMMSCs, after culture, were detached and resuspended in the culture medium and subsequently mixed with the xenograft in the BMSC group.

2.3. Lipectomy for Adipose Tissue Isolation

The adipose tissue was obtained from the back of all the 10 animals following the same general anesthesia protocol previously described by our group (Coelho de Faria et al.) [7].

The collected material of all the animals was immediately taken to the cell culture laboratory for tissue processing.

2.4. Culture of Adult Adipose Tissue-Derived Mesenchymal Stem Cells

The procedure to obtain the ATSCs followed the standard guidelines and was completely described in a previous publication of our group (Coelho de Faria et al.) [7].

The ATSCs, after culture, were detached and resuspended in the culture medium and subsequently mixed with the xenograft in the ATSC group.

2.5. Cell Adhesion Capability

Cell adhesion was analyzed using an inverted optical microscope 3 days after seeding the cells into the culture flask, and it was verified that the cells were plastic adherent when maintained under the standard culture conditions.

2.6. Differentiation Assays

Adipogenic, osteogenic, and chondrogenic differentiation assays were done, following the same methodology adopted previously by our group (Coelho de Faria et al.) [7].

2.7. Immunophenotypic Characterization

The bone marrow-derived and adipose tissue-derived stem cells from the second passage were used for immunophenotypic characterization, following the same methodology used previously by our group (Coelho de Faria et al.) [7]. The cells showed compatible immunophenotyping (CD16+, CD34−, CD45−, CD73+, CD90+, and CD105+).

2.8. Seeding Cells into the Scaffolds

In all the groups, 1 mL of the solution containing phosphate buffered saline (PBS) and 1×10^5 cells were seeded into the scaffolds. The solution was slowly pipetted onto the scaffold which, due to its characteristic, was fully absorbed. At the end of the procedure, the scaffolds containing the cells inside were ready to be inserted in the surgical site.

2.9. Experimental Design and Surgical Protocol

Ten adult male New Zealand rabbits aged between 10 and 12 months and weighing between 3.5 and 4 kg were selected. The animals were acclimatized in individual cages for 14 days, in a temperature-controlled room (18 °C to 20 °C), subjected to a 12-h light cycle. The animals were fed a commercial pelleted diet and allowed ad libitum access to water.

All animals were subjected to anesthesia following the same general anesthesia protocol previously described. The animals received two commercial xenogenous blocks of bovine origin (Baumer, Mogi Mirim, SP, Brazil). The blocks were placed on their parietal bones, bilaterally to the midline with the aid of one fixing screw, after performing five perforations into the cortical plate of the parietal bone to encourage bleeding and graft nutrition (Figure 1).

The xenograft blocks from group BMSC were combined with the autologous bone marrow-derived mesenchymal stem cells ($n = 10$) and those from group ATSC were combined with the autologous adipose tissue-derived mesenchymal stem cells ($n = 10$); 1 mL of phosphate buffered saline (PBS) solution (Sigma Aldrich, Darmstadt, Germany) containing 1×10^5 cells was used in both groups, and the respective stem cells were added dropwise to each block. Each animal received one block of each group (i.e., BMSC group and ATSC group). The block from the BMSC group was fixed on the right side of the calvaria and the block from the ATSC Group was fixed on the left side of the calvaria. The surgical wounds were then subjected to primary closure.

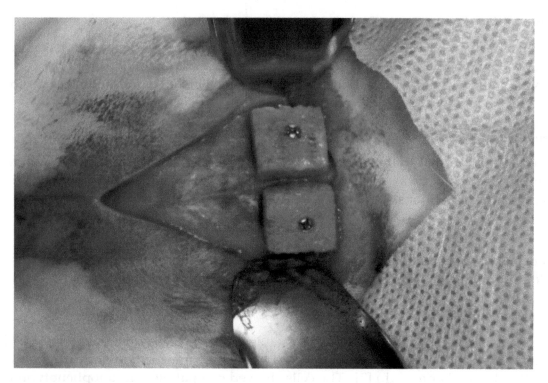

Figure 1. Xenograft blocks fixed on the rabbit's calvaria with titanium screws.

All animals were post-operatively medicated with benzylpenicillin (40,000 IU) and sodium dipyrone (0.25 mg/kg). The animals were sacrificed 8 weeks after surgery and their parietal bones were removed and processed for histological and histomorphometric evaluation.

2.10. Histological Preparation and Histomorphometric Evaluation

A portion of the parietal bone with an approximate area of 18 mm^2 containing the block at the center was removed using an oscillating saw. Samples were fixed in 10% formalin for 7 days and then decalcified in 10% EDTA for 6 days at room temperature and fixed with 10% buffered formaldehyde. The histological slices were prepared using a microtome to cut 5 μm transverse sections of the entire set, including the graft, from the center of the block (where the screw was positioned) up to 2 mm from the center of the block. The sections were stained with Masson's trichrome and assessed by optical microscopy (Nikon Eclipse C1, New York, NY, USA). A digital CCD camera was used to acquire images for the subsequent analyses (Infinity-1, Lumenera®, Ottawa, ON, Canada). All slides were analyzed in four areas (upper left, lower left, upper right, and lower right), which allowed the determination of tissue status in the interface, near the recipient bed (by using the lower left and lower right measurements) and also far from the recipient bed, at the block's surface (by using the upper left and upper right measurements). Then, the overall average was calculated for each slide. Each evaluated site had a dimension (area) of 1,347,442 μm^2. Two previously calibrated examiners assessed the specimens blindly and, in case of disagreement, the sample was reviewed to reach a consensus. An average of the measurements for each area obtained by the two examiners was recorded. The examiners traced all images using Infinity Analyse® (Lumenera Corporation, Ottawa, ON, Canada), measuring the following parameters: (1) newly formed bone (NFB), (2) xenogeneic residual particles (XRP), and (3) non-mineralized tissue (NMT). All results were obtained in μm^2 and expressed as percentage of the total area.

2.11. Statistical Analysis

Prior to the analyses, data from the newly formed bone (NFB), the xenogeneic residual particle (XRP) and the non-mineralized tissue (NMT) were evaluated for normality (Shapiro-Wilk tests) and homogeneity of variance (Levene tests), and it was verified that both were attended.

Analysis of variance with two criteria for randomized blocks (two-way ANOVA) was applied to investigate whether percentages of NFB, XRP, and NMT were influenced by independent variables of stem cell type (bone marrow/adipose tissue) and calvaria distance (near/far) or by the interaction of both. If there was a significant interaction, Tukey's test was used for multiple comparisons.

All quantitative data were analyzed by SPSS-V17® (SSPS Inc. 233, Chicago, IL, USA).

3. Results

Pearson's correlation test, which yielded a value of 0.99, was used to evaluate the measurements obtained from the two examiners. Therefore, we chose to use the mean measurements obtained by the two examiners. In low magnification (40×), the histological characteristics of the analyzed samples showed mineralized and non-mineralized tissues (Figure 2A). In higher magnification, both groups (BMSC and ATSC) showed areas of the newly formed bone, with a layer of osteoblasts adjacent to the reminiscent osseous trabeculae from xenograft blocks (Figure 2B,C, respectively). Variable quantities of the fibrovascular connective tissue were seen interspersed with the bone trabeculae (Figure 2B,C).

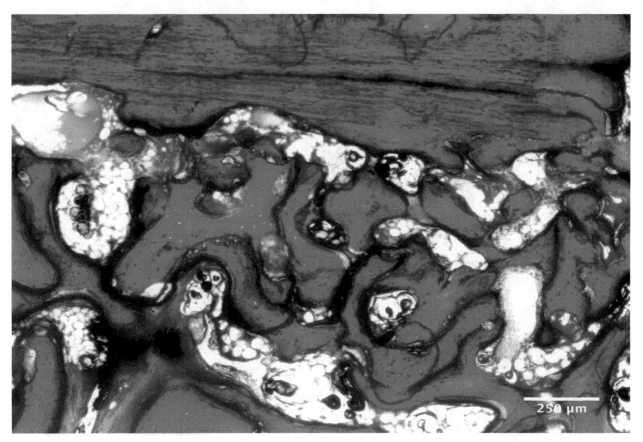

(A)

Figure 2. *Cont.*

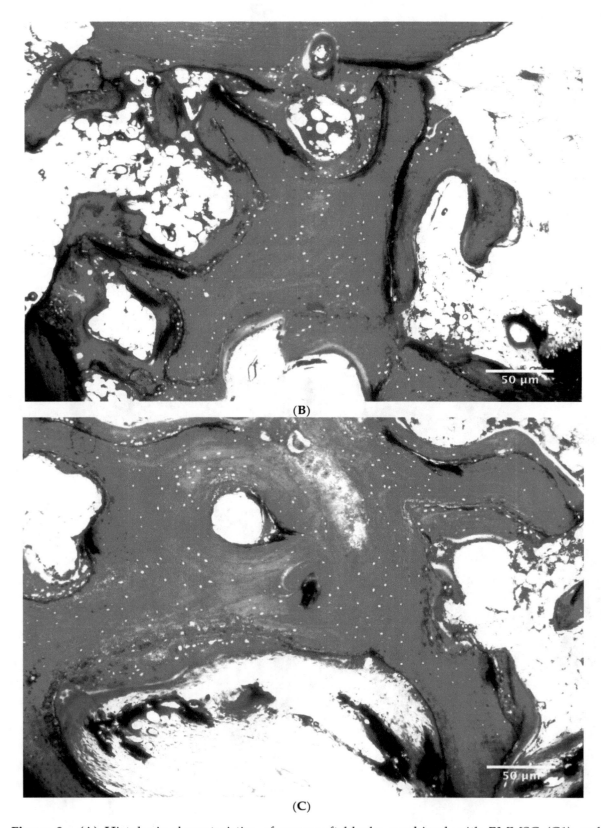

(B)

(C)

Figure 2. **(A)** Histologic characteristics of xenograft blocks combined with BMMSC (G1) and ATSC (adipose tissue stem cells) (G2). Histologic characteristics of a sample, in low magnification, showing native bone (above) and the grafted area, 40×. Stain, Masson's trichrome. **(B)** Higher magnification showing reminiscent bone trabeculae from G1 xenograft block surrounded by newly formed bone, 200×. Masson's trichrome. **(C)** Higher magnification showing reminiscent bone trabeculae from G2 xenograft block surrounded by the newly formed bone, 200×. Stain, Masson's trichrome.

For the newly formed bone (NFB) data, the two-way ANOVA showed no significant interaction between the concentrate type variables and the distance in the rabbit calvaria ($p = 0.356$). The results showed that the type of stem cell used significantly affected the percentage of the newly formed bone (NFB) ($p = 0.036$), a fact that occurred near (interface between the graft and the recipient bed) or far (graft's surface) from the recipient bed. Specifically, by Tukey's test, it was found that the impregnation of the xenograft block with the adipose tissue stem cells resulted in a percentage of newly formed bone (NFB) statistically lower than that observed for the group in which the bone marrow stem cells were used. Analysis of variance with two criteria for randomized blocks also indicated that in groups in which the xenograft block was impregnated with the adipose tissue stem cells or the bone marrow stem cells, the highest percentage of newly formed bone (NFB) was observed at a location near the recipient bed ($p = 0.003$).

For the percentage of xenogeneic residual particle (XRP), there was a significant interaction between both variables, type of cell and distance in rabbit calvaria ($p = 0.063$), as indicated by the analysis of variance with two criteria for randomized blocks. This test also identified no statistically significant difference ($p = 0.750$) between the groups (i.e., bone marrow and adipose tissue stem cells) in the percentage of xenogeneic residual particle (XRP). When the distances were compared, it was found that the percentage of xenogeneic residual particle (XRP) was significantly higher in the more distant location (i.e., far from the recipient bed) ($p = 0.002$).

Evaluating non-mineralized tissue (NMT), the two-way analysis of randomized blocks indicated a significant interaction between the stem cell type (i.e., BMSC and ATSC) and rabbit calvaria distance (i.e., near and far) ($p = 0.038$). Applying the Tukey's test, in close proximity to the calvaria, it was verified that the impregnation of the xenogeneic bone with the adipose tissue stem cells (ATSC) resulted in a greater percentage of non-mineralized tissue (NMT) in comparison to the group in which the impregnation occurred with the bone marrow stem cells (BMSC). In the more distant location, both groups did not differ significantly in relation to the percentage of non-mineralized tissue (NMT). The Tukey test also showed that the percentage of non-mineralized tissue (NMT) was higher in the distant location for the bone marrow stem cell group, whereas the adipose tissue stem cell group showed the highest percentage of non-mineralized tissue (NMT) at the nearest location. Table 1 shows the histomorphometric results and statistical comparisons.

Table 1. Histomorphometric results (mean and standard deviation) and statistical comparison between groups (in %)—BMSC, bone marrow stem cells group; ATSC, adipose tissue stem cells group; XRP, xenograft residual particles; NFB, newly formed bone; and NMT, non-mineralized tissue. Numbers inside the brackets are standard deviation and outside the brackets are mean. The mean values followed by different capital letters indicate statistically significant difference between the groups, within each column, considering separately each type of tissue. The mean values followed by different small letters indicate statistically significant difference between the sites, within each line, considering separately each type of tissue.

TISSUE	CELL SOURCE	DISTANCE-NEAR	DISTANCE-FAR	MEAN
NFB	BMSC	$16.0 \pm 6.1\%$	$7.8 \pm 6.7\%$	$11.9 \pm 7.5\%$ A
	ATSC	$9.9 \pm 5.4\%$	$5.3 \pm 5.2\%$	$7.6 \pm 5.6\%$ B
	MEAN	$12.9 \pm 6.4\%$ a	$6.6 \pm 5.9\%$ b	-
XRP	BMSC	$20.7 \pm 9.9\%$	$24.1 \pm 7.0\%$	$22.14 \pm 8.5\%$ A
	ATSC	$15.2 \pm 4.9\%$	$28.0 \pm 6.3\%$	$21.6 \pm 8.5\%$ A
	MEAN	$17.9 \pm 8.1\%$ a	$26.1 \pm 6.8\%$ b	-
NMT	BMSC	$63.4 \pm 10.5\%$ Bb	$68.3 \pm 10.3\%$ Aa	-
	ATSC	$74.8 \pm 7.4\%$ Aa	$66.7 \pm 7.4\%$ Ab	-

4. Discussion

There is consensus in the literature about the potential use of bone substitute materials to replace autogenous bone grafts in some clinical situations [20–22]. Nevertheless, in critical defects (e.g., vertical bone reconstruction), the lack of a cellular osteogenic component may limit the use of bone substitute biomaterials [11]. Therefore, the study of cell therapy is extremely important in order to remedy this situation.

As the adult mesenchymal stem cells have the capacity to differentiate into specialized cells of at least one mesenchymal lineage such as bone, cartilage, fat, or muscle [13], the use of these undifferentiated cells harvested from the adipose tissue and the bone marrow seems to have clinical applicability in regenerative medicine and, as far as the implant therapy is concerned, in bone reconstruction as well. The mesenchymal stem cells used in the present study fulfilled the minimal criteria proposed by the Mesenchymal and Tissue Stem Cell Committee of the International Society for Cellular Therapy (ISCT) position statement, which defined multipotent mesenchymal stromal cells [23]. These criteria were tested by cell adhesion, differentiation assays, and immunophenotypic analysis carried out as described in the Methods section. However, despite the fact the authors of the present study have used this standardization, SEM analysis was not performed to visualize the mesenchymal stem cells inside the scaffold.

In the present study, the percentage of newly formed bone was lower than in a previous study by our group [7], where we used a xenograft as a scaffold for the vertical bone construction on rabbit calvaria associated with the bone marrow-derived mesenchymal stem cells or the adipose tissue-derived stem cells. These differences in the levels of bone formation between the studies may have been caused by differences in (1) the characteristics of the scaffold and/or (2) the titanium device used to stabilize the scaffold. The presence of a particulate xenogenous graft in the first study could have contributed to a more adequate level of revascularization and, therefore, bone formation, when compared to the structured block graft of the present study. Moreover, the use of a titanium cylinder instead of a titanium screw certainly resulted in a larger titanium area in contact with the graft and bone in the previous study, which might have stimulated bone formation as titanium has a higher affinity for bone [24].

However, the XRP levels were similar between these two studies, with rates of 22.14 ± 8.5% and 21.6 ± 8.5% for the bone marrow-derived and the adipose tissue-derived mesenchymal stem cells, respectively, in the present study, and 23.31 ± 3.11% and 27.58 ± 3.98% for the bone marrow-derived and the adipose tissue-derived mesenchymal stem cells, respectively, in the previous study. Therefore, the use of a particulate or structured bone scaffold and the differences between the titanium areas probably did not have any influence. On the other hand, the NMT levels appear to be influenced by the scaffold characteristic and/or titanium area, since the percentage of this tissue in the group where the bone marrow-derived and the adipose tissue-derived stem cells were used was 65.8 ± 10.4% and 70.8 ± 7.4%, respectively, in the present study, and 50.23 ± 8.72% and 49.90 ± 8.76%, respectively, in the previous study. Therefore, the use of a particulate mineralized scaffold instead of a structured mineralized scaffold and the use of a larger area of titanium device to stabilize the scaffold may result in more newly formed bone and less soft tissue, which could contribute to an improved osseointegration when an implant is placed. However, it is important to state that the xenografts used in these two studies were not processed by the same company and, therefore, it might also contribute to different results.

Previous studies undertaken by our research group using the bone marrow-derived and the adipose tissue-derived mesenchymal stem cells in bone defects on rabbit calvaria showed the same tendency of higher levels of bone formation when using bone marrow stem cells (Pelegrine et al., 2014; Aloise et al., 2015; Zimmermann et al., 2015) [11,25,26]. Therefore, in both situations, onlay and inlay bone constructions, bone marrow may be considered a better choice for the tissue source of mesenchymal stem cells when compared to fat. The best results, in all studies, at the sites where the bone marrow-derived mesenchymal stem cells were used might be explained by the fact that cells from the bone marrow have a greater affinity for osteogenic differentiation, as stated before by our group [7]. Moreover, as mesenchymal stem cells are multipotent cells that are capable of multiple lineage differentiation due to the presence of inductive signals from the microenvironment [27,28], we hypothesize that the microenvironment of bone marrow present in the recipient bed had a more pronounced effect on the stem cells isolated from the bone marrow than on those obtained from the adipose tissue. This might also have repercussion in the higher levels of non-mineralized tissue at the interface between the recipient bed and the graft, as observed in the ATSC group. This finding represents a worse integration of the graft combined with the adipose tissue stem cells and, if proven by future clinical studies, could reflect in the implants' survival rates, as the dental implants are commonly installed in this interface area.

5. Conclusions

The bone marrow-derived mesenchymal stem cells seem to have a higher potential for bone formation compared with the adipose tissue-derived mesenchymal stem cells when used in combination with the xenogenous blocks in the vertical bone construction.

Author Contributions: Conceptualization, T.C.-A., A.A.P. and J.L.C.-G.; methodology, A.C.A.; software, T.C.-A.; validation, J.L.C.-G.; M.H.N.; formal analysis, A.C.A. and J.M.A.; investigation, C.E.S.d.C.; resources, A.C.A.; data curation, F.R.T.C.; writing—original draft preparation, F.P.-S.; writing—review and editing, F.R.T.C. and J.L.C.-G.; visualization, M.H.N.; supervision, A.A.P.; project administration, A.A.P.; and funding acquisition, A.A.P.

References

1. Sakkas, A.; Wilde, F.; Heufelder, M.; Winter, K.; Schramm, A. Autogenous bone grafts in oral implantology-is it still a "gold standard"? A consecutive review of 279 patients with 456 clinical procedures. *Int. J. Dent.* **2017**, *3*, 23. [CrossRef] [PubMed]

2. Laurie, S.W.; Kaban, L.B.; Mulliken, J.B.; Murray, J.E. Donor-site morbidity after harvesting rib and iliac bone. *Plast. Reconstr. Surg.* **1984**, *73*, 933–938. [CrossRef] [PubMed]

3. Hernigou, P.; Desroches, A.; Queinnec, S.; Lachaniette, C.H.F.; Poignard, A.; Allain, J.; Chevallier, N.; Rouard, H. Morbidity of graft harvesting versus bone marrow aspiration in cell regenerative therapy. *Int. Orthop.* **2014**, *38*, 1855–1860. [CrossRef] [PubMed]

4. Monaco, E.; Bionaz, M.; Hollister, S.J.; Wheeler, M.B. Strategies for regeneration of the bone using porcine adult adipose-derived mesenchymal stem cells. *Theriogenology* **2011**, *75*, 1381–1399. [CrossRef]

5. Fu, X.; Jin, L.; Ma, P.; Fan, Z.; Wang, G.S. Allogeneic stem cells from deciduous teeth in treatment for periodontitis in miniature swine. *J. Periodontol.* **2014**, *85*, 845–851. [CrossRef] [PubMed]

6. Yamada, Y.; Nakamura, S.; Ueda, M.; Ito, K. Papilla regeneration by injectable stem cell therapy with regenerative medicine: Long-term clinical prognosis. *J. Tissue Eng. Regener. Med.* **2015**, *9*, 305–309. [CrossRef] [PubMed]

7. Coelho de Faria, A.B.C.; Chiantia, F.B.; Teixeira, M.L.; Aloise, A.C.; Pelegrine, A.A. Comparative study between mesenchymal stem cells derived from bone marrow and from adipose tissue, associated with xenograft, in appositional reconstructions: Histomorphometric study in rabbits calvaria. *Int. J. Oral Maxillofac. Implants* **2016**, *31*, e155–e161. [CrossRef] [PubMed]

8. Katagiri, W.; Osugi, M.; Kawai, T.; Hibi, H. First-in-human study and clinical case reports of the alveolar bone regeneration with the secretive from human mesenchymal stem cells. *Head Face Med.* **2016**, *15*, 12–15.

9. Zhu, X.; Liu, J.; Yu, Z.; Chen, C.A.; Aksel, H.; Azim, A.A.; Huang, G.T. A Miniature Swine Model for Stem Cell-Based De Novo Regeneration of Dental Pulp and Dentin-Like Tissue. *Tissue Eng. Part. C Methods* **2018**, *24*, 108–120. [CrossRef]

10. Meschi, N.; Hilkens, P.; Lambrichts, I.; Van den Eynde, K.; Mavridou, A.; Strijbos, O.; De Ketelaere, M.; Van Gorp, G.; Lambrechts, P. Regenerative endodontic procedure of an infected immature permanent human tooth: An immunohistological study. *Clin. Oral. Investig.* **2016**, *20*, 807–814. [CrossRef]

11. Pelegrine, A.A.; Aloise, A.C.; Zimmermann, A.; de Mello e Oliveira, R.; Ferreira, L.M. Repair of critical-size bone defects using bone marrow stromal cells: A histomorphometric study in rabbit calvaria. Part I: Use of fresh bone marrow or bone marrow mononuclear fraction. *Clin. Oral Implants Res.* **2014**, *25*, 567–572. [CrossRef] [PubMed]

12. Victorelli, G.; Aloise, A.C.; Passador-Santos, F.; de Mello e Oliveira, R.; Pelegrine, A.A. Ectopic Implantation of Hydroxyapatite Xenograft Scaffold Loaded with Bone Marrow Aspirate Concentrate or Osteodifferentiated Bone Marrow Mesenchymal Stem Cells: A Pilot Study in Mice. *Int. J. Oral. Maxillofac. Implants* **2016**, *31*, e18–e23. [CrossRef] [PubMed]

13. Chamberlain, G.; Fox, J.; Ashton, B.; Middleton, J. Concise review: Mesenchymal stem cells: Their phenotype, differentiation capacity, immunological features, and potential for homing. *Stem Cells* **2007**, *25*, 2739–2749. [CrossRef] [PubMed]

14. Kawaguchi, H.; Hirachi, A.; Hasegawa, N.; Iwata, T.; Hamaguchi, H.; Shiba, H.; Takata, T.; Kato, Y.; Kurihara, H. Enhancement of periodontal tissue regeneration by transplantation of bone marrow mesenchymal stem cells. *J. Periodontol.* **2004**, *75*, 1281–1287. [CrossRef] [PubMed]

15. Moseley, T.A.; Zhu, M.; Hedrick, M.H. Adipose-derived stem and progenitor cells as fillers in plastic and reconstructive surgery. *Plast. Reconstr. Surg.* **2006**, *118* (Suppl. 3), 121S–128S. [CrossRef] [PubMed]

16. Machado, E.; Fernandes, M.H.; de Gomes, P.S. Dental stemcells for craniofacial tissue engineering. *Oral Surg. Oral Med. Oral Pathol. Oral Radiol.* **2012**, *113*, 728–733. [CrossRef] [PubMed]

17. Mitrano, T.I.; Grob, M.S.; Carrion, F.; Nova-Lamperti, E.; Luz, P.A.; Fierro, F.S.; Quintero, A.; Chaparro, A.; Sanz, A. Culture and characterization of mesenchymal stem cells from human gingival tissue. *J. Periodontol.* **2010**, *81*, 917–925. [CrossRef]

18. Man, Y.; Wang, P.; Guo, Y.; Xiang, L.; Yang, Y.; Qu, Y.; Gong, P.; Deng, L. Angiogenic and osteogenic potential of platelet-rich plasma and adipose-derived stem cell laden alginate microspheres. *Biomaterials* **2012**, *33*, 8802–8811. [CrossRef]

19. Kaully, T.; Kaufman-Francis, K.; Lesman, A.; Levenberg, S. Vascularization of the conduit to viable engineered tissues. *Tissue Eng. Part B Rev.* **2009**, *15*, 159. [CrossRef]

20. Araujo, D.B.; de Jesus Campos, E.; Oliveira, M.A.; Lima, M.J.; Martins, G.B.; Araujo, R.P. Surgical elevation of bilateral maxillary sinus floor with a combination of autogenous bone and lyophilized bovine bone. *J. Contemp. Dent. Pract.* **2013**, *14*, 445–450. [CrossRef]

21. Dottore, A.M.; Kawakami, P.Y.; Bechara, K.; Rodrigues, J.A.; Cassoni, A.; Figueiredo, L.C.; Piattelli, A.; Shibli, J.A. Stability of implants placed in augmented posterior mandible after alveolar osteotomy using resorbable nonceramic hydroxyapatite or intraoral autogenous bone: 12-month follow-up. *Clin. Implant Dent. Relat. Res.* **2014**, *16*, 330–336. [CrossRef]

22. Pang, C.; Ding, Y.; Zhou, H.; Qin, R.; Hou, R.; Zhang, G.; Hu, K. Alveolar ridge preservation with deproteinized bovine bone graft and collagen membrane and delayed implants. *J. Craniofac Surg.* **2014**, *25*, 1698–1702. [CrossRef]

23. Dominici, M.; Le Blanc, K.; Mueller, I.; Slaper-Cortenbach, I.; Marini, F.; Krause, D.; Deans, R.; Keating, A.; Prockop, D.J.; Horwitz, E. Minimal criteria for defining multipotent mesenchymal stromal cells. The International Society for Cellular Therapy position statement. *Cytotherapy* **2006**, *8*, 315–317. [CrossRef]

24. Brånemark, P.I. Osseointegration and its experimental background. *J. Prosthet. Dent.* **1983**, *50*, 399–410. [CrossRef]

25. Aloise, A.C.; Pelegrine, A.A.; Zimmermann, A.; de Mello e Oliveira Ferreira, L.M. Repair of Critical-Size Bone Defects Using Bone Marrow Stem Cells or Autogenous Bone with or Without Study in Rabbit Calvaria. *Int. J. Oral Maxillofac. Implants* **2015**, *30*, 208–215. [CrossRef] [PubMed]

26. Zimmermann, A.; Pelegrine, A.A.; Peruzzo, D.; Martinez, E.F.; de Mello e Oliveira, R.; Aloise, A.C.; Ferreira, L.M. Adipose mesenchymal stem cells associated with xenograft in a guided bone regeneration model: A histomorphometric study in rabbit calvaria. *Int. J. Oral Maxillofac. Implants* **2015**, *30*, 1415–1422. [CrossRef] [PubMed]

27. Mao, J.J.; Giannobile, W.V.; Helms, J.A.; Hollister, S.J.; Krebsbach, P.H.; Longaker, M.T.; Shi, S. Craniofacial tissue engineering by stem cells. *J. Dent. Res.* **2006**, *85*, 966–979. [CrossRef]

28. Zhang, L.; Feng, G.; Wei, X.; Huang, L.; Ren, A.; Dong, N.; Wang, H.; Huang, Q.; Zhang, Y.; Deng, F. The effects of mesenchymal stem cells in craniofacial tissue engineering. *Curr. Stem Cell Res. Ther.* **2014**, *9*, 280–289. [CrossRef]

6

Dental Implants with Different Neck Design: A Prospective Clinical Comparative Study with 2-Year Follow-Up

Pietro Montemezzi [1,2,*], Francesco Ferrini [1,2], Giuseppe Pantaleo [3], Enrico Gherlone [1,2] and Paolo Capparè [1,2]

1   Dental School, Vita-Salute San Raffaele University, 20132 Milan, Italy; ferrini.f@gmail.com (F.F.); gherlone.enrico@hsr.it (E.G.); cappare.paolo@hsr.it (P.C.)
2   Department of Dentistry, IRCCS San Raffaele Hospital, 20132 Milan, Italy
3   UniSR-Social.Lab (Research Methods), Faculty of Psychology, Vita-Salute San Raffaele University, 20132 Milan, Italy; pantaleo.giuseppe@hsr.it
*   Correspondence: m.montemezzi@libero.it

Abstract: The present study was conducted to investigate whether a different implant neck design could affect survival rate and peri-implant tissue health in a cohort of disease-free partially edentulous patients in the molar–premolar region. The investigation was conducted on 122 dental implants inserted in 97 patients divided into two groups: Group A (rough wide-neck implants) vs. Group B (rough reduced-neck implants). All patients were monitored through clinical and radiological checkups. Survival rate, probing depth, and marginal bone loss were assessed at 12- and 24-month follow-ups. Patients assigned to Group A received 59 implants, while patients assigned to Group B 63. Dental implants were placed by following a delayed loading protocol, and cemented metal–ceramic crowns were delivered to the patients. The survival rates for both Group A and B were acceptable and similar at the two-year follow-up (96.61% vs. 95.82%). Probing depth and marginal bone loss tended to increase over time (*follow-up*: t_1 = 12 vs. t_2 = 24 months) in both groups of patients. Probing depth (p = 0.015) and bone loss (p = 0.001) were significantly lower in Group A (3.01 vs. 3.23 mm and 0.92 vs. 1.06 mm; Group A vs. Group B). Within the limitations of the present study, patients with rough wide-neck implants showed less marginal bone loss and minor probing depth, as compared to rough reduced-neck implants placed in the molar–premolar region. These results might be further replicated through longer-term trials, as well as comparisons between more collar configurations (e.g., straight vs. reduced vs. wide collars).

Keywords: dental implants; dental implant neck design; peri-implant bone loss; peri-implant probing depth

1. Introduction

The scientific debate on dental implant macro-design is a well-known topic in the field of implant dentistry. The ideal fixture design should bring together the most suitable and distinctive characteristics for implant osseointegration, such as type of material (zirconium or titanium), body shape (cylindrical or conical), neck geometry (straight, reduced, or wide), threads depth, width, and pitch, as well as tapered or non-tapered apical portion, body length, and diameter. Although there is no perfect implant design [1,2], nor a best surface treatment [3], scientific evidence has consistently demonstrated that different dental implant macro-designs affect long-term implant success [4,5] and also accelerate the healing process, to allow implant therapy in the population of patients who are more prone to failure [6,7]. Implant collar, being the portion of the implant that connects the fixture with the oral cavity throughout a prosthetic device, is a very important feature related to the peri-implant tissue's health conditions.

Several studies about implant neck design and marginal bone loss can be found in the literature, but the results are controversial. In vivo animal studies reported a greater crestal bone height and thickness of surrounding implant tissue in dental implants with triangular neck designs [8]; smaller crestal bone loss but similar peri-implant tissue thickness in narrow ring extra-shorts implants [9]; and greater bone loss in dental implants with micro-rings on the neck, as compared to open-thread implant collars [10]. Human model studies reported improved biomechanical behavior for stress/strain distribution pattern in dental implants with divergent collar design [11]; no additional bone loss in non-submerged dental implants with a short smooth collar compared to similar but longer implant collar design [12].

Other clinical findings suggest that specific implant neck design might be suitable in anterior areas, where bone loss, even if acceptable, can lead to adverse aesthetic results [13,14].

The purpose of the present study is to compare peri-implant hard- and soft-tissue health conditions in partially edentulous patients who received the same dental implants but with two different implant neck designs, at a two-year follow-up. In this study, the null hypothesis led to the expectation of no differences in survival rate, probing depth, and marginal bone loss among patients who received dental implants with wide or reduced collar morphology.

2. Materials and Methods

2.1. Patients

Study participants were selected from patients who attended the Dental Department of IRCCS San Raffaele Hospital, Milan, Italy asking for partial fixed implant-prosthetic rehabilitation. Recruitment occurred from February 2016 to November 2017, and the investigation was conducted following all the ethical regulations related to the institution.

Patients had to meet the following inclusion criteria: (1) hopeless teeth to be extracted at least four months prior to surgery in molar/premolar region; (2) no previous dental implants already in place adjacent to surgical site; (3) natural antagonistic teeth (composite resin restorations allowed); (4) absence of diabetes, periodontitis, bruxism, and smoking; (5) absence of chemotherapy or radiation therapy of head and neck district, as well as anti-resorptive drug therapy (i.e., bisphosphonates); and (6) neither mucosal lesions (lichen planus, epulis fissuratum) nor bone lesions (i.e., simple bone cyst or odontomas). Eligible areas for surgery of edentulous maxilla or mandible were selected to receive 1 to a maximum of 3 dental implants. Participants were verbally informed about the purpose of the study but not assigned to a specific group, as they were randomly chosen either to receive a wide-neck implant (Group A) or a reduced-neck implant (Group B).

Patients were assigned to conditions according to a computer-generated random list, prescribing the use of the reduced vs. wide implant. Clinical measures (i.e., survival rate, peri-implant probing depth, and mean marginal bone loss) were taken at 12 and 24 months. Thus, the design amounted to a 2 (implant: wide vs. reduced) X 2 (time: 12 vs. 24 month follow-up) *mixed* factorial design, following the *Consolidated Standards of Reporting Trials* (CONSORT) guidelines available as supplementary material to this manuscript and on http://www.consort-statement.org/.

Written informed consent was signed before the start of the study; patients were allowed to leave the research at any time, without any consequence.

Implant macrogeometry regarding the two different collar designs used in the present study is shown in Figure 1 (CSR, Sweden & Martina, Due Carrare, Italy).

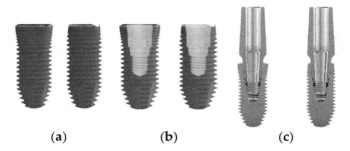

(a)   (b)   (c)

Figure 1. Image shows the CSR full-treatment ZirTi conical dental implant collar with different macro-design. (**a**) Rough wide neck compared with rough reduced neck; (**b**), wide-neck and reduced-neck designs with double conical implant–abutment connection with internal hexagon for prosthetic repositioning; and (**c**) wide-neck and reduced-neck designs with same contact length and tapered angles at the interface.

2.2. Implant Surgery

The study was based on a single blind design, with patients being unaware of which type of implant neck design (wide or reduced) was used for the therapy.

Local anesthesia was induced with local infiltration of lidocaine 20 mg/mL with 1:50.000 adrenaline (Ecocain, Molteni Dental, Firenze, Italy). A crestal horizontal incision was made, with buccal relieving incisions in the medial and distal portions of the main incision. A full-thickness flap was raised, and dental implants were placed in edentulous sites of 0.5 mm, subcrestally, with a minimum insertion torque of 35 Ncm. Cover screw was positioned, and a periosteal incision was performed in order to allow flap passivation in search for primary intention healing of the wound. Vertical mattress suturing technique was used with a 4-0 coated braided absorbable suture (Vicryl, ETHICON, Johnson & Johnson, New Brunswick, NJ, USA). Sterile dry gauze compression was performed on the wound to control post-operative bleeding. Ice packages were delivered to the patients immediately after surgery, with instruction to apply cold to the surgical area for the following 24 h. Semi-liquid cold diet was recommended for the first 48 h.

At-home pharmacological therapy prescribed was amoxicillin 1 g, every 12 hours, for six days, and non-steroid anti-inflammatory drug ibuprofen 400 mg, every 12 hours, for four days, post-operatively. All implants were loaded after a 4-month healing period, through a delayed loading protocol, with a composite resin temporary restoration, followed by metal–ceramic cemented crowns. Definitive abutments used for both Group A and B were the same and had conical connection with Double Action Tight (DAT), a system that presents a conical interface between the abutment and the implant, plus one more conical interface between the screw and the abutment.

Clinically, abutment screws were tightened at 25 Ncm by using a dental torque wrench.

2.3. Parameters

Dental implant survival rate was defined as the fixtures being osseointegrated and staying in situ; and capable to guarantee stability for prosthetic support along the 2-year observation period following the surgical placement. Peri-implant probing depth was estimated through a CP12 University of North Carolina color-coded periodontal probe (Hu Friedy, Chicago, IL, USA), in the mesial, distal, buccal, and lingual/palatal surfaces of the fixture. Distance in mm between the mucosal margin and the tip of the probe was considered as pocket depth.

Intraoral radiographs were taken, using extension cone paralleling system (XCP, Dentsply international, RINN), and mean marginal bone loss was calculated, using Digora Optime digital intraoral imaging system (Soredex, Tuusula, Finland).

A line was traced parallel to the long axis of the implant in order to measure in mm the distance between the crestal bone level at the margin of the implant neck and the top of the apical portion of the implant.

2.4. Statistical Analysis

All analyses were run at the implant level. Peri-implant probing depth and marginal bone loss were submitted to separate 2 (follow-up: $t_1 = 12$ vs. $t_2 = 24$ months) X 2 (*neck design*: reduced vs. wide) multivariate analyses of variance (MANOVA$_s$), in order to distinguish the effects of follow-up time, implant neck design, and additionally assess any interactive effect(s) of the two factors. Mean values were complemented by standard errors of the mean (*Se*) and 95% confidence intervals (CI).

3. Results

A total of 97 patients (56 men and 41 women) aged between 33 and 75 years (mean 58.2 ± 6.22 years) were selected for the present study. None of them withdrew from the research, and 122 fixtures were placed in the molar/premolar region.

Fixtures made of titanium grade 4 had a standard length (≥10 mm) and a diameter of 3.8 and 4.2 mm for wide-neck implants and 4.2 and 5.0 mm for reduced-neck ones. Dental implants received the same subtraction procedure, according to the Zir-Ti full-surface treatment (Zirconium Oxide Sand-Blasted and Acid Etched Titanium). The apical portion was tapered with 50° accentuated triangular threads and four longitudinal incisions, to increase penetration ability and anti-rotation features. Fifty patients formed Group A (rough wide-neck design) and received 59 implants. Group B (rough reduced-neck design) was composed of forty-eight patients, who received 63 implants.

The two groups were compared at one-year and two-year follow-ups. Survival rate, probing depth, and marginal bone loss were recorded through clinical and radiological checkups. Radiological records for different dental implants placed in Group A and B patients are shown in Figures 2 and 3.

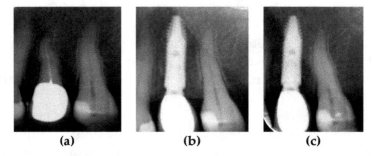

(a)   (b)   (c)

Figure 2. Periapical X-rays showing marginal bone level of CSR dental implant with a reduced neck. (**a**) Pre-operative X-ray; (**b**) post-operative follow-up at 12 months; and (**c**) post-operative follow-up at 24 months.

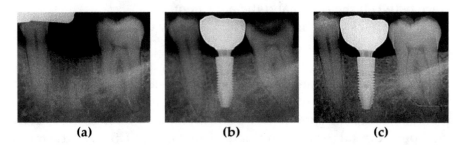

(a)   (b)   (c)

Figure 3. Periapical X-rays showing marginal bone level of CSR dental implant with a wide neck. (**a**) Pre-operative X-ray; (**b**) post-operative follow-up at 12 months; and (**c**) post-operative follow up at 24 months.

The overall survival rate of CSR dental implants at the two-year follow-up was 96.72% (four implant failures out of 122 implants placed). Both groups showed similar outcomes: At 12 months, survival rate was 98.30% for Group A and 98.41% for Group B, while it decreased at 96.61% for Group A and 96.82% for Group B at the 24-month follow-up.

Regarding peri-implant probing depth, a 2 (*follow-up*: t_1 = 12 vs. t_2 = 24 months) X 2 (*neck design*: reduced vs. wide) multivariate analysis of variance (MANOVA) affirmed a main effect of follow-up, F (1, 116) = 10.69, $p < 0.001$, such that probing depth was generally lower at 12 months (3.06 mm ± Se = 0.046; 95% CI = 2.96, 3.15) than at 24 months (3.18 mm ± Se = 0.050; 95% CI = 3.08, 3.28), independently of type of neck design. Furthermore, the analysis also revealed a main effect of neck design, F (1, 116) = 6.28, $p < 0.015$, such that probing depth was generally lower for wide (Group A: 3.01 mm ± Se = 0.063; 95% CI = 2.88, 3.13) than for reduced-neck implants (Group B: 3.23 mm ± Se = 0.061; 95% CI = 3.11, 3.35), independently of time of follow-up. More specifically, the difference between the two groups, considered at one and two years of follow-up were, respectively, as follows: Group A (one year): 2.93 mm ± Se = 0.07; 95% CI = 2.79, 3.07 vs. Group B (one year): 3.18 mm ± Se = 0.05; 95% CI = 3.07, 3.28 (p = 0.007); and Group A (two years): 3.09 mm ± Se = 0.07; 95% CI = 2.95, 3.24 vs. Group B (two years): 3.28 mm ± Se = 0.06; 95% CI = 3.15, 3.40 (p = 0.061). The interaction *follow-up* (t_1 = 12 vs. t_2 = 24 months) X *neck design* (reduced vs. wide) was not significant, F (1, 116) = 0.58, p = 0.45, n.s.

A 2 (*follow-up*: t_1 = 12 vs. t_2 = 24 months) X 2 (*neck design*: reduced vs. wide) multivariate analysis of variance (MANOVA) was also conducted for marginal bone loss and revealed a main effect of follow-up, F (1, 116) = 198.85, $p < 0.001$, such that marginal bone loss was generally lower at 12 months (0.89 mm ± Se = 0.02; 95% CI = 0.86, 0.93) than at 24 months (1.08 mm ± Se = 0.01; 95% CI = 1.06, 1.11), independently of type of neck design. Furthermore, the analysis also revealed a main effect of neck design, F (1, 116) = 34.04, $p < 0.001$, such that marginal bone loss was generally lower for wide (Group A: 0.92 mm ± Se = 0.02; 95% CI = 0.88, 0.95) than for reduced-neck implants (Group B: 1.06 mm ± Se = 0.02; 95% CI = 1.03, 1.10), independently of time of follow-up. More specifically, the difference between the two groups, considered at one and two years of follow-up, were, respectively, as follows: Group A (one year): 0.84 mm ± Se = 0.03; 95% CI = 0.78, 0.88 vs. Group B (one year): 0.95 mm ± Se = 0.02; 95% CI = 0.91, 0.99 (p = 0.001); and Group A (two years): 1.00 mm ± Se = 0.02; 95% CI = 0.97, 1.03 vs. Group B (two years): 1.17 mm ± Se = 0.02; 95% CI = 1.14, 1.20 (p = 0.001). Importantly, the two-way interaction *follow-up* (t_1 = 12 vs. t_2 = 24 months) X *neck design* (reduced vs. wide) was statistically significant, F (1, 116) = 3.91, p = 0.05, showing that the increase in bone loss for reduced-neck implants (Group B) was steeper than the increase observed for wide-neck implants.

4. Discussion

Our study focused on dental implants' macro-design, particularly on the clinical performance of the same type of fixture but with two different rough collar designs in partially edentulous patients, using a delayed loading protocol. Examined parameters were peri-implant probing depth, marginal bone loss, and survival rate at two-year follow-up. Both groups of patients showed an acceptable but almost similar implant survival rate. However, patients who received implants with a wide-neck design presented lower probing depth and minor marginal bone loss compared to reduced neck; thus, the null hypothesis of no differences between dental implants with different neck designs was partially rejected. From a clinical point of view, differences in probing depth and marginal bone loss between Group A and B were not relevant at the two-year follow-up. Since the absence of signs of soft-tissue inflammation and the absence of further additional bone loss following initial healing were found, according to peri-implant health definition by Renvert et al. [15], it can be affirmed that both groups of patients showed peri-implant tissue health conditions.

Implant therapy is a very helpful discipline when it comes to rehabilitating dental patients. Even if bone loss around oral implants is described to be an unavoidable and physiologic foreign-body reaction of bone against titanium [16–18], the key for success resides in the neutralization of risk factors at multiple levels: patient level, implant level, and prosthetic level.

Risk factors such as diabetes, periodontitis, bruxism, smoking, antidepressants intake, bone augmentation procedures, head and neck radiotherapy [19–22] play a principal role in long-term implants' outcome. These factors are found at the patient level, meaning that they are poorly controllable over time, as they can worsen along with local or systemic health conditions. Here, we must recall that patients included in the present study where disease-free individuals.

Other factors that are set at prosthesis level also interfere with the success of implant therapy and should not be underestimated. According to Vazquez-Alvarez et al. [23], the distance between the implant platform and the horizontal component of the prosthesis has a significant influence on peri-implant bone loss, and to be adequate, it should range from 3.3 to 6 mm. According to Lemos et al. [24], the retention system for implant-supported prostheses may lead to a different bone-loss pattern, as cement-retained restorations showed less marginal bone loss than screw-retained restorations, and implant survival rate was in favor of cement-retained prosthesis.

Restorations for the present study were cemented crowns where a minimum distance of 3.5 mm was kept between implant-abutment junction and horizontal prosthetic component, and where extreme attention was payed to remove any cement excess that could be found underneath them.

Accuracy of dental impression used, whether traditionally or digitally taken, may lead to differences in the fit of the definitive restoration [25]. In our case, prosthetic rehabilitations were performed by passing through light and putty consistency polyvinylsiloxane materials.

The type of prosthetic material itself is described to be capable of having an effect on the peri-implant tissues [26]. In this study, the decision for metal–ceramic crowns was supported by appropriate biomechanical properties, as it was demonstrated in the literature [27–29].

Occlusal forces were exerted against natural antagonistic teeth in the molar/premolar region, to standardize the procedure and avoid contact with previously installed dental restorations made of unknown or undefined material properties (e.g., a preexisting zirconium-based bridge in the antagonistic region).

Finally, implant therapy risk factors are also found at the implant level, being the fixture macro-design capable to affect the osseointegration process, as reported by several authors [4,5,30–33]. Fixture micro- and macro-designs can be adequately selected before treatment, and with the ideal concept design, implant success rate would be more predictable.

Starting from the type of material from which implants are manufactured, different osseointegration processes (amount of bone attachment to the surface and strength of the bone-surface interaction) may occur at the bone level.

Recently reported by Taek-Ka et al. [34], a qualitative different osseointegration was found through higher bone-surface interaction in commercially pure titanium grade 2 implants compared to grade 4. Apart from titanium, zirconia has also been proposed as an alternative material for oral fixtures. At the moment, despite its optimal biocompatibility, no definitive decision is available on the clinical performance of such implants [35,36].

Back to implant collar, the manner in which it is configured appears to be of relevant interest: The maximum loading stress distribution in bone is localized at the neck of the implants, as described by Anitua et al. [37] and Huang et al. [38]. Several studies are available in the literature, but no consensus on which collar design is more suitable for osseointegration was agreed on by the authors.

Our study would qualify rough wide-neck implants to reduce bone loss over time, being conscious that a longer follow-up period is necessary to confirm these findings. This may be related to the platform-switching concept, which has been described to be beneficial for osseointegration [39–43]. In fact, even in the case that a platform-matched abutment is used in such implants, a minimal effect of switching platform still exists, being that the neck of the implant is wider in diameter with respect to the main body. Otherwise, reduced-neck implants are less likely to benefit from the platform-switching effect because of their narrower platform.

According to Eshkol-Yogev et al. [44], round neck implants may significantly increase primary stability when compared to triangular neck design. In a paper by Mendoca et al. [45], bone remodeling showed to be of benefit around implants with rough collar design, in mandible but not in maxilla, if compared to machined collar surface implants. In a review by Koodaryan et al. [46], rough-surfaced micro-threaded neck implants appeared to lose less bone compared to polished and rough-surfaced neck implants.

CSR implants placed in this study had roughened surface collars with no microthreads at the bone cervical region. Presence or absence of microthreads, as well as the amount of surface roughness, may have an effect on bone preservation. Despite that an implant collar with a microthread can help in the maintenance of peri-implant bone against prosthetic loading, [47] this study was focused on conventional rough-surface dental implants, not to add confounding aspects related to numerous available surface topography (e.g., smooth, polished neck vs. machined surface vs. microthread design). Furthermore, CSR implants had a moderate degree of roughness, as no beneficial effect seemed to be associated with an increase in surface roughness. In fact, a 20-year follow-up clinical trial by Donati et al. [48] reported no peri-implant bone preservation related to implants with an increased surface roughness.

Another relevant issue to consider is the implant–abutment connection system. Implants in the present study were provided with DAT connection. Consisting of a double conical interface and internal hexagon for prosthetic repositioning, this type of connection follows the recent literature's outcomes. According to Caricasulo et al. [49], internal connection, particularly conical interfaces seem to better maintain crestal bone level around dental implants.

As stated by Kim et al. [50], transmission of the occlusal load from the restoration to the implant, and then from the implant to the surrounding bone, is essential to stimulate osteoblasts activity. This is to say, to avoid minimum but regular and continuous bone resorption, described to be around 1 mm for the first year and of 0.2 mm per year thereafter [51], bone deposition must be encouraged.

The concept of biocompatibility related to implant-prosthetic rehabilitation can be considered as the ultimate key for success: proper design of the fixture, together with a correct function of the implant–abutment connection, and optimal adaptation of the prosthetic restoration generates a self-defensive mechanism that guarantees long-term survival rates.

Considering multiple and confounding aspects which affect implant failure, with risk factors set at patient, implant, and prosthetic level, it is important to affirm that bone loss in not solely determined by collar morphology. Further studies should be conducted on multiple heterogeneous implant collar design in different populations (e.g., diabetic vs. nondiabetic) and with different prosthetic restorations (e.g., screwed vs. cemented). Longer follow-up periods could highlight the enhancement of the clinical performance of dental implants with specific neck configurations.

5. Conclusions

Within the limitations of the present prospective clinical comparative study, peri-implant probing depth and marginal bone level around dental implants placed in edentulous sites in molar/premolar region were affected by different neck designs. Patients who received implants with rough wide-neck design presented lower probing depth and minor marginal bone loss compared to patients with rough reduced-neck implants.

Reduced-neck implants showed a tendency to lose comparatively more bone over time if compared with wide-neck implants.

However, dental implants' survival rate was acceptable and satisfactory for both groups of patients and showed no differences at the two-year follow-up.

Author Contributions: P.M.: conceptualization, writing-original draft preparation; F.F.: investigation, data curation; G.P.: study design, research methodology, statistical analysis, drafting and final approval of the manuscript; E.G.: supervision, project administration; P.C.: conceptualization, investigation. All authors have read and agreed to published version of the manuscript.

References

1. Steigenga, J.T.; Al-Shammari, K.F.; Nociti, F.H.; Misch, C.E.; Wang, H.L. Dental implant design and its relationship to long-term implant success. *Implant Dent.* **2003**, *12*, 306–317. [CrossRef] [PubMed]

2. Ogle, O.E. Implant surface material, design, and osseointegration. *Dent. Clin. N. Am.* **2015**, *59*, 505–520. [CrossRef] [PubMed]

3. Rupp, F.; Liang, L.; Geis-Gerstorfer, J.; Scheideler, L.; Huttig, F. Surface characteristics of dental implants: A review. *Dent. Mater.* **2018**, *34*, 40–57. [CrossRef]

4. Spies, B.C.; Bateli, M.; Ben Rahal, G.; Christmann, M.; Vach, K.; Kohal, R.J. Does oral implant design affect marginal bone loss? Results of a parallel group randomized controlled equivalence trial. *BioMed Res. Int.* 2018. [CrossRef] [PubMed]

5. Ormianer, Z.; Matalon, S.; Block, J.; Kohen, J. Dental implant thread design and the consequences on long-term marginal bone loss. *Implant Dent.* **2016**, *25*, 471–477. [CrossRef] [PubMed]

6. Lesmes, D.; Laster, Z. Innovations in dental implant design for current therapy. *Oral. Maxillofac. Surg. Clin. N. Am.* **2011**, *23*, 193–200. [CrossRef]

7. Boyan, B.D.; Cheng, A.; Olivares-Navarrete, R.; Schwartz, Z. Implant surface design regulates mesenchymal stem cell differentiation and maturation. *Adv. Dent. Res.* **2016**, *28*, 10–17. [CrossRef]

8. Perez-Albacete, M.A.; Perez-Albacete, C.; Mate-Sanchez de Val, J.E.; Ramos-Oltra, M.L.; Fernandez-Dominguez, M.; Calvo-Guirado, J.L. Evaluation of a new dental implant cervical design in comparison with a conventional design in an experimental american foxhound model. *Materials* **2018**, *11*, 462. [CrossRef]

9. Calvo-Guirado, J.L.; Morales-Melendez, H.; Perez-Martinez, C.; Morales-Schwarz, D.; Kolerman, R.; Fernandez-Dominguez, M.; Gehrke, S.A.; Mate-Sanchez de Val, J.E. Evaluation of the surrounding ring of two different extra-short implant designs in crestal bone maintenance: A histologic study in dogs. *Materials* **2018**, *11*, 1630. [CrossRef]

10. Calvo-Guirado, J.L.; Jimenez-Soto, R.; Perez-Martinez, C.; Fernandez-Dominguez, M.; Gehrke, S.A.; Mate-Sanchez de Val, J.E. Influence of implant neck design on peri-implant tissue dimensions: A comparative study in dogs. *Materials* **2018**, *11*, 2007. [CrossRef]

11. Shen, W.L.; Chen, C.S.; Hsu, M.L. Influence of implant collar design on stress and strain distribution in the crestal compacte bone: A three-dimensional finite element analysis. *Int. J. Oral Maxillofac. Implant.* **2010**, *25*, 901–910. [PubMed]

12. Hanggi, M.P.; Hanggi, D.C.; Schoolfield, J.D.; Meyer, J.; Cochran, D.L.; Hermann, J.S. Crestal bone changes around titanium implants. Part I: A retrospective radiographics evaluation in humans comparing two non-submerged implant designs with different machined collar lengths. *J. Periodontol.* **2005**, *76*, 791–802. [CrossRef] [PubMed]

13. Crespi, R.; Capparè, P.; Polizzi, E.; Gherlone, E. Fresh-Socket implants of different collar length: Clinical evaluation in the aesthetic zone. *Clin. Implant. Dent. Relat. Res.* **2015**, *17*, 871–878. [CrossRef] [PubMed]

14. Chappuis, V.; Bornstein, M.M.; Buser, D.; Belser, U. Influence of implant neck design on facial bone crest dimensions in the esthetic zone analyzed by cone beam CT: A comparative study with a 5-to-9-year follow-up. *Clin. Oral Implant. Res.* **2016**, *27*, 1055–1064. [CrossRef] [PubMed]

15. Renvert, S.; Person, G.R.; Pirih, F.Q.; Camargo, P.M. Peri-implant health, peri implant mucositis, and peri-implantitis: Case definitions and diagnostic considerations. *J. Periodontol.* **2018**, *89*, s304–s312. [CrossRef]

16. Albrektsson, T.; Dahlin, C.; Jemt, T.; Sennerby, L.; Turri, A.; Wennerberg, A. Is marginal bone loss around dental implants the result of a provoked foreign body reaction? *Clin. Implant Dent. Relat. Res.* **2014**, *16*, 155–165. [CrossRef]

17. Albrektsson, T.; Canullo, L.; Cochran, D.; De Bruyn, H. Peri-implantitis: A complication of a foreign body or a man-made "Disease". Facts and fiction. *Clin. Implant Dent. Relat. Res.* **2016**, *18*, 840–849. [CrossRef]

18. Buser, D.; Sennerby, L.; De Bruyn, H. Modern implant dentistry based on osseointegration: 50 years of progress, current trends and open questions. *Periodontol* **2000**, *73*, 7–21. [CrossRef]

19. Tecco, S.; Grusovin, M.G.; Sciara, S.; Bova, F.; Pantaleo, G.; Capparè, P. The association between three attitude-related indexes of oral hygiene and secondary implant failures: a retrospective longitudinal study. *Int. J. Dent. Hyg.* **2018**, *16*, 372–379. [CrossRef]

20. Kandasamy, B.; Kaur, N.; Tomar, G.K.; Bharadwaj, A.; Manual, L.; Chauhan, M. Long-term retrospective study based on implant succes rate in patients with risk factor: 15-year follow-up. *J. Contemp. Dent. Pract.* **2018**, *19*, 90–93. [CrossRef]

21. Chrcanovic, B.R.; Kisch, J.; Albrektsson, T.; Wennerberg, A. Factors influencing early dental implant failures. *J. Dent. Res.* **2016**, *95*, 995–1002. [CrossRef] [PubMed]

22. Gherlone, E.F.; Capparè, P.; Tecco, S.; Polizzi, E.; Pantaleo, G.; Gastaldi, G.; Grusovin, M.G. A prospective longitudinal study on implant prosthetic rehabilitation in controlled HIV-positive patients with 1-year follow-up: The role of CD4+ level, smoking habits, and oral hygiene. *Clin. Implant Dent. Relat. Res.* **2016**, *18*, 955–964. [CrossRef] [PubMed]

23. Vazquez-Alvarez, R.; Perez-Sayans, M.; Gayoso-Diz, P.; Garcia-Garcia, A. Factors affecting peri-implant bone loss: A post-five-year retrospective study. *Clin. Oral Implant. Res.* **2015**, *26*, 1006–1014. [CrossRef] [PubMed]

24. Lemos, C.A.; de Souza Batista, V.E.; Almeida, D.A.; Santiago Junior, J.F.; Verri, F.R.; Pellizzer, E.P. Evaluation of cement-retained versus screw-retained implant-supported restorations for marginal bone loss: A systematic review and meta-analysis. *J. Prosthet. Dent.* **2016**, *115*, 419–427. [CrossRef] [PubMed]

25. Cappare, P.; Sannino, G.; Minoli, M.; Montemezzi, P.; Ferrini, F. Conventional versus digital impression for full arch screw-retained maxillary rehabilitations: A randomized clinical trial. *Int. J. Environ. Res. Public Health* **2019**, *16*, 829. [CrossRef] [PubMed]

26. Maminskas, J.; Puisys, A.; Kuoppala, R.; Raustia, A.; Juodzbalys, G. The prosthetic influence and biomechanics on peri-implant strain: A systematic literature review of finite element studies. *J. Oral Maxillofac. Res.* **2016**, *7*, e4. [CrossRef] [PubMed]

27. Augustin-Panadero, R.; Soriano-Valero, S.; Labaig-Rueds, C.; Fernandez-Estevan, L.; Sola-Ruiz, M.F. Implant-supported metal-ceramic and resin.modified ceramic crowns: A 5-year prospective clinical study. *J. Prosthet. Dent.* **2019**. [CrossRef]

28. Schwartz, S.; Schroder, C.; Hassel, A.; Bomicke, W.; Rammelsber, P. Survival and chipping of zirconia-based and metal-ceramic implant-supported single crowns. *Clin. Oral Implant. Res.* **2012**, *14*, e119–e125. [CrossRef]

29. Pjetursson, B.E.; Valente, N.A.; Strasding, M.; Zwahlen, M.; Liu, S.; Sailer, I. A systematic review of the survival and complication rates of zirconia-ceramic and metal-ceramic single crowns. *Clin. Oral Implant. Res.* **2018**, *16*, 199–214. [CrossRef]

30. Vivan-Cardoso, M.; Vandamme, K.; Chaudhari, A.; De Rycker, J.; Van Meerbeek, B.; Naert, I.; Duyck, J. Dental implant macro-design features can impact the dynamics of osseointegration. *Clin. Implant Dent. Relat. Res.* **2015**, *17*, 639–645. [CrossRef]

31. Lima de Andrade, C.; Carvalho, M.A.; Bordin, D.; da Silva, W.J.; Del Bel Cury, A.A.; Sotto-Maior, B.S. Biomechanical behavior of the dental implant macrodesign. *Int. J. Oral Maxillofac. Implant.* **2017**, *32*, 264–270. [CrossRef] [PubMed]

32. Jimbo, R.; Tovar, N.; Marin, C.; Teixera, H.S.; Anchieta, R.B.; Silveira, L.M.; Janal, M.N.; SHibli, J.A.; Coelho, P.G. The impact of a modified cutting flute implant design on osseointegration. *Int. J. Oral Maxillofac. Surg.* **2014**, *43*, 883–888. [CrossRef] [PubMed]

33. Triplett, R.G.; Frohberg, U.; Sykaras, N.; Woody, R.D. Implant materials, design, and surface topographies: The influence on osseointegration of dental implants. *J. Long Term Eff. Med. Implant.* **2003**, *13*, 485–501. [CrossRef]

34. Taek-Ka, K.; Jung-Yoo, C.; Jae-Il, P.; In-Sung, L.Y. A clue to the existence of bonding between bone and implant surface: An in vivo study. *Materials* **2019**, *12*, 1187. [CrossRef]

35. Hashim, D.; Cionca, N.; Courvoisier, D.S.; Mombelli, A. A systematic review of the clinical survival of zirconia implants. *Clin. Oral Investig.* **2016**, *20*, 1403–1417. [CrossRef] [PubMed]

36. Cionca, N.; Hashim, D.; Mombelli, A. Zirconia dental implants: Where are we now, and where are we heading? *Periodontol* **2000**, *73*, 241–258. [CrossRef]

37. Anitua, E.; Tapia, R.; Luzuriaga, F.; Orive, G. Influence of implant length, diameter, and geometry on stress distribution: A finite element analysis. *Int. J. Periodontics Restor. Dent.* **2010**, *30*, 89–95.

38. Huang, Y.M.; Chou, I.C.; Jiang, C.P.; Wu, Y.S.; Lee, S.Y. Finite element analysis of dental implant neck effects on primary stability and osseointegration in a type IV bone mandible. *Bio Med. Mater. Eng.* **2014**, *24*, 1407–1415. [CrossRef]

39. Salamanca, E.; Lin, J.C.; Tsai, C.Y.; Hsu, Y.S.; Huang, H.M.; Teng, N.C.; Wang, P.D.; Feng, S.W.; Chen, M.S.; Chang, W.J. Dental implant surrounding marginal bone level evaluation: Platform switching versus platform matching-one-year retrospective study. *BioMed Res. Int.* 2017. [CrossRef]

40. Santiago, J.J.F.; Batista, V.E.; Verri, F.R.; Honorio, H.M.; de Mello, C.C.; Almeida, D.A.; Pellizzer, E.P. Platform-switching implants and bone preservation: A systematic review and meta-analysis. *Int. J. Oral Maxillofac. Surg.* **2016**, *45*, 332–345. [CrossRef]

41. Rocha, S.; Wagner, W.; Wiltfang, J.; Nicolau, P.; Moergel, M.; Messias, A.; Behrens, E.; Guerra, F. Effect of platform switching on crestal bone levels around implants in the posterior mandible: 3 years results from a multicentre randomized clinical trial. *J. Clin. Periodontol.* **2016**, *43*, 374–382. [CrossRef] [PubMed]

42. Strietzel, F.P.; Neumann, K.; Hertel, M. Impact of platform switching on marginal peri-implant bone-level changes. Asystematic review and meta-analysis. *Clin. Oral Implant. Res.* **2015**, *26*, 342–358. [CrossRef] [PubMed]

43. Bouazza-Juanes, K.; Martinez-Gonzalez, A.; Peiro, G.; Rodenas, J.J.; Lopez-Molla, M.V. Effect of platform switching on the peri-implant bone: A finite element study. *J. Clin. Exp. Dent.* **2015**, *7*, e483–e488. [CrossRef] [PubMed]

44. Eshkol-Yogev, I.; Tandlich, M.; Shapira, L. Effect of implant neck design on primary and secondary implant stability in the posterior maxilla: A prospective randomized controlled study. *Clin. Oral Implant. Res.* **2019**. [CrossRef] [PubMed]

45. Mendoca, J.A.; Senna, P.M.; Francischone, C.E.; Francischone Junior, C.E.; de Souza Picorelli Assis, N.M.; Sotto-Maior, B. Retrospective evaluation of the influence of the collar surface topography on peri-implant bone preservation. *Int. J. Oral Maxillofac. Implant.* **2017**, *32*, 858–863. [CrossRef] [PubMed]

46. Koodaryan, R.; Hafezeqoran, A. Evaluation of implant collar surfaces for marginal bone loss: A systematic review and meta-analysis. *BioMed Res. Int.* **2016**. [CrossRef]

47. Lee, D.W.; Choi, Y.S.; Park, K.H.; Kim, C.S.; Moon, I.S. Effect of microthread on the maintenance of marginal bone level: A 3-year prospective study. *Clin. Oral Implant. Res.* **2007**, *18*, 465–470. [CrossRef]

48. Donati, M.; Ekestubbe, A.; Lindhe, J.; Wennstrom, J.L. Marginal bone loss at implants with different surface characteristics: A 20-year follow-up of a randomized controlled clinical trial. *Clin. Oral Implant. Res.* **2018**, *29*, 480–487. [CrossRef]

49. Caricasulo, R.; Malchiodi, L.; Ghensi, P.; Fantozzi, G.; Cucchi, A. The influence of implant-abutment connection to peri-implant bone loss: A systematic review and meta-analysis. *Clin. Implant Dent. Relat. Res.* **2018**, *20*, 653–664. [CrossRef]

50. Kim, J.J.; Lee, J.H.; Kim, J.C.; Lee, J.B.; Yeo, I.L. Biological responses to the transitional area of dental implants: Material and structure dependent responses of peri-implant tissue to abutments. *Materials* **2019**, *13*, 72. [CrossRef]

51. Albrektsson, T.; Zarb, G.; Worthington, P.; Eriksson, A.R. The long-term efficacy of currently used dental implants: A review and proposed criteria of success. *Int. J. Oral Maxillofac. Implant.* **1986**, *1*, 11–25.

7

Improvement in Fatigue Behavior of Dental Implant Fixtures by Changing Internal Connection Design: An In Vitro Pilot Study

Nak-Hyun Choi [1,†], Hyung-In Yoon [2,†], Tae-Hyung Kim [3] and Eun-Jin Park [1,*]

[1] Department of Prosthodontics, School of Medicine, Ewha Womans University, Seoul 07985, Korea; hyun_bc@naver.com
[2] Department of Prosthodontics, School of Dentistry and Dental Research Institute, Seoul National University, Seoul 03080, Korea; prosyhi@naver.com
[3] Kim and Lee Dental Clinic, Seoul 06626, Korea; kthrock@nate.com
*   Correspondence: prosth@ewha.ac.kr
†   These authors contributed equally to this work.

Abstract: (1) Background: The stability of the dental implant–abutment complex is necessary to minimize mechanical complications. The purpose of this study was to compare the behaviors of two internal connection type fixtures, manufactured by the same company, with different connection designs. (2) Methods: 15 implant–abutment complexes were prepared for each group of Osseospeed® TX (TX) and Osseospeed® EV (EV): 3 for single-load fracture tests and 12 for cyclic-loaded fatigue tests (nominal peak values as 80%, 60%, 50%, and 40% of the maximum breaking load) according to international standards (UNI EN ISO 14801:2013). They were assessed with micro-computed tomography (CT), and failure modes were analyzed by scanning electron microscope (SEM) images. (3) Results: The maximum breaking load [TX: 711 ± 36 N (95% CI; 670–752), EV: 791 ± 58 N (95% CI; 725–857)] and fatigue limit (TX: 285 N, EV: 316 N) were higher in EV than those in TX. There was no statistical difference in the fracture areas ($P > 0.99$). All specimens with 40% nominal peak value survived 5×10^6 cycles, while 50% specimens failed before 10^5 cycles. (4) Conclusions: EV has improved mechanical properties compared with TX. A loading regimen with a nominal peak value between 40% and 50% is ideal for future tests of implant cyclic loading.

Keywords: dental implants; fracture strength; mechanical stress; fatigue; dental implant–abutment connection; dental implant–abutment design

1. Introduction

Dental implants have been a fairly reliable and predictable treatment option for edentulous patients since their introduction [1]. In previous systematic reviews, a 5-year survival rate of 95.6–97.2% and 10-year survival rate of 93.1% in implants supporting fixed partial dentures were reported, implying that implants have a high survival rate [2–4]. Although dental implants have been clinically and scientifically studied as a viable treatment option to restore the edentulous area [5–7], complications remain a big concern for clinicians. Complication of dental implants can be mainly classified as either biological or mechanical. Biological complications include early loss of osseointegration, marginal bone loss, and peri-implantitis, eventually leading to the implants failing and falling out. Mechanical complications include loose abutment or screw, veneer or ceramic fracture, loss of retention, sinking down of abutment, and fracture of implant fixture, abutment, or screw [2]. Previous reports have demonstrated incidence rates of implant fixture fracture of 0.2–1.1% and abutment or screw fracture of 0.7–2.3% [2]. In particular, fracture of implant fixture is a catastrophic complication, which requires extensive surgical treatments. To overcome mechanical failure of dental implants and guarantee long-term clinical success, the stability of the implant–abutment connection to withstand a masticatory load is important [4,8]. The mechanical stability of the connection may be affected by modifying the implant–abutment connection design as well as by improving material properties of the components [9]. Recently, manufacturers of dental implant systems such as Astra Tech Dental have introduced a modified connection design of the dental implant fixture to improve its mechanical properties. To date, however, only a few studies have demonstrated the effect of different connection designs on the mechanical properties of the implant fixtures [10].

Fatigue is the process of localized, permanent structural change of a material under fluctuating stress [11]. Mechanical complications of implants are generally caused by fatigue stress related to mechanical overload [12]. The interpretation of fatigue limit in implants is slightly different from general mechanics. The fatigue limit of dental implants is defined as "the maximum loading value that can withstand 5×10^6 cycles", contrary to the general definition in mechanics: "the maximum loading value that can withstand infinite cycles" [11,13]. To evaluate fatigue stress in the laboratory, finite element analysis and cyclic loading can be utilized [14–16]. While finite element analysis is considered to simulate fairly reliable results, cyclic loading is used as a method to observe the mechanical properties of actual specimens [16]. To standardize the testing method in the laboratory, ISO 14801 was suggested to simulate a "worst-case scenario" applied on an implant–abutment assembly and consists of sinusoidally curved cyclic loading [13]. These methods can be utilized to substitute in vivo tests, and while a generalized clinical conclusion may not be drawn, a tendency can be observed to provide insight to researchers and clinicians.

The purpose of this study was to compare the mechanical behaviors of two internal connection type dental implant fixtures with different connection designs manufactured by a single manufacturer. By strictly adhering to the procedures considered as the norm, it may provide data on implant systems widely used on the market, and moreover, supply background for additional protocols to the universal standard. The null hypothesis was that the fatigue behavior including the mode of failure of the dental implant–abutment complex is not affected by the modification of the connection design of the dental implant fixture.

2. Materials and Methods

2.1. Preparation of Specimens

The fixtures and abutments tested in this study are listed in Table 1 and the flow of the experiment is shown in Figure 1. A total of 30 implant–abutment assemblies were prepared for test and control groups (n = 15 per group): Osseospeed® EV (EV) and Osseospeed® TX (TX) (Astra Tech Dental, Dentsply Sirona Implants, Mölndal, Sweden). Among the 15 specimens, 3 were tested for single-load fracture tests to identify the maximum fracture load and the other 12 specimens were divided into 4 groups (n = 3 each) for fatigue test under cyclic loading. Each specimen was marked with an indelible marker indicating where the load would be applied to analyze the fractured surface with a scanning electron microscope (SEM). Each implant and abutment was connected with a torque of 25 N cm, as recommended by the manufacturer.

2.2. Micro-CT Image Observation

The implant–abutment assemblies were scanned with micro-computed tomography (CT) scanner (SkyScan 1172, Bruker, Kontich, Belgium) to obtain a series of detailed structural images prior to cyclic loading. The samples were firmly fixed to a full 360° rotational inspection jig. The frame rate was four frames per rotational step of 0.5°, for a total of 2880 images per specimen.

Table 1. Materials used in this study. All fixtures and abutments were composed of commercially pure grade 4 titanium.

Components	Test Group	Control Group
Implant Fixture	OsseoSpeed® EV (4.2 mm × 11 mm)	OsseoSpeed® TX (4.0 mm × 11 mm)
Abutment	TiDesign® EV Abutment height: 5.5 mm Gingival height: 2.5 mm	TiDesign® Abutment height: 5.5 mm Gingival height: 1.5 mm

Manufacturer: Dentsply Sirona Implants, Mölndal, Sweden.

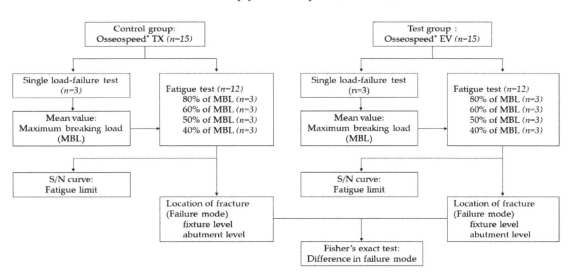

Figure 1. Overall flow of the experiment.

2.3. Single-Load Failure Test and Fatigue

All mechanical tests were performed according to ISO 14801:2013 (Figure 2). The testing apparatus should impose a force within ± 5% of the maximum error range of the nominal peak value with constant frequency. The testing apparatus should also be able to monitor maximum and minimum load values and to stop when the specimen fractures. A servo-hydraulic test system (MTS Landmark, Minneapolis, MN, USA) under load control was used. Single-load failure tests and fatigue tests were conducted in an atmospheric environment of 20 °C ± 5 °C. Each implant–abutment assembly was inserted in a custom stainless-steel jig and collet up to the first thread of the implant fixture (approximately 3.0 mm). The collets were then held at a 30° off-axis angle and fixed to the jig and testing machine. A hemispherical cap was engaged to the implant–abutment assembly, contacting the flat head of the universal testing machine. Compressive load increasing at a speed of 1mm/min was applied to the implant–abutment assembly until fracture or deformation occurred. Three implants from each group were tested and their maximum fracture load values were recorded. The average value of maximum fracture load of the tested implants served as the nominal peak value for the fatigue test.

For the fatigue testing under cyclic loading, we applied a sinusoidal oscillation with 15 Hz frequency between a nominal peak level (maximum) and a 10% value of the nominal peak level (minimum) to the implant–abutment assembly. The cyclic loading was conducted until the fracture occurred. If fracture did not occur, the cyclic loading was conducted up to a maximum number of 5×10^6 cycles. The nominal peak levels of 80%, 60%, 50%, and 40% of the maximum fracture load from the previous single-load-to-failure test were selected. Three samples for each nominal peak level group were tested and the number of cycles in which fracture occurred was recorded. If the implant–abutment assembly survived the entire loading cycle, 5×10^6 cycles were recorded. The results were then plotted on an S/N curve, which is a plot of the magnitude of an alternating stress versus the number of cycles to failure for a given material. The S/N curves were estimated by a logarithmic linear regression model utilizing the least squares method. The fatigue limit of the tested dental implant was defined as the maximum fracture load value which can withstand 5×10^6 cycles [13].

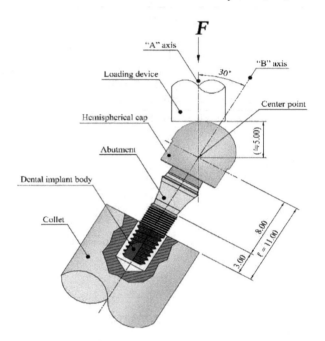

Figure 2. Schematic diagram of the loading test device according to ISO 14801:2013.

2.4. Failure Modes and Microscopic Observation

The fractured area of each implant–abutment assembly was microscopically observed and divided into three categories of failures: fixture-level, abutment-level, and screw-level. Two representative specimens were randomly selected before fatigue testing to examine the connection area of the intact implant–abutment assembly using a field emission scanning electron microscope (SEM) (S-4700, Hitachi, Tokyo, Japan). The specimens were inspected one more time after fatigue testing. The frontal and coronal sectional views of fractured specimens were microscopically examined with 15.0 kV accelerating voltage at ×25 and ×30. For the frontal view, specimens were aligned to show the loading direction from left to right. The abutment and fixture cross-sectional views were symmetrically aligned such that the loading direction could be observed from 12 o'clock and 6 o'clock respectively.

2.5. Statistical Analysis

Mean values and standard deviations of the maximum breaking loads and mean values of the performed cycle from the fatigue tests were calculated. Fisher's exact test was used to analyze the numbers of each type of failure to evaluate the difference of failure modes (fixture-level, abutment-level, and screw-level failure). All statistical analyses were performed using SAS® version 9.4 (SAS Institute, Cary, NC, USA).

3. Results

3.1. Micro-CT Image Observation

Frontal and coronal cross-sectional views of micro-CT showed the detailed design of TX and EV (Figure 3). The thinnest areas, excluding the most coronal portion of the fixture, were expected to be the initiation point of the crack; however, the initiation point was the first thread under the microthread, which does not coincide with the thinnest part.

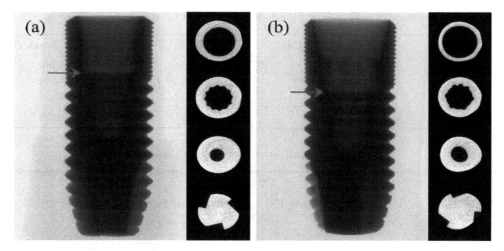

Figure 3. Frontal and cross-sectional micro-CT view: (**a**) TX, (**b**) EV; red arrow = location of the thinnest part of the implant fixture.

3.2. Maximum Breaking Load and Fatigue Limit

The TX samples that underwent single-load failure tests showed a mean maximum breaking load of 711 ± 36 N (95% CI; 670–752), and the EV samples showed an average value of 791 ± 58 N (95% CI; 725–857) (Table 2). The trend of the load and fracture of the specimens was plotted on a time–load diagram, the peak being the point when deformation occurs on the implant–abutment complex (Figure 4). Fatigue testing results are shown in Table 3 and were plotted on an S/N curve with the logarithmic values of the cycles endured on the X-axis and nominal peak level on the Y-axis (Figure 5). All three TX samples of 40% nominal peak level of 285 N endured 5×10^6 cycles, whereas the other nine specimens failed to resist breaking. The fatigue limit was 285 N to withstand 5×10^6 cycles. However, all three EV samples of 40% nominal peak level of 316 N endured 5×10^6 cycles, while the other nine samples failed. The fatigue limit was 316 N to withstand 5×10^6 cycles.

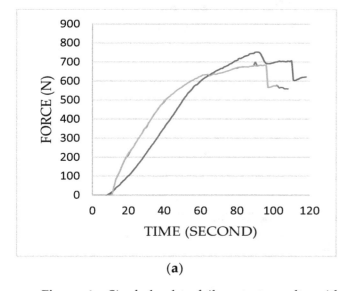

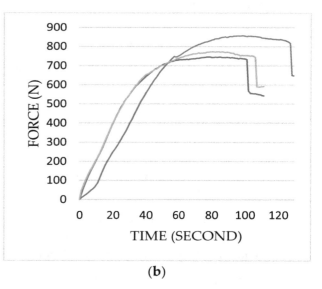

(**a**)   (**b**)

Figure 4. Single-load-to-failure test results with two different implant fixtures: (**a**) TX, (**b**) EV. Compressive load increasing at a speed of 1mm/min was applied. The peak indicates when deformation starts to occur on the implant–abutment assembly, which is the maximum breaking load. The average maximum breaking load of TX = 711 ± 36 N; EV = 791 ± 58 N.

Table 2. Values of the maximum breaking loads in single-load failure tests on three specimens each.

TX Ø4.0	Load at Break (N)	EV Ø4.2	Load at Break (N)
	698 N		856 N
	684 N		772 N
	752 N		745 N
Mean ± SD	711 ± 36 N	**Mean ± SD**	791 ± 58 N

Table 3. Values of the Fatigue Tests.

TX Ø4.0			
Loading Level (%)	**Sinusoidal Loading (N)**	**Number of Performed Cycles**	**Mean**
80	57–569	3209; 4369; 3851	3810
60	43–426	25,884; 14,353; 13,742	17,993
50	36–355	19,549; 66,014; 61,825	49,129
40	29–285	5,000,000; 5,000,000; 5,000,000	5,000,000
EV Ø4.2			
Loading Level (%)	**Sinusoidal Loading (N)**	**Number of Performed Cycles**	**Mean**
80	63–632	6696; 8567; 9333	8199
60	47–474	16,118; 39,423; 11,219	22,253
50	40–395	75,210; 23,584; 47,651	48,815
40	32–316	5,000,000; 5,000,000; 5,000,000	5,000,000

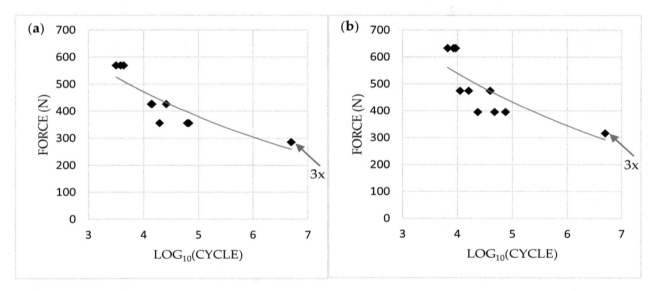

Figure 5. Plotted S/N curves from cyclic loading tests results: (**a**) TX, (**b**) EV. The x-axis represents the logarithmic value of the number of cycles performed. The loading level represents the maximum of the sinusoidal loading level; red arrow = 3 dots overlapped.

3.3. Failure Modes

Failure modes were observed to speculate the fracture mechanism of the TX and EV samples and are shown in Table 4. For the TX groups, every tested assembly except one, which showed abutment-level failure at the 80% loading level, exhibited failure at the fixture level. For the EV groups, two tested assemblies appeared to have torn-out fixtures at the 80% loading level, which were designated as fixture-level failures. The other assemblies exhibited fixture-level fractures occurring between the first and second threads. All fractures of the specimens were accompanied by screw fractures. There was no statistical difference between fractured areas between the TX and EV groups ($P > 0.99$).

Table 4. Fisher's exact test showed no difference between fractured areas ($P > 0.99$).

Fractured Area	Failure Aspect (TX Ø4.0)		Failure Aspect (EV Ø4.2)	
	Static Load	Cyclic Load	Static Load	Cyclic Load
Abutment Fracture	0	1	0	0
Fixture Fracture	3	8	3	9

3.4. Microscopic Observation

Based on the SEM examination, all the samples, except one TX sample which had an abutment-level fracture, showed a tendency of fixture-level fracture around the first and second threads apical to the microthread area. The thinnest part at the implant–abutment interface and the fractured area did not correspond for TX specimens (Figure 6). For the EV specimens, the 50% loading-level group was characterized with a clean-cut fracture tendency at the first thread level. The other groups showed a tendency to be torn out in a wavy pattern apical and coronal to the first thread. The fractured area was almost at the same level as the thinnest part of the fixture itself (Figure 7). Therefore, from the results, the null hypothesis was accepted.

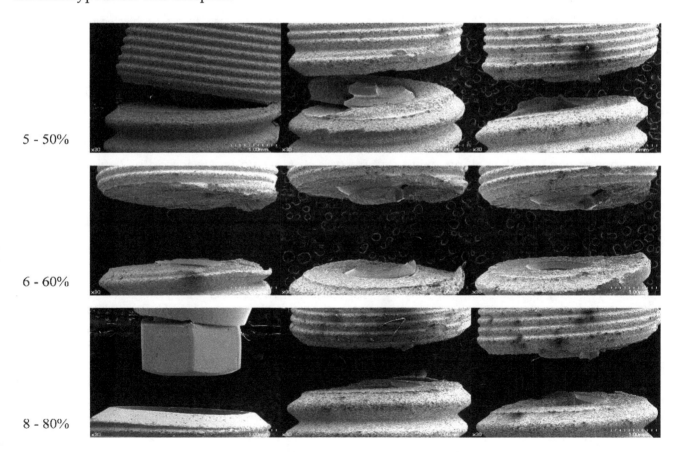

5 - 50%

6 - 60%

8 - 80%

Figure 6. Frontal view of TX samples (×30). Fixtures are aligned to represent a load subjected from left to right.

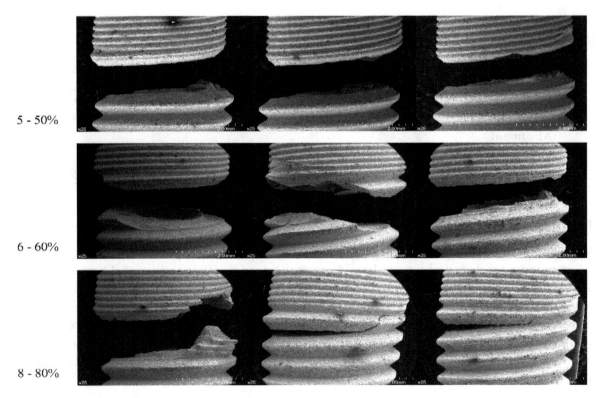

5 - 50%

6 - 60%

8 - 80%

Figure 7. Frontal view of EV samples (×25). Fixtures are aligned to represent a load subjected from left to right.

4. Discussion

During masticatory function, the dental implant fixture and abutment complex should withstand high axial and lateral force of the jaw [17]. An average value of the axial direction force on a single molar implant restoration was previously reported as 120 N [18]. The reported values of maximum loads ranged from 108 to 299 N in the incisor region and from 216 to 847 N in the molar region [18–21]. In previous research, Park et al. have reported fracture strength under static loading between 799 and 1255 N in the grade 4 titanium implant–abutment assemblies with a diameter close to 4.0 mm [22]. Marchetti et al. have reported fracture strength of 430 N and a fatigue limit of 172 N (i.e., 40% of the maximum breaking load) in a grade 4 titanium implant fixture with a diameter of 3.8 mm [23]. Although a direct comparison between current findings and previous results was impossible due to the difference in the loading conditions between the studies, a similar tendency could be observed. Both TX and EV systems used in this study could overcome the normative requirements, and could be characterized by stable mechanical properties. Furthermore, the calculated fatigue strength proportion between TX and EV in our study was approximately 11%. A study conducted by Johansson and Hellqvist has previously reported that the EV system had 11–20% superior fatigue resistance compared to the TX system, which was consistent with the current findings [24]. The increased strength of EV may be the result of a more apically-located implant–abutment joint area, leading to a better stress distribution, which can be speculated from the micro-CT images. Even with similar chemical compositions, the geometry of the implant–abutment connection can affect the mechanical performance in dental implants. Therefore, the clinician should consider the mechanical properties of implant systems in the treatment planning phase, especially in locations where intraoral conditions may be harsh.

Although ISO 14801 provides a standardized protocol for cyclic loading, it does not provide a loading regimen other than starting at a nominal peak value of 80%, and so one must design the interval between the loading values. This leaves the researcher to guess a nominal peak value that can withstand 5×10^6 cycles, which in this case was 40%. However, a 50% nominal peak value seems to be too high a value to accurately estimate the fatigue limit. The 40% groups of TX and EV in this study that endured 5×10^6 cycles are equivalent to 20 years of service time in the mouth. Previous studies have shown that humans have an average of 250,000 mastication cycles per year [25,26]. Therefore, it can be assumed that 5×10^6 cycles are equivalent to 20 years of service time in the mouth. As the worst-case scenario simulates the harshest environment, it can also be assumed that both specimens can successfully survive intraoral clinical conditions. In contrast, the 50% groups fractured before an average of 50,000 cycles, which is equivalent to less than three months of service time. This "extreme" loading could have affected the failure modes as well as the estimated fatigue limit. Therefore, a loading regimen that includes a nominal peak value between 40% and 50% is recommended for future implant cyclic loading tests. In addition, we speculate that extrapolation to a clinical situation of extreme loading is less applicable for the interpretation of the 50% peak value.

The observation of fractured areas is also important in understanding the fracture mechanism in dental implants. With the advance of technology, micro-CT can be used in observing possible deformations of the dental implant [27]. In this study, the micro-CT images taken before the loading test revealed design differences between the two fixtures. The thinnest part, excluding the coronal portion of the fixture, of TX was located at the microthread area, which was approximately 0.5–1 mm coronal to the first thread of the implant fixture. The thinnest part of EV was located at the first thread of the implant fixture. The thinnest areas of each fixture are shown in Figure 4 and were expected to be the mechanically weakest parts, eventually being the fracture-prone area. However, the fracture lines initiated around the first thread of the fixture in this study. The first thread area was at the same level as the thinnest part in the EV fixture, while they were not at the same level in the TX. This suggested that the weakest part, not necessarily the thinnest part, of the TX and EV fixtures was located around the first thread area. These findings are consistent with a previous study by Shemtov-Yona et al. who tested a conical 13 mm dental implant made of titanium alloy. Three different diameters (3.3, 3.75, and 5 mm) at the implant neck were tested for fatigue performance under cyclic loading. All 5 mm implants fractured at the abutment neck and screw, while all 3.3 and 3.75 mm implants fractured at the implant body. As the implants became thinner, they showed a tendency to fracture more apically than thicker samples [10]. While the results of this study showed no statistical difference between the fracture modes of two groups in the present study ($p > 0.99$), the one sample that fractured at the abutment level may have been affected by the diameter of the implant, and not solely from the design of the connection.

A limitation of this study is the relatively small size of the samples, three specimens for each group. While ISO 14801:2013 states that at least three specimens for each group is required, the small size of samples may not be enough to extract a general conclusion. However, the tendency of the results may provide a surmise on how different implant–abutment complexes react to fatigue. Also, another limitation of this study is that loading conditions such as the number of cycles, loading force, and loading angle were not similar to intraoral masticatory conditions. However, to the best of our knowledge, no testing apparatus or protocol currently can perfectly mimic the function of physiologic mastication. Additional research with large sample size and long-term cyclic loading program is required in the future. Also, a standardized testing protocol with further detail may be a prerequisite to the research.

5. Conclusions

Within the limitation of this study, we conclude the following:

1. While both implant–abutment complexes are suitable for intraoral use, the EV fixtures in this study performed better than the TX fixtures, which indicates possible differentiation between the two implant–abutment complex designs.

2. Since all specimens with a 40% nominal peak value survived 5×10^6 cycles and 50% specimens failed before 10^5 cycles, a loading regimen with nominal peak value between 40% and 50% may be recommended for future testing of cyclic loading for the dental implant fixture.

3. The weakest parts of the tested fixtures were located at the first thread area, which happens to be the area directly coronal to the fixation simulating a 3 mm bone loss, and not necessarily the thinnest part.

From these conclusions, future researchers and implant manufacturers may benefit from starting cycling loading at the loading regimen and by considering the weakest part presented when designing an implant. On the other hand, clinicians should consider the mechanical properties of the implants they plan to use.

Author Contributions: Conceptualization, H.-I.Y., T.-H.K., E.-J.P.; methodology, H.-I.Y., T.-H.K., E.-J.P.; validation, H.-I.Y., E.-J.P.; formal analysis, N.-H.C., H.-I.Y., T.-H.K., E.-J.P.; investigation, N.-H.C.; resources, N.-H.C., H.-I.Y.; data curation, N.-H.C.; writing—original draft preparation, N.-H.C.; writing—review and editing, H.-I.Y., T.-H.K., E.-J.P.; visualization, N.-H.C.; supervision, H.-I.Y., E.-J.P.; project administration, E.-J.P.; funding acquisition, H.-I.Y., T.-H.K., E.-J.P.

Acknowledgments: This study was funded in part by Dentsply Sirona Implants (Mölndal, Sweden) and Yuhan Co. (Seoul, S. Korea). The authors would like to thank Hong-Seok Lim of Dongguk University who helped with the collection of data.

References

1.   Buser, D.; Janner, S.F.M.; Wittneben, J.G.; Brägger, U.; Ramseier, C.A.; Salvi, G.E. 10-Year Survival and Success Rates of 511 Titanium Implants with a Sandblasted and Acid-Etched Surface: A Retrospective Study in 303 Partially Edentulous Patients. *Clin. Implant Dent. Relat. Res.* **2012**, *14*, 839–851. [CrossRef] [PubMed]

2.   Pjetursson, B.E.; Thoma, D.; Jung, R.; Zwahlen, M.; Zembic, A. A Systematic Review of the Survival and Complication Rates of Implant-Supported Fixed Dental Prostheses(FDPs) after a Mean Observation Period of at Least 5 Years. *Clin. Oral Implants Res.* **2012**, *23*, 22–38. [CrossRef] [PubMed]

3.   Jung, R.E.; Zembic, A.; Pjetursson, B.E.; Zwahlen, M.; Thoma, D.S. Systematic Review of the Survival Rate and the Incidence of Biological, Technical, and Aesthetic Complications of Single Crowns on Implants Reported in Longitudinal Studies with a Mean Follow-up of 5 Years. *Clin. Oral Implants Res.* **2012**, *23*, 2–21. [CrossRef] [PubMed]

4.   Jung, R.E.; Pjetursson, B.E.; Glauser, R.; Zembic, A.; Zwahlen, M.; Lang, N.P. A Systematic Review of the 5-Year Survival and Complication Rates of Implant-Supported Single Crowns. *Clin. Oral Implants Res.* **2008**, *19*, 119–130. [CrossRef] [PubMed]

5.   Åstrand, P.; Ahlqvist, J.; Gunne, J.; Nilson, H. Implant Treatment of Patients with Edentulous Jaws: A 20-Year Follow-Up. *Clin. Implant Dent. Relat. Res.* **2008**, *10*, 207–217. [CrossRef] [PubMed]

6.   Blanes, R.J.; Bernard, J.P.; Blanes, Z.M.; Belser, U.C. A 10-Year Prospective Study of ITI Dental Implants Placed in the Posterior Region. I: Clinical and Radiographic Results. *Clin. Oral Implants Res.* **2007**, *18*, 699–706. [CrossRef] [PubMed]

7.   Lekholm, U.; Gröndahl, K.; Jemt, T. Outcome of Oral Implant Treatment in Partially Edentulous Jaws Followed 20 Years in Clinical Function. *Clin. Implant Dent. Relat. Res.* **2006**, *8*, 178–186. [CrossRef] [PubMed]

8.   Tabrizi, R.; Behnia, H.; Taherian, S.; Hesami, N. What Are the Incidence and Factors Associated With Implant Fracture? *J. Oral Maxillofac. Surg.* **2017**, *75*, 1866–1872. [CrossRef]

9.   Balik, A.; Karatas, M.O.; Keskin, H. Effects of Different Abutment Connection Designs on the Stress Distribution Around Five Different Implants: A 3-Dimensional Finite Element Analysis. *J. Oral Implantol.* **2012**, *38*, 491–496. [CrossRef]

10. Shemtov-Yona, K.; Rittel, D.; Levin, L.; Machtei, E.E. Effect of Dental Implant Diameter on Fatigue Performance. Part I: Mechanical Behavior. *Clin. Implant Dent. Relat. Res.* **2014**, *16*, 172–177. [CrossRef]

11. ASTM. *ASTM E1823-10-Standard Terminology Relating to Fatigue and Fracture Testing*; ASTM International: West Conshohocken, PA, USA, 2010.

12. Imakita, C.; Shiota, M.; Yamaguchi, Y.; Kasugai, S.; Wakabayashi, N. Failure Analysis of an Abutment Fracture on Single Implant Restoration. *Implant Dent.* **2013**, *22*, 326–331. [CrossRef] [PubMed]

13. ISO14801. *Fatigue Test for Endosseous Dental Implants*; International Organization for Standardization: Geneva, Switzerland, 2013.

14. Kelly, J.R.; Benetti, P.; Rungruanganunt, P.; Bona, A.D. The Slippery Slope-Critical Perspectives on in Vitro Research Methodologies. *Dent. Mater.* **2012**, *28*, 41–51. [CrossRef] [PubMed]

15. Chieruzzi, M.; Pagano, S.; Cianetti, S.; Lombardo, G.; Kenny, J.M.; Torre, L. Effect of Fibre Posts, Bone Losses and Fibre Content on the Biomechanical Behaviour of Endodontically Treated Teeth: 3D-Finite Element Analysis. *Mater. Sci. Eng. C* **2017**, *74*, 334–346. [CrossRef] [PubMed]

16. Geng, J.P.A.; Tan, K.B.C.; Liu, G.R. Application of Finite Element Analysis in Implant Dentistry: A Review of the Literature. *J. Prosthet. Dent.* **2001**, *85*, 585–598. [CrossRef] [PubMed]

17. van der Bilt, A. Assessment of Mastication with Implications for Oral Rehabilitation: A Review. *J. Oral Rehabil.* **2011**, *38*, 754–780. [CrossRef] [PubMed]

18. Richter, E.-J. In Vivo Vertical Forces on Implants. *Int. J. Oral Maxillofac. Implants* **1995**, *10*, 99–108. [PubMed]

19. Gibbs, C.H.; Mahan, P.E.; Mauderli, A.; Lundeen, H.C.; Walsh, E.K. Limits of Human Bite Strength. *J. Prosthet. Dent.* **1986**, *56*, 226–229. [CrossRef]

20. Helkimo, E.; Carlsson, G.E.; Helkimo, M. Bite Forces Used during Chewing of Food. *J. Dent. Res.* **1959**, *29*, 133–136.

21. Waltimo, A.; Könönen, M. A Novel Bite Force Recorder and Maximal Isometric Bite Force Values for Healthy Young Adults. *Eur. J. Oral Sci.* **1993**, *101*, 171–175. [CrossRef]

22. Park, S.-J.; Lee, S.-W.; Leesungbok, R.; Ahn, S.-J. Influence of the Connection Design and Titanium Grades of the Implant Complex on Resistance under Static Loading. *J. Adv. Prosthodont.* **2016**, *8*, 388–395. [CrossRef]

23. Marchetti, E.; Ratta, S.; Mummolo, S.; Tecco, S.; Pecci, R.; Bedini, R.; Marzo, G. Mechanical Reliability Evaluation of an Oral Implant-Abutment System According to UNI En ISO 14801 Fatigue Test Protocol. *Implant Dent.* **2016**, *25*, 613–618. [CrossRef] [PubMed]

24. Johansson, H.; Hellqvist, J. Functionality of a Further Developed Implant System: Mechanical Integrity. *Clin. Oral Implants Res.* **2013**, *24*, 166.

25. Sakaguchi, R.L.; Douglas, W.H.; DeLong, R.; Pintado, M.R. The Wear of a Posterior Composite in an Artificial Mouth: A Clinical Correlation. *Dent. Mater.* **1986**, *2*, 235–240. [CrossRef]

26. DeLong, R.; Douglas, W.H. Development of an Artificial Oral Environment for the Testing of Dental Restoratives: Bi-Axial Force and Movement Control. *J. Dent. Res.* **1983**, *62*, 32–36. [CrossRef] [PubMed]

27. Stimmelmayr, M.; Edelhoff, D.; Güth, J.-F.; Erdelt, K.; Happe, A.; Beuer, F. Wear at the Titanium–Titanium and the Titanium–Zirconia Implant–Abutment Interface: A Comparative in Vitro Study. *Dent. Mater.* **2012**, *28*, 1215–1220. [CrossRef]

8

Fracture Resistance of Zirconia Oral Implants In Vitro

Annalena Bethke [1], Stefano Pieralli [1,2], Ralf-Joachim Kohal [2], Felix Burkhardt [1,2], Manja von Stein-Lausnitz [1], Kirstin Vach [3] and Benedikt Christopher Spies [1,2,*]

[1] Department of Prosthodontics, Geriatric Dentistry and Craniomandibular Disorders, Charité—Universitätsmedizin Berlin, corporate member of Freie Universität Berlin, Humboldt-Universität zu Berlin, and Berlin Institute of Health, Aßmannshauser Str. 4-6, 14197 Berlin, Germany; a.k.bethke@web.de (A.B.); stefano.pieralli@charite.de (S.P.); felix.burkhardt@charite.de (F.B.); manja.von-stein-lausnitz@charite.de (M.v.S.-L.)

[2] Department of Prosthetic Dentistry, Faculty of Medicine, Center for Dental Medicine, Medical Center—University of Freiburg, Hugstetter Str. 55, 79106 Freiburg, Germany; ralf.kohal@uniklinik-freiburg.de

[3] Institute of Medical Biometry and Statistics, Faculty of Medicine, Medical Center—University of Freiburg, University of Freiburg, Stefan-Meier-Str. 26, 79104 Freiburg, Germany; kv@imbi.uni-freiburg.de

* Correspondence: benedikt.spies@charite.de

Abstract: Various protocols are available to preclinically assess the fracture resistance of zirconia oral implants. The objective of the present review was to determine the impact of different treatments (dynamic loading, hydrothermal aging) and implant features (e.g., material, design or manufacturing) on the fracture resistance of zirconia implants. An electronic screening of two databases (MEDLINE/Pubmed, Embase) was performed. Investigations including > 5 screw-shaped implants providing information to calculate the bending moment at the time point of static loading to fracture were considered. Data was extracted and meta-analyses were conducted using multilevel mixed-effects generalized linear models (GLMs). The Šidák method was used to correct for multiple testing. The initial search resulted in 1864 articles, and finally 19 investigations loading 731 zirconia implants to fracture were analyzed. In general, fracture resistance was affected by the implant design (1-piece > 2-piece, $p = 0.004$), material (alumina-toughened zirconia/ATZ > yttria-stabilized tetragonal zirconia polycrystal/Y-TZP, $p = 0.002$) and abutment preparation (untouched > modified/grinded, $p < 0.001$). In case of 2-piece implants, the amount of dynamic loading cycles prior to static loading ($p < 0.001$) or anatomical crown supply ($p < 0.001$) negatively affected the outcome. No impact was found for hydrothermal aging. Heterogeneous findings of the present review highlight the importance of thoroughly and individually evaluating the fracture resistance of every zirconia implant system prior to market release.

Keywords: dental implant; zirconia; ceramics; aging; artificial mouth; fracture load; fatigue; chewing simulation; meta-analysis

1. Introduction

To date, titanium can be considered the gold standard material in oral implantology [1]. However, due to increasing esthetic standards and a discussed impact of metal/titanium particle release on the pathogenesis of peri-implant bone loss [2,3], a renaissance of ceramic oral implants can be observed in dental media. Nowadays, the market share of zirconia oral implants seems to be increasing, even if still comparatively small compared to conventional titanium implants.

Nonetheless, the superiority of ceramic oral implants regarding esthetics and biocompatibility, or, as an example, the frequently claimed patients' demand for metal-free implantology are still not soundly scientifically evidenced. Nevertheless, the majority of dental experts are of the opinion that zirconia oral implants will be coexistent with titanium implants in the near future [4].

When zirconium dioxide (zirconia, ZrO_2) was introduced as ceramic implant material, research focused to evaluate and improve its osseointegrative potential by creating a microroughened surface topography [5]. In the first instance, parameters like bone-to-implant contact (BIC), push-in values and removal torque were assessed in animal experiments. As a result, zirconia implants with various surface modifications (additive by sintering a porous ceramic layer, subtractive by sandblasting and/or acid-etching or, for example, by texturing the inner surface of a mold in case of an injection-molded implant) can nowadays be considered comparable to titanium implants by means of osseointegration in preclinical studies [6]. This finding was confirmed in clinical trials, however limited to short- and mid-term observation periods and the replacement of up to three adjacent missing teeth (single-tooth restorations and three-unit fixed dental prostheses) using one-piece ceramic implants [7].

From a technical point of view, such a 1-piece design, comprising the abutment and endosseous part in a single piece, might benefit from increased fracture resistance and reduced susceptibility for low-temperature degradation or so-called "aging" (by exposing a reduced total surface area to aging by inducing oral fluids), compared to 2-piece ceramic implants. Furthermore, 1-piece implants do not have a micro-gap in between the assembled implant and abutment. One might consider the absence of such a micro-gap beneficial, since it is capable in hosting bacteria, potentially resulting in marginal inflammation and consecutive bone resorption [8]. However, no advantage of a monobloc design was found for "seamless", 1-piece implants made from titanium [9]. Moreover, from a practitioner's point of view, a 1-piece implant design is associated with several surgical and prosthodontic shortcomings [10]. As an example, submerged implant healing is hardly possible, since the transmucosal part of a 1-piece implant cannot be detached. If no sufficient primary stability can be attained or guided bone regeneration is necessary, a missing option for wound closure might be considered disadvantageous. Furthermore, there is only a limited potential to compensate for mal-positioned implants with the provisional and final restoration. When trying to remove subsections in case of misaligned implants to support a bridge, intra-oral grinding of the zirconia abutment is necessary [11]. This, however, might have an impact upon the osseointegration (due to potential heat development or the displacement of zirconia particles in surrounding tissues) and fracture resistance of the implant [12]. Therefore, a two-piece design represents the favorable option for daily clinical use. Today, several two-piece zirconia implants are available on the market. In these systems, implant-abutment assembly is mostly realized by either luting the abutment to the implant or by screw-retention [13]. Luting the abutment to the implant seals the micro-gap, and allows for initial but irreversible correction of the implant angulation, but misses flexibility for future restorations of the implant. On the other hand, when going for screw-retention, several ceramic implants are still assembled with a titanium screw, and therefore, still not metal-free in the proper sense.

Even if the market share of zirconia dental implants increases, concerns regarding their fracture resistance are still present, and standardized testing protocols for zirconia implants adequately addressing the aging behavior of the final product are still missing [14]. To overcome this, different treatments were proposed to mimic intraoral conditions to the extent possible for the evaluation of ceramic implants. These treatments included thermal aging (high-temperature conditions or thermal cycling) [15,16] and/or dynamic loading procedures (various exposure times and different applied loading modes) [12,17]. Zirconia implants evaluated regarding their fracture resistance in the literature comprised a heterogeneous range of features like material selection (yttria-stabilized tetragonal zirconia polycrystal, Y-TZP or alumina-toughened zirconia, ATZ) [18], design (1- or 2-piece) [13], manufacturing (subtractive or by ceramic injection molding, CIM) [19], restoration (anatomical crown, hemisphere or no restoration) [20,21], abutment preparation (in the case of 1-piece implants) [22], or assembly (in the case of 2-piece implants) [13].

Therefore, the objective of the present systematic review was to evaluate the influence of the aforementioned treatments and features on the fracture resistance of zirconia oral implants in different preclinical studies. The null hypothesis supposed no distinction between treatments and features in relation to bending moment when statically loading the implant to fracture.

2. Materials and Methods

2.1. Study Design

To determine a selection of comparable studies on the question of zirconia implant fracture resistance, the preferred reporting items for systematic reviews and meta-analyses (PRISMA) statement of 2009 was applied [23]. Therefore, this report takes the appropriate Enhancing the Quality and Transparency of health Research (EQUATOR) (http://www.equator-network.org) guidelines into account.

2.2. Focused Question

Is there a variable significantly affecting the fracture resistance of 1- and 2-piece zirconia implants in preclinical in-vitro studies?

2.3. Search Strategy

Two databases, namely the Medical Literature Analysis and Retrieval System Online (MEDLINE) (PubMed) and Embase (accessed via Ovid), were screened for relevant articles. The database specific search strategies consisted of a combination of subject headings and free text words. Data was extracted from the databases on 3rd December 2019 without applying any time restrictions. Thereafter, references of included articles were screened for further records satisfying the inclusion criteria (cross-referencing). In case of the availability of the full methodological procedures in the literature and accessibility of information regarding the included samples, unpublished data of the authors of the present review was likewise included. The resulting studies were imported and stored in a reference managing program (EndNote X9; Clarivate Analytics, Philadelphia, PA, USA). Articles written in English and the German language were considered.

2.4. Screening Process

To build up the search terms, three categories addressing the samples (dental implants), materials (zirconia ceramics) and outcome (fracture load) were combined ("AND"). These categories consisted of combinations ("OR") of free text words and indexed vocabulary (MEDLINE: MeSH terms, Embase: Emtree terms). An asterisk was used in combination with some free text words as a truncation symbol (e. g. "ceramic *") to allow for the so-called "wildcard search".

Pubmed search term:

> *(((((dental implant [MeSH Terms]) OR ((((oral) AND ((implant) OR implants))) OR ((dental) AND ((implant) OR implants))))) AND (((zircon *) OR ceramic *) OR ceramics[MeSH Terms])) AND ((((((ageing) OR aging) OR artificial mouth) OR fracture resistance) OR load *)*

Embase search term:

> *('tooth implant'/exp OR (oral AND implant) OR (dental AND implant)) AND (zircon * OR ceramic * OR 'ceramics'/exp) AND (ageing OR aging OR (artificial AND mouth) OR (fracture AND resistance) OR load *)*

2.5. Eligibility Criteria

Studies to be included in this systematic review needed to fulfill the following inclusion criteria:

-      Language: English or German

- Samples: Screw-shaped, ceramic oral implants containing a minimum of 50% *v/v* ZrO_2 within the bulk material
- Outcome: Static loading to fracture
- Outcome measure: Bending moment [Ncm or Nmm] or fracture load [N] allowing to calculate the bending moment (e.g., by adopting ISO 14801 or providing data to calculate the lever arm) was provided
- Sample size: Minimum of five samples tested

2.6. Selection of Studies

Concerning the inclusion criteria, both the first author and the senior author of this manuscript (A.B. and B.C.S.) independently screened the titles and abstracts of the extracted data in the reference management program. If sufficient information needed for inclusion or exclusion was not provided within the title or abstract, the corresponding full texts were read. In case of disagreement, a third author (S.P.) was consulted for final decision making.

2.7. Data Extraction

Besides the total number of samples within one study, the number of implants made from different materials (Y-TZP, ATZ), processing routes (subtractive, injection molding), design (1- and 2-piece) and diameters were retrieved. Further features like restoration mode (anatomical crown, hemisphere or no reconstruction), abutment preparation (yes/no in case of 1-piece implants), implant-abutment connection (screwed/bonded in case of 2-piece implants), thermal aging (thermal cycling, high temperature, no aging) or dynamic loading (yes/no), dynamic loading conditions (exerted load and amount of cycles), crosshead speed during static fracture, and angulation, were likewise extracted. This allowed us to group the implants finally subjected to static loading within the included studies in cohorts. For standardization purposes, the bending moment at the time point of fracture [Ncm] was considered the outcome measure of interest, and the corresponding authors of the articles to be included were contacted by email in case of solely providing fracture load values [N] without mentioning the lever arm. Extracted cohorts were subdivided into groups subjected to comparable treatments:

1. No dynamic loading
2. 1–1.2 million loading cycles (50 N)
3. 1–1.2 million loading cycles (100 N)
4. 3.5–5 million loading cycles (100 N)
5. 5 million loading cycles (>500 N)
6. 10 million loading cycles (100 N)

2.8. Statistical Analysis

From the included nineteen studies/datasets, two to twelve observations were extracted each. One observation consisted of the mean bending moment and standard deviation (at the time point of fracture) and/or mean fracture load and standard deviation (including additional information allowing us to calculate the bending moment) of a specific cohort of implants (comprising the same type of implant subjected to the same treatment) extracted from one included study. These observations had sample sizes of 2 to 12 implants. To analyze the effect of specific treatments of features (as indicated in 2.7) on the bending moment, a multilevel mixed-effects generalized linear model was used for each outcome, with each investigation as random effect to cluster observations by the respective studies. The Šidák method was used to correct for multiple testing. The level of significance was set at $p < 0.05$.

In order to compare the aforementioned groups (1–6, depending on load and cycles) for heterogeneity of the data, both inter- and intra-standard deviations with 95% confidence intervals (Cis) were computed. In addition, the cohort-specific standard error of the bending moment was used for weighting. Furthermore, box plots were created for visualization of the data. The data were analyzed with STATA 16.1 (StataCorp LLC, Texas, TX, USA).

3. Results

3.1. Screening Process/Included Data

Screening of two databases using the aforementioned specifically adapted search terms resulted in a total of 1864 records. After the removal of 622 duplicates, another 1202 records were withdrawn for analyses by screening the titles and abstracts. After reading the full texts of the remaining 40 studies, a further 23 manuscripts were excluded (Figure 1). Detailed reasons for exclusion can be found in Table A1. In general, the most frequent reasons for exclusion were the fracture of zirconia abutments assembled with titanium implants (mostly excluded by title and abstract) and the fracture on the restoration level using zirconia one-piece implants as support (mostly excluded during full-text screening). When only the fracture load [N] during static loading was reported, three options allowed for the calculation of the bending moment: (1) embedding was described to fully respect ISO 14801 (prescribing a lever arm of 5.5 mm allowing for the calculation of the bending moment), (2) all details regarding the embedding were provided in the manuscript (e.g., by providing a scheme) or (3) the bending moment and/or lever arm were provided by the authors upon request. As an example, six of the included studies adopted ISO 14801 for embedding [15,17,21,24–26], whereas three provided all necessary information [19,27,28] allowing us to calculate the bending moment (embedding level, angulation, total sample length, point of loading). In the remaining cases the bending moment was reported [13,20,22] or sent by the authors [12,18,29,30]. Finally, 17 full-texts were analyzed in the present systematic review (Table 1). In addition, the datasets of two finalized projects, currently under review and in preparation of the manuscript, were included. Two authors of the present review (R.K. and B.C.S.) were involved in both of these two investigations, and were able to access the full data. The applied materials and methods were already described in detail in precedent publications [21,26]. Since available on the market, the material composition of the included implant systems is likewise available and accessible. In detail, three zirconia implant systems (1-piece: Straumann PURE Ceramic, Straumann AG, Basel, CH; 2-piece: 5s-50-10, Z-Systems AG, Oensingen, CH and Ceralog Hexalobe Implant, Axis biodental, Les Bois, CH) were subjected to identical treatments and fracture load measurements, as described in two of the included studies [21,26]. In the case of Straumann 1-piece (as-received: 609 ± 20 Ncm; loaded/aged: 557 ± 36 Ncm) and Z-Systems 2-piece implants (as-received: 463 ± 21 Ncm; loaded/aged: 443 ± 39 Ncm), aging/loading (as described in [21,26]) did not affect the fracture resistance to a statistically significant level ($p = 0.171$). In contrast, the fracture resistance of 2-piece Ceralog Hexalobe Implants (as-received: 547 ± 89 Ncm; loaded/aged: 413 ± 127 Ncm) was significantly affected ($p = 0.046$) by aging/loading (as described in [21,26]).

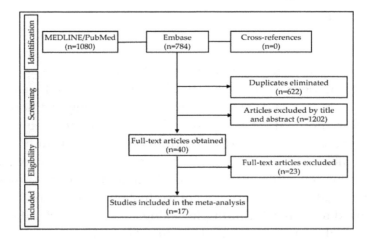

Figure 1. Flowchart according to the preferred reporting items for systematic reviews and meta-analyses (PRISMA) guidelines.

Table 1. A total of 731 one- and two-piece implants made from yttria-stabilized tetragonal zirconia polycrystal (Y-TZP) and alumina-toughened zirconia (ATZ), extracted from 17 studies and two unpublished datasets, subjected to different dynamic loading and thermal aging conditions prior to static loading to fracture, were finally included in meta-analyses.

First Author	Year	Ref.	n	Material	Pieces	Loading Cycles ($\times 10^6$)	Thermal Aging
Andreiotelli	2009	[29]	88	Y-TZP	1	0, 1.2	TC, none
Kohal	2009	[30]	32	Y-TZP	2	0, 1.2	TC, none
Kohal	2010	[18]	72	ATZ, Y-TZP	1	0, 1.2, 5	TC, none
Kohal	2011	[12]	48	Y-TZP	1	0, 1.2, 5	TC, none
Rosentritt	2014	[28]	36	Y-TZP	1, 2	1.2	TC
Kohal	2015	[20]	48	Y-TZP	1	0, 5, 10	TC, none
Sanon	2015	[25]	30	Y-TZP	1	0	HT
Spies	2015	[22]	48	ATZ	1	0, 1.2, 5	TC, none
Kammermeier	2016	[27]	30	Y-TZP	1, 2	0, 3.6	TC, none
Preis	2016	[19]	32	ATZ, Y-TZP	2	1	TC, none
Spies	2016	[13]	48	ATZ, Y-TZP	1, 2	0, 10	HT, none
Joda	2017	[24]	11	ATZ	2	0	none
Spies	2017	[21]	28	Y-TZP	2	0, 10	HT, none
Ding	2018	[17]	29	Y-TZP	1	0, 5	none
Spies	2018	[26]	14	ATZ	2	0, 10	HT, none
Monzavi	2019	[15]	60	Y-TZP	1	0	HT, none
Stimmelmayr	2019	[16]	36	Y-TZP	2	1.2	TC
Kohal	2020	*	28	Y-TZP	1, 2	0, 10	HT, none
Zhang	2020	*	13	Y-TZP	2	0, 10	HT, none

* Unpublished data, Ref. = Reference, n = total number of included implants, TC = thermal cycling, HT = high temperature.

3.2. Meta-Analyses

All 17 articles published between 2009 [29] and 2019 [15,16] were included and analyzed in the present meta-analysis. Moreover, unpublished data of two projects currently under review and in preparation of the manuscript were included (Table 1). From the included articles/datasets, 114 observations were extracted or calculated (mean bending moment), comprising different implant features (e.g., diameter, material, crown supply, abutment preparation or implant-abutment-connection) or treatments (e.g., thermal aging or dynamic loading). One observation consisted of the mean bending moment and standard deviation (SD) of up to 12 included implants.

In order to evaluate the impact of different dynamic loading procedures (implants were subjected to prior to fracture loading) on the outcome (bending moment), groups as indicated in Section 2.7 were analyzed for heterogeneity. As a result, standard deviation as a measure of variation within and in between the included studies revealed to be within the same range (Table 2). No heterogeneity of the bending moments for groups 1–6 was found, even if a decreased mean value for group 3 was calculated ($p = 0.612$). This did not change when stratifying the implants according to their design (1-piece: $p = 0.951$; 2-piece: $p = 0.056$).

Table 2. Groups 1–6 (as indicated in 2.7) were tested for heterogeneity regarding the outcome.

Groups	Overall	1	2	3	4	5	6
Effect [1]	395.27	407.42	397.99	262.17	400.73	579.96	448.94
95% CI	330.2–460.3	338.4–476.4	272.1–523.9	195.0–329.3	249.2–552.2	521.8–638.0	373.7–524.1
Intra [2]	103.57	110.07	74.58	100.30	150.33	46.64	57.59
95% CI	89.4–120.0	89.3–135.7	42.4–131.0	61.4–163.8	95.8–235.8	18.2–119.7	28.5–116.4
Inter [3]	126.06	126.92	133.58	$1.670 \times e^{-15}$	146.81	$4.690 \times e^{-18}$	77.72
95% CI	86.5–183.8	82.1–196.2	65.5–272.3	$-\infty - +\infty$	59.0–365.5	$-\infty - +\infty$	33.9–178.2

[1] Mean bending moment [Ncm], [2] Standard deviation/variation within included studies, [3] Standard deviation/variation in between included studies.

3.3. Outcomes

Outcomes extracted from the 17 included studies and the two unpublished datasets were calculated and stratified for the material selection, manufacturing, implant diameter, anatomical crown supply, abutment preparation (1-piece implants), implant-abutment-connection (IAC; 2-piece implants), thermal aging procedure prior to static loading (none; TC = thermal cycling, mostly in between 5–55 °C; HT = high temperature, mostly in between 60–134 °C) and/or dynamic loading in a chewing simulation device applying different loads (ranging from 50 to > 500 N) for a different amount of cycles (ranging from 1 to 10 millions). In total, 731 implants were available for analyses, revealing a mean bending moment at the time point of fracture of 386.4 ± 167.6 Ncm. Furthermore, the outcome was stratified for 1- and 2-piece implants. Mean bending moments, standard deviations and the included number of implants are listed in Table 3. Significance (linear mixed models, level of significance $p < 0.05$) calculated for differences regarding the implant design, different covariables and treatments can be found in Table 4.

Table 3. Calculated mean bending moment (in Ncm) and standard deviation depending on the implant design, several covariables and treatments.

	Overall [1]			1-Piece			2-Piece		
	n	Mean	SD	*n*	Mean	SD	*n*	Mean	SD
Overall	731	386.4	167.6	495	431.9	151.0	236	291.7	162.4
Material									
Y-TZP	577	378.7	160.1	383	422.2	143.4	194	284.3	155.7
ATZ	154	418.7	106.0	112	475.8	180.7	42	318.6	194.0
Manufacturing									
Subtractive	591 [2]	397.5	177.4	417	457.4	154.4	174	260.1	149.6
Injection molded	120 [2]	364.8	116.7	70	329.4	73.7	50	426.8	154.4
Implant diameter									
3.0–3.3 mm	15	207.2	14.3	9	215.0	6.7	6	191.6	-
3.8–4.4 mm	675	394.9	170.4	463	441.3	152.7	212	293.6	165.0
4.5–5.0 mm	41	349.4	125.4	23	388.0	59.4	18	301.2	178.0
Anatomical crown supply									
Yes	209	237.5	96.6	74	327.0	65.4	135	186.9	71.4
No	522	455.2	147.7	421	453.2	154.8	101	463.9	114.2
Abutment preparation									
Yes	-	-	-	112	411.3	126.2	-	-	-
No	-	-	-	383	436.5	156.5	-	-	-
Implant-Abutment-Connection									
Screw-retained	-	-	-	-	-	-	159	327.5	179.0
Bonded	-	-	-	-	-	-	77	217.0	86.0
Thermal aging									
Thermal cycling	310	355.5	171.7	218	426.5	149.4	92	174.6	41.1
High temperature	124	392.9	115.9	75	362.6	96.4	49	453.4	135.1
None	297	406.2	180.4	202	464.0	163.2	95	299.9	164.6
Dynamic loading									
Yes	391	389.4	169.2	250	447.7	146.6	141	279.2	156.5
No/Group 1	340	383.2	166.3	245	417.7	153.6	95	303.5	171.2
Group 2	86	258.1	111.5	66	362.6	59.4	20	174.4	50.2
Group 3	76	394.7	211.2	40	457.3	188.1	36	144.4	15.0
Group 4	132	379.6	159.7	96	437.8	140.5	36	205.1	20.5
Group 5	17	580.8	55.7	17	580.8	55.7	-	-	-
Group 6	80	435.1	108.3	31	420.2	93.0	49	443.6	122.5

n = number of included implants, SD = standard deviation, [1] 1- and 2-piece implants pooled together, [2] the authors of one included study could not provide the manufacturing mode for all included implants [28].

Table 4. Significance (linear mixed models (LMMs), level of significance $p < 0.05$) was calculated for differences regarding the implant design, different covariables and treatments.

Parameter	Options	Significance (p)		
		Overall [1]	1-Piece	2-Piece
Implant design	1-piece, 2-piece	0.004	-	-
Material	Y-TZP, ATZ	0.002	0.001	0.282
Manufacturing	Subtractive, injection-molded	0.749	0.076	0.095
Implant diameter	Range: 3.3–5.0 mm	0.327	0.273	0.191
Anatomical crown	Yes/No	<0.0001	0.080	<0.0001
Abutment preparation	Yes/No	-	<0.0001	-
Connection type	Screw-retained, bonded	-	-	0.584
Thermal aging	TC, HT, none	0.446	0.538	0.776
	Yes/No	0.410	0.559	0.474
Dynamic loading	Applied load [range: 50–500 N]	0.050	0.181	0.202
	Amount of cycles [range: $1–10 \times 10^6$]	0.238	0.971	<0.0001
	Groups 1–6 [as indicated in 2.7]	0.612	0.951	0.056
Angulation	Range: 30–45°	0.215	0.671	0.003
Crosshead speed	Range: 0.5–10 mm/s	0.261	0.562	<0.0001

[1] 1- and 2-piece implants pooled together, TC = thermal cycling, HT = high temperature.

3.3.1. Implant Design

Eight studies [12,15,17,18,20,22,25,29] focused on 1-piece zirconia implants, whereas six studies solely included 2-piece implants [16,19,21,24,26,30]. The remaining investigations evaluated a mixture of both 1- and 2-piece implants [13,27,28]. Regardless of all other variables, 1-piece implants (431.9 ± 151.0 Ncm) were found to be more fracture resistant than 2-piece implants (291.7 ± 162.4 Ncm, $p = 0.004$; Figure 2).

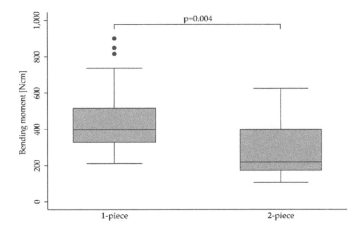

Figure 2. Boxplot showing the bending moment at the time point of fracture for 1- and 2-piece zirconia implants. Whiskers are used to represent all samples lying within 1.5 times the interquartile range (IQR). Dots represent outliers. Detailed data can be found in Tables 3 and 4.

3.3.2. Material

Material selection of the included studies is listed in Table 1. Of the included implants, 577 were made from Y-TZP, whereas 154 were manufactured from ATZ [13,18,19,22,24,26]. When pooling the outcome for 1- and 2-piece zirconia implants, the bending moment at the time point of implant fracture was significantly affected by the material ($p = 0.002$; Table 4). In detail, implants made from alumina-toughened zirconia (ATZ, 418.7 ± 106.0 Ncm) were more fracture-resistant compared to implants made from yttria-stabilized tetragonal zirconia polycrystals (Y-TZP, 378.7 ± 160.1 Ncm,

$p = 0.002$). When stratifying the outcome for 1- and 2-piece implants, however, material selection only affected 1-piece implants ($p = 0.001$, Figure 3a), whereas 2-piece implants performed the same, regardless of the material selection ($p = 0.282$, Figure 3b).

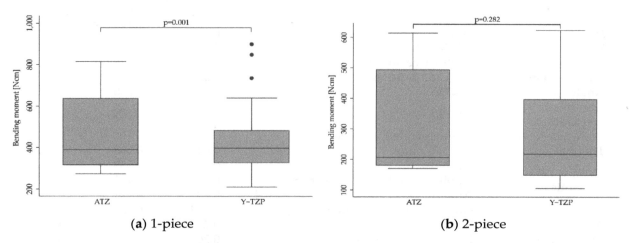

(a) 1-piece   (b) 2-piece

Figure 3. Boxplots showing the bending moment at the time point of fracture depending on the material selection for 1- (**a**) and 2-piece (**b**) zirconia implants. Whiskers are used to represent all samples lying within 1.5 times the interquartile range. Dots represent outliers. Detailed data can be found in Tables 3 and 4.

3.3.3. Manufacturing

Manufacturing was mostly subtractive ($n = 591$ implants), but ceramic injection-molding (CIM) was likewise used for the production ($n = 120$ implants) [15,19,21,25]. There was no statistically significant difference in the fracture resistance of implants when manufacturing method (subtractive: 397.5 ± 177.4 Ncm, CIM: 364.8 ± 116.7 Ncm) was regarded ($p > 0.095$). Boxplots can be seen in Figure 4.

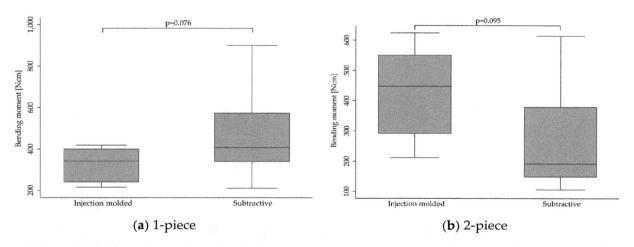

(a) 1-piece   (b) 2-piece

Figure 4. Boxplots showing the bending moment at the time point of fracture depending on the manufacturing method for 1- (**a**) and 2-piece (**b**) zirconia implants. Whiskers are used to represent all samples lying within 1.5 times the interquartile range. Detailed data can be found in Tables 3 and 4.

3.3.4. Implant Diameter

No statistically significant difference could be calculated for the bending moment at the time point of fracture regarding the implant diameter ranging from 3 to 5 mm ($p = 0.327$). This did not change when stratifying the outcome for 1- ($p = 0.273$) and 2-piece ($p = 0.191$) implants. However, the included studies evaluated only very few implants in the range of 3 mm (range: 3.0–3.3 mm; $n = 15$, 207.2 ± 14.3 Ncm) [24,27] and 5 mm (range: 4.5–5.0 mm; $n = 41$, 349.4 ± 125.4 Ncm) [15,19,27,28], whereas the majority of implants had a diameter in the range of 4 mm (range: 3.8–4.4 mm; $n = 675$, 394.9 ± 170.4 Ncm). Boxplots can be seen in Figure 5.

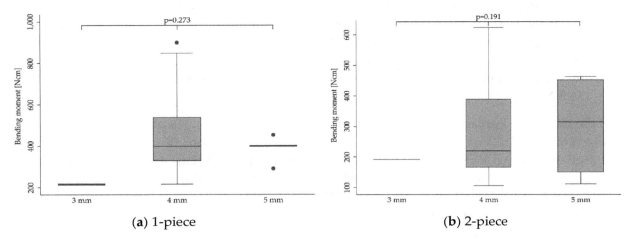

Figure 5. Boxplots showing the bending moment at the time point of fracture depending on the implant diameter for 1- (**a**) and 2-piece (**b**) zirconia implants. Whiskers are used to represent all samples lying within 1.5 times the interquartile range. Dots represent outliers. Detailed data can be found in Tables 3 and 4.

3.3.5. Anatomical Crown Supply

Of the included 731 implants, 209 were restored with an anatomically shaped crown, mostly made from ceramic materials. Most of the crowns were designed to replace maxillary central incisors but also some premolar reconstructions were included. The remaining 522 implants did not receive any reconstruction and were directly loaded to the abutment or were equipped with a non-anatomical stainless-steel hemisphere according to ISO 14801. When pooling the data for 1- and 2-piece implants, anatomical crown supply (237.5 ± 96.6 Ncm) negatively affected the outcome compared to implants with no crowns or equipped with a hemisphere (455.2 ± 147.7 Ncm, $p < 0.0001$). When stratifying for 1- and 2-piece implants (Figure 6), statistical significance was only reached for the group of 2-piece implants ($p < 0.0001$), likewise revealing an inferior outcome for implants restored with anatomical crowns. Fracture resistance of 1-piece implants was not affected by crown supply ($p = 0.080$).

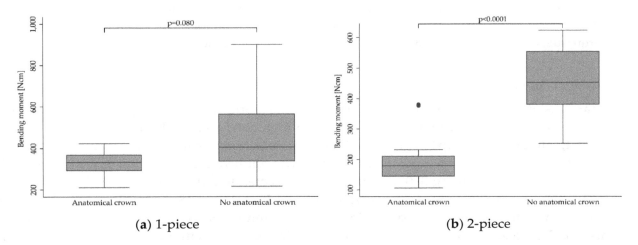

Figure 6. Boxplots showing the bending moment at the time point of fracture depending on the crown supply for 1- (**a**) and 2-piece (**b**) zirconia implants. Whiskers are used to represent all samples lying within 1.5 times the interquartile range. Dots represent outliers. Detailed data can be found in Tables 3 and 4.

3.3.6. Abutment Preparation and Implant-Abutment-Connection (IAC)

Of the 1-piece implants (n = 495), 112 abutments were prepared/modified by grinding [12,18,22,29], whereas 383 abutments remained untouched until fracture. In most cases, abutment preparation should simulate a clinically relevant situation of a 1-piece implant installed in anterior regions of the mouth. In both groups, some implants were restored with anatomically shaped incisor crowns, and some did not receive any reconstruction. Grinding of the abutment (411.3 ± 126.2 Ncm) resulted in a significantly reduced bending moment at the time point of fracture compared to non-grinded implants (436.5 ± 156.5 Ncm, p < 0.0001; Figure 7a).

Of the two-piece implants included in the present review (n = 236), 159 abutments were assembled by screw retention [13,16,19,21,24,26]. Most screws were made from titanium, but also gold and polyetheretherketone (PEEK; in one study, carbon-fiber-reinforced [26]) were used. The remaining 77 two-piece implants were irreversibly assembled by adhesive bonding [13,19,27,28,30]. The type of abutment retention (screw-retained: 327.5 ± 179.0 Ncm, bonded: 217.0 ± 86.0 Ncm) did not affect the fracture resistance (p = 0.584; Figure 7b).

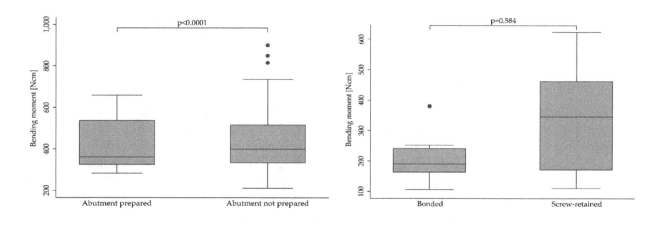

(a) Abutment preparation: 1-piece

(b) IAC: 2-piece

Figure 7. Boxplots showing the bending moment at the time point of fracture depending on the abutment preparation for 1-piece (**a**) and depending on the implant-abutment-connection (IAC) for 2-piece (**b**) zirconia implants. Whiskers are used to represent all samples lying within 1.5 times the interquartile range. Dots represent outliers. Detailed data can be found in Tables 3 and 4.

3.3.7. Thermal Aging

Regardless of the implant design, in 297 implants, no aging was induced prior to static loading to fracture, whereas 124 implants were subjected to a high temperature (HT) treatment in a humid environment, ranging from 60 up to 134 °C for different time periods lasting from 5–30 h (134 °C) [15,25] to 60 days (85 °C) [21,26]. High temperature treatment was applied in combination or during dynamic loading or alone. The remaining 310 implants were subjected to a thermal cycling (TC) procedure, exposing the samples to a changing water bath set at 5 and 55 °C [12,16,18–20,22,27–30]. The latter was mostly performed during dynamic loading in a chewing simulation device. Compared to untreated implants (406.2 ± 180.4 Ncm), neither HT treatment (392.9 ± 115.9 Ncm) nor TC (355.5 ± 171.7 Ncm) did affect the fracture resistance (p = 0.446). This did not change when calculating the outcome for 1- (p = 0.538) and 2-piece implants (p = 0.776) separately (Figure 8).

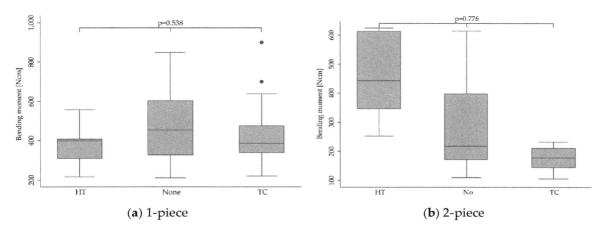

(a) 1-piece

(b) 2-piece

Figure 8. Boxplots showing the bending moment at the time point of fracture, depending on the thermal aging conditions (none, HT = high temperature, TC = thermal cycling) for 1- (**a**) and 2-piece (**b**) zirconia implants. Whiskers are used to represent all samples lying within 1.5 times the interquartile range. Dots represent outliers. Detailed data can be found in Tables 3 and 4.

3.3.8. Dynamic Loading

The effect of dynamic loading was evaluated from different perspectives. The simplest one assigned the included implants to two categories subjected to either no dynamic loading procedure ("No") or those being subjected to dynamic loading ("Yes"; Figure 9, Table 4). Furthermore, the effect of dynamic loading was evaluated regarding the dynamically "applied load", ranging from 45 [30] up to more than 500 N [17], or regarding the "amount of cycles" ranging from 1.2 [12,16,18,22,28–30] to 10 million [13,20,21,26] loading cycles. Finally, a combination of "applied load" and "amount of cycles" was used to from six groups, as mentioned in Section 2.7 (Figure 10).

When pooling the extracted data for 1- and 2-piece implants, dynamic loading did not affect the fracture resistance (dynamically-loaded implants showed a mean bending moment at the time point of fracture of 389.4 ± 169.2 Ncm compared to 383.2 ± 166.3 Ncm calculated for non-loaded implants ($p = 0.410$)). This did not change when evaluating 1- and 2-piece implants separately ($p > 0.474$). Solely the category "applied load" was close to statistical significance ($p = 0.05$). However, none of the multiple pairwise comparisons comparing different dynamically applied loads showed a statistically significant difference ($p > 0.07$). When solely evaluating 2-piece implants, "amount of cycles" significantly affected the fracture resistance ($p < 0.0001$), whereas "applied load" ($p = 0.202$) and groups 1–6 respecting the applied load and the amount of cycles ($p = 0.056$) did not affect the outcome.

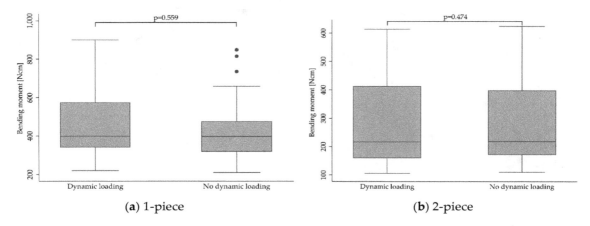

(a) 1-piece

(b) 2-piece

Figure 9. Boxplots showing the bending moment at the time point of fracture depending on dynamic loading (Yes: Implants were subjected to dynamic loading, No: Implants were not dynamically loaded) for 1- (**a**) and 2-piece (**b**) zirconia implants. Whiskers are used to represent all samples lying within 1.5 times the interquartile range. Dots represent outliers. Detailed data can be found in Tables 3 and 4.

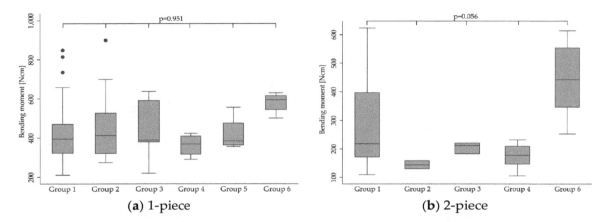

(a) 1-piece   **(b)** 2-piece

Figure 10. Boxplots showing the bending moment at the time point of fracture depending on dynamic loading conditions respecting the applied load and amount of cycles (as categorized in Section 2.7) for 1- (**a**) and 2-piece (**b**) zirconia implants. Whiskers are used to represent all samples lying within 1.5 times the interquartile range. Dots represent outliers. Detailed data can be found in Tables 3 and 4. No 2-piece implants were allocated to group 5.

4. Discussion

The present systematic review and meta-analysis included the data of 17 studies and two unpublished datasets. To be finally able to compare the outcomes of the included data, it was necessary to extract or calculate the bending moment at the time point of implant fracture [Ncm], since the mostly reported fracture load values [N] do not respect the leverage (length of the lever arm) and are therefore, if not considering a rigorously standardized embedding procedure as described in ISO 14801, not comparable to each other. Of the included 19 investigations/datasets, three studies reported the bending moment individually calculated for each included implant [13,20,22], whereas six studies [15,17,21,24–26] and the two included unpublished datasets fully respected ISO 14801 for embedding. Fully respecting this ISO implies the fixation of the endosseous part in a rigid clamping device or embedding in a material with a modulus of elasticity higher than 3 GPa. Moreover, the embedding/clamping level should respect a distance of 3.0 ± 0.5 mm apically from the nominal bone level, as specified in the manufacturer's instructions for use. Furthermore, implant abutments need to be equipped with a non-anatomical hemisphere designed to realize a distance of $l = 11.0 \pm 0.5$ mm from the center of the hemisphere to the embedding level (Figure 11).

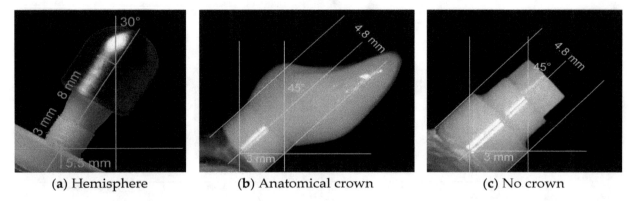

(a) Hemisphere   **(b)** Anatomical crown   **(c)** No crown

Figure 11. Exemplary schemes of embedded implants according to ISO 14801 (**a**) [21], equipped with an anatomically shaped incisor crown (**b**) or without any restorative supply (**c**) [20]. When embedding the samples according to ISO 14801, the lever arm measures 5.5 mm. In the latter two cases, the lever arm needs to be individually calculated and reported.

When loading such samples with an angle of $\alpha = 30°$ to the vertical, the lever arm (y) or bending moment (M) for this configuration can be calculated with the reported fracture load (F) by using Equation (1).

$$M = y \cdot F = sin\ \alpha \cdot l \cdot F \qquad (1)$$

This results in $y = 0.55$ cm when embedding according to ISO 14801. For the aforementioned publications/datasets fully respecting ISO 14801 for embedding and reporting the fracture load values [N], the bending moment was therefore calculated by multiplying the fracture load with 0.55. Interestingly, some of the included investigations reported embedding according to ISO 14801, but solely adopted the embedding level (simulation of a bony recession of 3 mm), and sometimes the angulation (30°), but did not use a loading hemisphere, finally resulting in a lever arm different to 5.5 mm, as proposed by the ISO standard [16,19,27,28]. In most cases, anatomical crowns (maxillary premolars or incisors) made from ceramic materials were used instead of the hemisphere, finally resulting in altered lever arms and loading conditions. In the investigations of one group, the crown design and embedding procedure were described in detail (l, α and F were reported), allowing us to calculate y and M [19,27,28]. To calculate the bending moment for the remaining studies, authors needed to provide the necessary data upon request or standardized photographs provided in the publications, or by the authors needed to allow the approximation of the lever arm by using an image analysis software (ImageJ, National Institutes of Health, Bethesda, MD, USA) [12,16,18,29,30]. In order to be able to compare the outcome of preclinical studies evaluating the fracture resistance of dental implants, it is therefore recommended to either fully adopt an ISO standard for the embedding procedure or to provide the bending moment additionally to the fracture load. Considering different lever arms due to different embedding procedures for the implants included in this systematic review and meta-analysis, one needs to keep in mind that dynamic loading prior to static loading to fracture can result in altered fatigue, even if the applied load was the same.

The heterogeneity of the included samples comprising a mixture of market-available products (finally sterilized and incorporating a micro-roughened surface) [15,16,22,24,26] but also prototype implants (e.g., with or without any surface post-processing) [13,19,21,25,28,30] represents a major limitation of the present systematic review and meta-analysis. However, it was shown that, for example, surface modifications like micro-roughening to enhance osseointegration or steam-sterilization can significantly compromise fracture strength and ageing kinetics [31,32].

Another shortcoming of this systematic review presents the fact that of the 19 included datasets, more than half (nine published and two unpublished studies) were at least partially authored by the collaborates of the current paper. This might be considered a reasonable risk of bias. However, the present review was conducted according to standardized guidelines, and the available literature was systematically screened on the basis of predefined search terms and inclusion criteria. Modifying the search strategy, outcome measure or inclusion criteria in consequence of unexpected or homogeneously authored findings would likewise present a source of bias.

Regarding the treatments, the included samples have been subjected to prior to loading, and six groups (representing different categories of loading conditions as indicated in Section 2.7) have been evaluated for heterogeneity of the outcome. As a result, no heterogeneity of the bending moments for groups 1–6 was found ($p = 0.612$). This did not change when stratifying the implants according to their design (1-piece: $p = 0.951$; 2-piece: $p = 0.056$). Therefore, it was decided to pool the data of all groups for any further calculations, and yet still, one can hardly generalize the present findings and apply them to a specific zirconia implant system.

No statistically significant influence of hydrothermal aging on the fracture resistance of zirconia implants was calculated in the present review. It is important to note that aging or so-called low-temperature degradation (LTD) can, depending upon the sample quality and surface conditions, result in both increased [21,25] and decreased [33] fracture load. This might be explained by the following: Assuming a zirconia sample surface with various process-related defects/impurities, the largest defects/impurities are thought to act as "locus minoris resistentiae", and can thereby be considered representative for the fracture resistance of this sample. Increased fracture load of such zirconia samples after a hydrothermal aging procedure is thought to be attributed to a transformed layer at the sample surface, inducing a compressive stress on the surface, tending to close a potential advancing crack at such existing defects/impurities located on the surface. This phenomenon is liable to cause an increase in the strength of the material, and was described for the first time three decades ago [34]. On the other side, at some point when the degradation process penetrates deeper into the material, the contribution from the aging may instead cause the strength of the same sample to be decreased, since once transformed to the monoclinic, zirconia grains cannot exhibit stress-induced phase transformation toughening anymore [33]. As an example, in the included investigation of Monzavi and co-workers [15] the effect of artificial aging on the mechanical resistance and micromechanical properties of commercially- and noncommercially-available zirconia dental implants was evaluated. In this study, the bending moment was significantly increased after aging for three of six groups, whereas two groups showed no influence of the aging procedure, and one group was negatively affected in terms of fracture resistance by the treatment [15]. When pooling the outcomes of the included studies showing positive, negative or no effects of LTD on the fracture resistance of zirconia implants in one dataset, as happened in the present meta-analyses, no effect of hydrothermal aging on the bending moment at the time point of fracture was calculated ($p > 0.446$). This, however, might be misleading, since several of the included studies indeed showed that aging can significantly affect the fracture resistance. However, due to the explanation given at the beginning of this paragraph, both in a negative or positive way. Therefore, missing significance, as calculated for pooled data in this review, should not be interpreted as an argument to refrain from aging tests of a zirconia implant system prior to market release. Therefore, pooling the data from different studies using the different conditions of thermal aging needs to be considered a limitation of the present review. It is discussed in the literature that the present amount of transformation to the monoclinic on the surface of as-delivered zirconia implants can be decisive for the ongoing fracture resistance after further hydrothermal aging procedures. In detail, implants showing no or very limited transformation to the monoclinic when released to the market (e.g., due to final temperature annealing [35] or manufacturing by ceramic injection-molding [21,25]) were observed to be less fracture-resistant in the original as-delivered state, but significantly gained fracture resistance due to increasing compressive stress at the sample surface after transformation to the monoclinic occurred. In contrast, samples already revealing a transformed layer of several micrometers (e.g., due to subtractive manufacturing or post-processing steps like sandblasting in order to roughen the surface to enhance osseointegration [26]) mostly do not benefit from further aging by means of an increased fracture resistance. Besides the amount of already transformed grains, implant surface topography showed to have a significant impact on aging susceptibility and its impact on fracture resistance [32,36]. As an example, implants structured with porous or alveolar surfaces were more likely to be negatively affected by aging procedures due to interconnected porosities in the surface layer, offering a path for the transformation to start at every surface accessible by water [25]. Finally, a layer structured in this way can be transformed in a shorter period of time.

Of the implants included in the present investigation, 209 of 731 were restored with anatomically-shaped crowns [16,19,20,27–30]. Most of these crowns were designed as maxillary central incisors, and were manufactured from: lithium disilicate [20], veneered [29] or monolithic [19,27,28] zirconia, or porcelain fused to metal [30]. Another included study restored the implants with maxillary first premolar restorations made from lithium disilicate [16], whereas Joda and collaborates restored the implants with non-anatomical hemispheres likewise made from lithium disilicate [24].

Most of the included studies not restoring the implants with anatomically-shaped crowns were conducted by adopting ISO 14801. According to this standard, the loading force shall be applied to the hemispherical loading surface, by a loading device with a plane surface normal to the loading direction of the machine, without additional horizontal loading forces. In contrast, especially incisor crowns present an inclined plane when loaded during the dynamic and finally static loading procedure, resulting in an increased shear force. Additionally, some investigations applied horizontal forces during the dynamic loading procedure (as it happens in the oral cavity), causing further fatigue of the sample [20,29,30]. Therefore, not the restoration itself, but the altered investigational setup, resulting in increased shear forces and fatigue during static loading, and in some cases, precedent chewing simulation might be considered responsible for decreased fracture resistance. Nonetheless, this finding should be taken into account when drafting international standards in order to guarantee clinical safety, since the anatomical reconstruction of zirconia oral implants and horizontal shear forces during loading represent clinical reality. Regarding the nature or location of failure, 1-piece implants mostly fractured at the embedding level or slightly below, with crack initiation on the tensile side of the implant. As described in the included studies, it seems that the fracture mode was not affected by crown supply. In 2-piece implants, fracture modes were generally observed to be highly heterogeneous, depending on the mode of assembly and the materials used.

When it comes to clinical reality, the fracture resistance of a zirconia implant should finally withstand the maximum voluntary bite forces of the patients. Nonetheless, one cannot find the definition of any indication specific (e.g., for implants installed in anterior or posterior regions) minimum value for the fracture strength of a zirconia implant in ISO 14801. This, as an example, is provided in detail in ISO 6872 for ceramic materials used for reconstructions (e.g., crowns, bridges) in dentistry [37]. Taking the highest bending moment measured in vivo (95 Ncm) with the help of strain gauge abutments into account [38], and applying a safety buffer of 100%, one might consider a minimum fracture resistance of 200 Ncm sufficient to guarantee clinical safety. When applying this requirement to the included studies, mostly 2-piece prototype implants and implants with a reduced diameter ($\leq$ 3.3 mm) did not meet this demand [19,24,27,28,30].

Of the zirconia implants included in the present investigation, 577 were manufactured from Y-TZP and 154 from ATZ. Overall, implant stability was significantly affected by the material, in favor of ATZ ($p = 0.002$). When evaluating 1- and 2-piece implants separately, however, only 1-piece implants made from ATZ performed better ($p = 0.001$), whereas 2-piece implants performed the same, regardless of the material selection ($p = 0.282$). This might be explained by the fact that 1-piece zirconia implants or even, as an example, 2-piece titanium implants are mostly made from one single material (in the case of titanium: the implant, the abutment and the abutment screw are mostly fabricated from titanium). In contrast, most of the available 2-piece zirconia systems represent a multi-material complex comprising at least two or sometimes even three different materials. In some cases, only the implant body is manufactured from zirconia, whereas the screw (e.g., titanium or PEEK) and/or abutment (e.g., glass-fiber or polyetherketoneketone/PEKK) might be manufactured from different materials revealing different aging or degradation behavior during treatments (hydrothermal aging, dynamic loading), precedent to final static loading to fracture. To date, sound correlations to approximate intraoral aging conditions in an accelerated way in the dental laboratory are mostly available for zirconia ceramics, but missing for screw and abutment materials prone to degradation in aqueous environments, like e.g., polyetherketones [39,40]. In consequence, no standardized testing procedures were proposed to the present date, sufficiently evaluating multi-material, 2-piece implants regarding their fracture resistance, and individually respecting the degradation behavior of several included components. Regrettably, the sample size and heterogeneity of the extracted data gathered from 2-piece implants included in the present review did not allow for the statistical evaluation of a potential impact of the screw or abutment material on the fracture resistance of 2-piece zirconia implants. In one of the included studies, the aim was to measure the abutment rotation and fracture load of 2-piece zirconia implants screwed with three different abutment screw materials [16]. Implants and abutments of the included system were assembled with screws made from gold, titanium and PEEK.

As a result, no significant differences were found for these three materials, even if PEEK screws showed inferior results. When choosing PEEK as an abutment screw material, the incorporation of continuous carbon fibers proved to positively affect the maximum tensile strength of the screw [41]. However, a strengthening effect on the entire implant-abutment complex in case of zirconia implants still needs to be evidenced. In one of the included studies [26], a 2-piece ATZ implant system assembled with a carbon-fiber-reinforced abutment screw showed to be non-inferior compared to a market-established 2-piece titanium implant of a highly comparable design regarding its fracture resistance.

5. Conclusions

The null hypothesis of the present review, supposing no distinction between treatments and features in relation to bending moment when statically loading a zirconia implant to fracture, needs to be partially rejected. The focused question can be answered as follows: In general, 1-piece implants can be considered more fracture resistant than 2-piece implants, even if some of the included studies showed very promising results for 2-piece zirconia implants. When focusing on 1-piece implants, implants made from ATZ are more fracture resistant than implants made from Y-TZP. Due to its negative impact on fracture resistance, abutment preparation of 1-piece zirconia implants should be avoided. When drafting international standards to guarantee clinical safety, one should keep in mind that the loading of anatomically shaped crowns might result in the decreased fracture resistance of zirconia implants compared to non-anatomical loading hemispheres, as mentioned in ISO 14801. Further research is needed to define adequate hydrothermal aging and dynamic loading conditions for 2-piece ceramic implants, nowadays mostly comprising a multi-material complex.

Author Contributions: Conceptualization, B.C.S.; methodology, B.C.S. and A.B.; validation, S.P., M.v.S.-L., F.B. and K.V.; statistical analysis, K.V.; writing—original draft preparation, B.C.S. and A.B.; writing—review and editing, S.P., K.V., R.-J.K., F.B. and M.v.S.-L. All authors have read and agreed to the published version of the manuscript.

Acknowledgments: We acknowledge support from the German Research Foundation (DFG) and the Open Access Publication Fund of Charité—Universitätsmedizin Berlin.

Appendix A

Table A1. Articles excluded after screening of the full-texts.

First Author	Year	Ref.	Reason for Exclusion
Young	1972	[42]	Narrative review
Kohal	2006	[43]	Root analogue implants
Silva	2009	[44]	No static loading to fracture (step-stress fatigue)
Silva	2011	[45]	No static loading to fracture (pendulum impact tester)
Van Dooren	2012	[46]	Narrative review and case report
Iijima	2013	[47]	No evaluation of dental implants (discs)
Mobilio	2013	[48]	No static loading to fracture (strain measurements), <5 samples
Sanon	2013	[36]	No static loading to fracture (step-stress fatigue)
Cattani-Lorente	2014	[31]	No evaluation of dental implants (bar-shaped samples)
Rohr	2015	[49]	Fracture on the restoration level
Kamel	2017	[50]	Calculation of bending moment not possible, no author response
Karl	2017	[51]	No static loading to fracture (insertion torque measurements)
Korabi	2017	[52]	No static loading to fracture (finite element analysis)
Monzavi	2017	[53]	No static loading to fracture (accelerated aging only)
Zietz	2017	[54]	No zirconia implants
Baumgart	2018	[55]	No static loading to fracture
Rohr	2018	[56]	Fracture on the restoration level
Zaugg	2018	[57]	Fracture on the restoration level
Faria	2019	[58]	No evaluation of dental implants (discs)
Nueesch	2019	[59]	Fracture on the restoration level
Rohr	2019	[60]	Fracture on the restoration level
Scherrer	2019	[61]	Fractographic analysis of clinically fractured zirconia implants
Siddiqui	2019	[62]	Cyclic fatigue w/o subsequent fracture loading

References

1. Bosshardt, D.D.; Chappuis, V.; Buser, D. Osseointegration of titanium, titanium alloy and zirconia dental implants: Current knowledge and open questions. *Periodontol. 2000* **2017**, *73*, 22–40. [CrossRef] [PubMed]

2. Kniha, K.; Kniha, H.; Grunert, I.; Edelhoff, D.; Holzle, F.; Modabber, A. Esthetic Evaluation of Maxillary Single-Tooth Zirconia Implants in the Esthetic Zone. *Int. J. Periodontics Restor. Dent.* **2019**, *39*, e195–e201. [CrossRef] [PubMed]

3. Fretwurst, T.; Nelson, K.; Tarnow, D.P.; Wang, H.L.; Giannobile, W.V. Is Metal Particle Release Associated with Peri-implant Bone Destruction? An Emerging Concept. *J. Dent. Res.* **2018**, *97*, 259–265. [CrossRef] [PubMed]

4. Sanz, M.; Noguerol, B.; Sanz-Sanchez, I.; Hammerle, C.H.F.; Schliephake, H.; Renouard, F.; Sicilia, A.; Cordaro, L.; Jung, R.; Klinge, B.; et al. European Association for Osseointegration Delphi study on the trends in Implant Dentistry in Europe for the year 2030. *Clin. Oral Implant. Res.* **2019**, *30*, 476–486. [CrossRef]

5. Sennerby, L.; Dasmah, A.; Larsson, B.; Iverhed, M. Bone tissue responses to surface-modified zirconia implants: A histomorphometric and removal torque study in the rabbit. *Clin. Implant. Dent. Relat. Res.* **2005**, *7*, S13–S20. [CrossRef]

6. Pieralli, S.; Kohal, R.-J.; Lopez Hernandez, E.; Doerken, S.; Spies, B.C. Osseointegration of zirconia dental implants in animal investigations: A systematic review and meta-analysis. *Dent. Mater.* **2018**, *34*, 171–182. [CrossRef]

7. Pieralli, S.; Kohal, R.J.; Jung, R.E.; Vach, K.; Spies, B.C. Clinical Outcomes of Zirconia Dental Implants: A Systematic Review. *J. Dent. Res.* **2017**, *96*, 38–46. [CrossRef]

8. Prithviraj, D.R.; Gupta, V.; Muley, N.; Sandhu, P. One-piece implants: Placement timing, surgical technique, loading protocol, and marginal bone loss. *J. Prosthodont.* **2013**, *22*, 237–244. [CrossRef]

9. Östman, P.O.; Hellman, M.; Albrektsson, T.; Sennerby, L. Direct loading of Nobel Direct and Nobel Perfect one-piece implants: A 1-year prospective clinical and radiographic study. *Clin. Oral Implant. Res.* **2007**, *18*, 409–418. [CrossRef]

10. Cionca, N.; Hashim, D.; Mombelli, A. Zirconia dental implants: Where are we now, and where are we heading? *Periodontol. 2000* **2017**, *73*, 241–258. [CrossRef]

11. Spies, B.C.; Witkowski, S.; Vach, K.; Kohal, R.J. Clinical and patient-reported outcomes of zirconia-based implant fixed dental prostheses: Results of a prospective case series 5 years after implant placement. *Clin. Oral Implant. Res.* **2018**, *29*, 91–99. [CrossRef] [PubMed]

12. Kohal, R.J.; Wolkewitz, M.; Tsakona, A. The effects of cyclic loading and preparation on the fracture strength of zirconium-dioxide implants: An in vitro investigation. *Clin. Oral Implant. Res.* **2011**, *22*, 808–814. [CrossRef] [PubMed]

13. Spies, B.C.; Nold, J.; Vach, K.; Kohal, R.J. Two-piece zirconia oral implants withstand masticatory loads: An investigation in the artificial mouth. *J. Mech. Behav. Biomed. Mater.* **2016**, *53*, 1–10. [CrossRef] [PubMed]

14. Frigan, K.; Chevalier, J.; Zhang, F.; Spies, B.C. Is a Zirconia Dental Implant Safe When It Is Available on the Market? *Ceramics* **2019**, *2*, 44. [CrossRef]

15. Monzavi, M.; Zhang, F.; Meille, S.; Douillard, T.; Adrien, J.; Noumbissi, S.; Nowzari, H.; Chevalier, J. Influence of artificial aging on mechanical properties of commercially and non-commercially available zirconia dental implants. *J. Mech. Behav. Biomed. Mater.* **2020**, *101*, 103423. [CrossRef]

16. Stimmelmayr, M.; Lang, A.; Beuer, F.; Mansour, S.; Erdelt, K.; Krennmair, G.; Guth, J.F. Mechanical stability of all-ceramic abutments retained with three different screw materials in two-piece zirconia implants-an in vitro study. *Clin. Oral Investig.* **2019**. [CrossRef]

17. Ding, Q.; Zhang, L.; Bao, R.; Zheng, G.; Sun, Y.; Xie, Q. Effects of different surface treatments on the cyclic fatigue strength of one-piece CAD/CAM zirconia implants. *J. Mech. Behav. Biomed. Mater.* **2018**, *84*, 249–257. [CrossRef]

18. Kohal, R.J.; Wolkewitz, M.; Mueller, C. Alumina-reinforced zirconia implants: Survival rate and fracture strength in a masticatory simulation trial. *Clin. Oral Implant. Res.* **2010**, *21*, 1345–1352. [CrossRef]

19. Preis, V.; Kammermeier, A.; Handel, G.; Rosentritt, M. In vitro performance of two-piece zirconia implant systems for anterior application. *Dent. Mater.* **2016**, *32*, 765–774. [CrossRef]

20. Kohal, R.J.; Kilian, J.B.; Stampf, S.; Spies, B.C. All-Ceramic Single Crown Restauration of Zirconia Oral Implants and Its Influence on Fracture Resistance: An Investigation in the Artificial Mouth. *Materials* **2015**, *8*, 1577–1589. [CrossRef]

21. Spies, B.C.; Maass, M.E.; Adolfsson, E.; Sergo, V.; Kiemle, T.; Berthold, C.; Gurian, E.; Fornasaro, S.; Vach, K.; Kohal, R.J. Long-term stability of an injection-molded zirconia bone-level implant: A testing protocol considering aging kinetics and dynamic fatigue. *Dent. Mater.* **2017**, *33*, 954–965. [CrossRef] [PubMed]

22. Spies, B.C.; Sauter, C.; Wolkewitz, M.; Kohal, R.J. Alumina reinforced zirconia implants: Effects of cyclic loading and abutment modification on fracture resistance. *Dent. Mater.* **2015**, *31*, 262–272. [CrossRef] [PubMed]

23. Moher, D.; Liberati, A.; Tetzlaff, J.; Altman, D.G. Preferred Reporting Items for Systematic Reviews and Meta-Analyses: The PRISMA Statement. *PLoS Med.* **2009**, *6*, e1000097. [CrossRef] [PubMed]

24. Joda, T.; Voumard, B.; Zysset, P.K.; Bragger, U.; Ferrari, M. Ultimate force and stiffness of 2-piece zirconium dioxide implants with screw-retained monolithic lithium-disilicate reconstructions. *J. Prosthodont. Res.* **2018**, *62*, 258–263. [CrossRef] [PubMed]

25. Sanon, C.; Chevalier, J.; Douillard, T.; Cattani-Lorente, M.; Scherrer, S.S.; Gremillard, L. A new testing protocol for zirconia dental implants. *Dent. Mater.* **2015**, *31*, 15–25. [CrossRef]

26. Spies, B.C.; Fross, A.; Adolfsson, E.; Bagegni, A.; Doerken, S.; Kohal, R.J. Stability and aging resistance of a zirconia oral implant using a carbon fiber-reinforced screw for implant-abutment connection. *Dent. Mater.* **2018**, *34*, 1585–1595. [CrossRef]

27. Kammermeier, A.; Rosentritt, M.; Behr, M.; Schneider-Feyrer, S.; Preis, V. In vitro performance of one- and two-piece zirconia implant systems for anterior application. *J. Dent.* **2016**, *53*, 94–101. [CrossRef]

28. Rosentritt, M.; Hagemann, A.; Hahnel, S.; Behr, M.; Preis, V. In vitro performance of zirconia and titanium implant/abutment systems for anterior application. *J. Dent.* **2014**, *42*, 1019–1026. [CrossRef]

29. Andreiotelli, M.; Kohal, R.-J. Fracture Strength of Zirconia Implants after Artificial Aging. *Clin. Implant. Dent. Relat. Res.* **2009**, *11*, 158–166. [CrossRef]

30. Kohal, R.; Finke, H.C.; Klaus, G. Stability of Prototype Two-Piece Zirconia and Titanium Implants after Artificial Aging: An In Vitro Pilot Study. *Clin. Implant. Dent. Relat. Res.* **2009**, *11*, 323–329. [CrossRef]

31. Cattani-Lorente, M.; Scherrer, S.S.; Durual, S.; Sanon, C.; Douillard, T.; Gremillard, L.; Chevalier, J.; Wiskott, A. Effect of different surface treatments on the hydrothermal degradation of a 3Y-TZP ceramic for dental implants. *Dent. Mater.* **2014**, *30*, 1136–1146. [CrossRef] [PubMed]

32. Chevalier, J.; Loh, J.; Gremillard, L.; Meille, S.; Adolfson, E. Low-temperature degradation in zirconia with a porous surface. *Acta Biomater.* **2011**, *7*, 2986–2993. [CrossRef] [PubMed]

33. Kim, H.T.; Han, J.S.; Yang, J.H.; Lee, J.B.; Kim, S.H. The effect of low temperature aging on the mechanical property & phase stability of Y-TZP ceramics. *J. Adv. Prosthodont.* **2009**, *1*, 113–117. [CrossRef] [PubMed]

34. Virkar, A.V.; Huang, J.L.; Cutler, R.A. Strengthening of oxide ceramics by transformation-induced stress. *J. Am. Ceram. Soc.* **1987**, *70*, 164–170. [CrossRef]

35. Fischer, J.; Schott, A.; Martin, S. Surface micro-structuring of zirconia dental implants. *Clin. Oral Implants Res.* **2016**, *27*, 162–166. [CrossRef]

36. Sanon, C.; Chevalier, J.; Douillard, T.; Kohal, R.J.; Coelho, P.G.; Hjerppe, J.; Silva, N.R. Low temperature degradation and reliability of one-piece ceramic oral implants with a porous surface. *Dent. Mater.* **2013**, *29*, 389–397. [CrossRef]

37. Peixoto, H.E.; Bordin, D.; Cury, A.A.D.B.; Da Silva, W.J.; Faot, F. The role of prosthetic abutment material on the stress distribution in a maxillary single implant-supported fixed prosthesis. *Mater. Sci. Eng. C* **2016**, *65*, 90–96. [CrossRef]

38. Morneburg, T.R.; Pröschel, P.A. In vivo forces on implants influenced by occlusal scheme and food consistency. *Int. J. Prosthodont.* **2003**, *16*, 481–486.

39. Aversa, R.; Apicella, A. Osmotic Tension, Plasticization and Viscoelastic response of amorphous Poly-Ether-Ether-Ketone (PEEK) equilibrated in humid environments. *Am. J. Eng. Appl. Sci.* **2016**, *9*, 565–573. [CrossRef]

40.	Chevalier, J.; Cales, B.; Drouin, J.M. Low-Temperature Aging of Y-TZP Ceramics. *J. Am. Ceram. Soc.* **1999**, *82*, 2150–2154. [CrossRef]

41.	Schwitalla, A.D.; Abou-Emara, M.; Zimmermann, T.; Spintig, T.; Beuer, F.; Lackmann, J.; Muller, W.D. The applicability of PEEK-based abutment screws. *J. Mech. Behav. Biomed. Mater.* **2016**, *63*, 244–251. [CrossRef] [PubMed]

42.	Young, F.A., Jr. Ceramic tooth implants. *J. Biomed. Mater. Res.* **1972**, *6*, 281–296. [CrossRef] [PubMed]

43.	Kohal, R.J.; Klaus, G.; Strub, J.R. Zirconia-implant-supported all-ceramic crowns withstand long-term load: A pilot investigation. *Clin. Oral Implant. Res.* **2006**, *17*, 565–571. [CrossRef] [PubMed]

44.	Silva, N.R.; Coelho, P.G.; Fernandes, C.A.; Navarro, J.M.; Dias, R.A.; Thompson, V.P. Reliability of one-piece ceramic implant. *J. Biomed. Mater. Res. B Appl. Biomater.* **2009**, *88*, 419–426. [CrossRef]

45.	Silva, N.R.; Nourian, P.; Coelho, P.G.; Rekow, E.D.; Thompson, V.P. Impact Fracture Resistance of Two Titanium-Abutment Systems Versus a Single-Piece Ceramic Implant. *Clin. Implant. Dent. Relat. Res.* **2011**, *13*, 168–173. [CrossRef]

46.	Van Dooren, E.; Calamita, M.; Calgaro, M.; Coachman, C.; Ferencz, J.L.; Pinho, C.; Silva, N.R. Mechanical, biological and clinical aspects of zirconia implants. *Eur. J. Esthet. Dent.* **2012**, *7*, 396–417. [PubMed]

47.	Iijima, T.; Homma, S.; Sekine, H.; Sasaki, H.; Yajima, Y.; Yoshinari, M. Influence of surface treatment of yttria-stabilized tetragonal zirconia polycrystal with hot isostatic pressing on cyclic fatigue strength. *Dent. Mater. J.* **2013**, *32*, 274–280. [CrossRef] [PubMed]

48.	Mobilio, N.; Stefanoni, F.; Contiero, P.; Mollica, F.; Catapano, S. Experimental and numeric stress analysis of titanium and zirconia one-piece dental implants. *Int. J. Oral Maxillofac. Implant.* **2013**, *28*, e135–e142. [CrossRef] [PubMed]

49.	Rohr, N.; Coldea, A.; Zitzmann, N.U.; Fischer, J. Loading capacity of zirconia implant supported hybrid ceramic crowns. *Dent. Mater.* **2015**, *31*, e279–e288. [CrossRef]

50.	Kamel, M.; Vaidyanathan, T.K.; Flinton, R. Effect of Abutment Preparation and Fatigue Loading in a Moist Environment on the Fracture Resistance of the One-Piece Zirconia Dental Implant. *Int. J. Oral Maxillofac. Implant.* **2017**, *32*, 533–540. [CrossRef]

51.	Karl, M.; Scherg, S.; Grobecker-Karl, T. Fracture of Reduced-Diameter Zirconia Dental Implants Following Repeated Insertion. *Int. J. Oral Maxillofac. Implant.* **2017**, *32*, 971–975. [CrossRef] [PubMed]

52.	Korabi, R.; Shemtov-Yona, K.; Rittel, D. On stress/strain shielding and the material stiffness paradigm for dental implants. *Clin. Implant. Dent. Relat. Res.* **2017**, *19*, 935–943. [CrossRef] [PubMed]

53.	Monzavi, M.; Noumbissi, S.; Nowzari, H. The Impact of In Vitro Accelerated Aging, Approximating 30 and 60 Years In Vivo, on Commercially Available Zirconia Dental Implants. *Clin. Implant. Dent. Relat. Res.* **2017**, *19*, 245–252. [CrossRef] [PubMed]

54.	Zietz, C.; Vogel, D.; Mitrovic, A.; Bader, R. Mechanical investigation of newly hybrid dental implants. *Biomedizinische Technik* **2017**, *62* (Suppl. 1), S447.

55.	Baumgart, P.; Kirsten, H.; Haak, R.; Olms, C. Biomechanical properties of polymer-infiltrated ceramic crowns on one-piece zirconia implants after long-term chewing simulation. *Int. J. Implant. Dent.* **2018**, *4*, 16. [CrossRef] [PubMed]

56.	Rohr, N.; Martin, S.; Fischer, J. Correlations between fracture load of zirconia implant supported single crowns and mechanical properties of restorative material and cement. *Dent. Mater. J.* **2018**, *37*, 222–228. [CrossRef]

57.	Zaugg, L.K.; Meyer, S.; Rohr, N.; Zehnder, I.; Zitzmann, N.U. Fracture behavior, marginal gap width, and marginal quality of vented or pre-cemented CAD/CAM all-ceramic crowns luted on Y-TZP implants. *Clin. Oral Implant. Res.* **2018**, *29*, 175–184. [CrossRef]

58.	Faria, D.; Pires, J.M.; Boccaccini, A.R.; Carvalho, O.; Silva, F.S.; Mesquita-Guimaraes, J. Development of novel zirconia implant's materials gradated design with improved bioactive surface. *J. Mech. Behav. Biomed. Mater.* **2019**, *94*, 110–125. [CrossRef]

59.	Nueesch, R.; Conejo, J.; Mante, F.; Fischer, J.; Martin, S.; Rohr, N.; Blatz, M.B. Loading capacity of CAD/CAM-fabricated anterior feldspathic ceramic crowns bonded to one-piece zirconia implants with different cements. *Clin. Oral Implant. Res.* **2019**, *30*, 178–186. [CrossRef]

60.	Rohr, N.; Balmer, M.; Muller, J.A.; Martin, S.; Fischer, J. Chewing simulation of zirconia implant supported restorations. *J. Prosthodont. Res.* **2019**, *63*, 361–367. [CrossRef]

61. Scherrer, S.S.; Mekki, M.; Crottaz, C.; Gahlert, M.; Romelli, E.; Marger, L.; Durual, S.; Vittecoq, E. Translational research on clinically failed zirconia implants. *Dent. Mater.* **2019**, *35*, 368–388. [CrossRef] [PubMed]
62. Siddiqui, D.A.; Sridhar, S.; Wang, F.; Jacob, J.J.; Rodrigues, D.C. Can Oral Bacteria and Mechanical Fatigue Degrade Zirconia Dental Implants in Vitro? *ACS Biomater. Sci. Eng.* **2019**, *5*, 2821–2833. [CrossRef]

9

The Effect of Ultraviolet Photofunctionalization on a Titanium Dental Implant with Machined Surface: An In Vitro and In Vivo Study

Jun-Beom Lee [1], Ye-Hyeon Jo [2], Jung-Yoo Choi [3], Yang-Jo Seol [1], Yong-Moo Lee [1], Young Ku [1], In-Chul Rhyu [1],* and In-Sung Luke Yeo [2],*

[1]   Department of Periodontology, Seoul National University School of Dentistry, Seoul 03080, Korea
[2]   Department of Prosthodontics, School of Dentistry and Dental Research Institute, Seoul National University, Seoul 03080, Korea
[3]   Dental Research Institute, Seoul National University, Seoul 03080, Korea
*   Correspondence: icrhyu@snu.ac.kr (I.-C.R.); pros53@snu.ac.kr (I.-S.L.Y.)

Abstract: Ultraviolet (UV) photofunctionalization has been suggested as an effective method to enhance the osseointegration of titanium surface. In this study, machined surface treated with UV light (M + UV) was compared to sandblasted, large-grit, acid-etched (SLA) surface through in vitro and in vivo studies. Groups of titanium specimens were defined as machined (M), SLA, and M + UV for the disc type, and M + UV and SLA for the implant. The discs and implants were assessed using scanning electron microscopy, confocal laser scanning microscopy, electron spectroscopy for chemical analysis, and the contact angle. Additionally, we evaluated the cell attachment, proliferation assay, and real-time polymerase chain reaction for the MC3T3-E1 cells. In a rabbit tibia model, the implants were examined to evaluate the bone-to-implant contact ratio and the bone area. In the M + UV group, we observed the lower amount of carbon, a 0°-degree contact angle, and enhanced osteogenic cell activities ($p < 0.05$). The histomorphometric analysis showed that a higher bone-to-implant contact ratio was found in the M + UV implant at 10 days ($p < 0.05$). In conclusion, the UV photofunctionalization of a Ti dental implant with M surface attained earlier osseointegration than SLA.

Keywords: dental implants; titanium; osseointegration; photofunctionalization; ultraviolet light; surface treatment

1. Introduction

Dental implant restorations to replace missing teeth have become a routine practice in dental clinics. Using the implants as a prosthesis helps patients feel more comfortable and these implants are more functional compared to the traditional removable dentures [1–3]. For successful implant restorations, osseointegration must be achieved between the bone and the implant. Osseointegration is the direct structural and functional connection between living bone and the surface of a load-carrying implant [4], and it is an essential factor in achieving a successful implant. Generally, it is necessary to wait for several months after implant placement for osseointegration to be achieved [5]. Unsuccessful osseointegration leads to the early failure of implants, meaning that the implants cannot endure masticatory forces, resulting in implant mobility or pain [6,7]. This includes other time-consuming situations, such as an edentulous area with limited bone quantity, or problems in patients with osteoporosis, diabetes, cancer, irradiation, old age, and heavy smokers [8–10].

The original implant surface was a smooth machined surface, with an approximate Sa value of 0.5 μm [11,12]. This machined surface has certain advantages, including a simple manufacturing process (turning and polishing) and the ability to maintain a good hygienic state, resulting in a low incidence of peri-implant disease [12,13]. However, implants with a machined surface have shown a low bone-to-implant contact ratio (BIC) and a frequent failure of osseointegration before loading [14]. To enhance the osseointegration process, various surface modifying techniques have since been developed, where a roughened surface has demonstrated the best clinical long-term results. There are various roughening techniques, although the sandblasted, large-grit, acid-etched (SLA) surface is the most widely used and reported technique. The SLA surface sufficiently differentiates the pre-osteoblastic cells, enhances the osseointegration process, and leads to a higher BIC compared to the machined surface [15,16]. However, the roughened surface has been reported to accelerate plaque accumulation, wherein it is more difficult to remove plaque on the roughened surface than on the machined surface [12]. In this regard, reports show a greater incidence of peri-implant disease stemming from the use of the roughened surface compared to the machined surface [17].

Meanwhile, the photofunctionalization of implants using ultraviolet (UV) light has been highlighted as a simple and effective method to stimulate osseointegration in machined surfaces [18–20]. UV photofunctionalization is a phenomenon of changes occurring in titanium (Ti) surfaces after UV treatment. The process was discovered in 1977, where UV treatment transforms the natural hydrophobic properties of Ti surfaces into superhydrophilic properties by altering the physicochemical properties of the Ti. The process has been applied in environmental engineering and microbiology [21,22]. UV treatment creates the hydrophilic phase on the surface structure, thereby transforming the surface into a hydrophilic surface [23]. Photofunctionalization is also reported to enhance biological capabilities [18,19]. Consequently, the purpose of this study was to evaluate the effect of UV photofunctionalization on implants with a machined surface compared to the SLA surface, using an in vitro and in vivo study.

2. Materials and Methods

2.1. Ti Samples, Surface Analysis, and UV Treatment

2.1.1. Preparation of the Ti Disc and Implant

In this experiment, commercially pure grade 4 Ti was tested in the shape of a disc (10 mm in diameter and 1 mm in thickness) and a screw-shaped implant (3.3 mm in diameter and 7 mm in length). The surface of the specimen was treated using the following methods: (a) M: The machined surface was turned and polished using sandpaper (600–1000 times); (b) SLA: The surface was sandblasted with alumina (Al_2O_3) particles, which were 50 μm in size and acid-etched, using hydrochloric acid and sulfuric acids (SLA surface; Point Implant Co., Seoul, Korea); and (c) M + UV: Machined surface treated with ultraviolet (UV) light. For the disc type, all the three surface treatments were examined for a negative control (M), a positive control (SLA), and an experimental group (M + UV). For the implant type sample, two surface treatments, i.e., the control (SLA) and the experimental group (M + UV), were investigated.

2.1.2. Surface Analysis

Three samples were used in each group for each examination. We performed field emission scanning electron microscopy (FE–SEM; Hitachi S-4700, Hitachi, Tokyo, Japan) for a qualitative evaluation of the overall surface image. This was followed by a confocal laser scanning microscope (CLSM; LSM 800, Carl Zeiss AG, Oberkochen, Germany), where the surface roughness was quantitatively measured. The surface roughness parameters—arithmetical mean height (Sa), root mean square height (Sq), and developed interfacial area ratio (Sdr)—were measured at three randomly selected points in each sample. In addition, the chemical composition was analyzed using electron spectroscopy for chemical analysis (Sigma Probe, Thermo VG, East Grinstead, UK). Furthermore, the surface wettability of the Ti discs was examined using the contact angle from the sessile drop method, as measured by a contact angle meter (Pheonix 150, SEO, Kyunggido, Korea). All the procedures were performed under controlled conditions of 20 °C temperature and 46% humidity.

2.1.3. UV Light Treatment

UV light treatment was achieved by irradiating the Ti discs in a specially manufactured generator using four 15 W bactericidal lamps (G15T8, Sankyo Denki, Tokyo, Japan), for at least 48 h. The intensity was approximately 5 mW/cm^2 ($\lambda = 254 \pm 20$ nm).

2.2. In Vitro Experiment

2.2.1. Cell Culture

Murine pre-osteoblast MC3T3-E1 cells were purchased from ATCC (American Type Culture Collection; Manassas, VA, USA). The cells were seeded onto the discs (1×10^4 cells/well) in a 12-well culture plate (Nunc, Roskilde, Denmark), and then cultured in α-minimum essential medium (α-MEM; Thermo Fisher Scientific, Waltham, MA, USA) supplemented with a 10% fetal bovine serum (FBS) and 1% penicillin/streptomycin. The cells were incubated at 37 °C under a humidified atmosphere of 95% air and 5% CO_2. The culture medium was replaced every three days, and the osteogenic medium contained 10 mM β-glycerophosphate and 50 µg/mL ascorbic acid in the α-MEM.

2.2.2. Cell Attachment

At 24 h after being seeded, the cell attachment was dual-stained using fluorescent dyes: 4′,6-diamidino-2-phenylindole (DAPI; Invitrogen, Carlsbad, CA, USA) and Alexa Fluor 568 phalloidin (Invitrogen, Carlsbad, CA, USA) to detect the nucleus and actin filaments, respectively. Fluorescence was visualized by a CLSM (LSM 800, Carl Zeiss AG, Oberkochen, Germany), and analyzed with the ZEN2010 software (Carl Zeiss, Oberkochen, Germany).

2.2.3. Cell Proliferation

The proliferative activity of cells was measured using a methyl thiazolyl tetrazolium (MTT) assay (Sigma-Aldrich, St. Louis, MO, USA) at 1, 3, and 7 days after being seeded. The culture media was replaced with an MTT solution and incubated for 3 h at 37 °C. After removing the MTT solution, 0.5 mL of 10% dimethyl sulfoxide in isopropanol (iDMSO) was added for 30 min at 37 °C. Then, the proliferation rate was assessed by its optical density (OD) at 570 nm. The value of the OD was measured using a microplate reader (BioTek, Winooski, VT, USA).

2.2.4. Cell Differentiation

Total RNA in the cell cultures was extracted using the TRIzol method described by Chomczynski at 1, 4, 7, 10, and 14 days after osteoblast differentiation [24]. A reverse transcriptase–polymerase chain reaction (RT–PCR) was performed with primer sets for type I collagen (Col), alkaline phosphatase (Alp), and osteocalcin (Ocn), as described in Table 1. Quantitative real-time PCR was performed using a Takara SYBR premix Ex Taq (Takara Bio, Kusatsu, Japan) on a 7500 real-time PCR system (Applied Biosystems, Foster City, CA, USA). Each primer contained a final concentration of 200 nM, and a quantity of cDNA corresponding to 50 ng of total RNA. The PCR primers were synthesized using Integrated DNA Technology (Coralville, IA, USA). According to the manufacturer's instructions, the PCR cycling conditions comprised 40 cycles at 95 °C for 5 s, and 60 °C for 34 s after denaturation at 95 °C for 30 s. The cycle threshold (Ct) values were acquired using the automated threshold analysis in the Sequence Detection software version 1.4 (Applied Biosystems, Foster, CA USA). Each target mRNA expression was calculated using the comparative cycle threshold method according to the manufacturer's instructions. The relative mRNA expression levels were normalized to glyceraldehyde-3-phosphate dehydrogenase (GAPDH). The GAPDH mRNA expression levels remained steady during the osteoblast differentiation, showing similar Ct values.

Table 1. Primer sequences for the reverse transcriptase–polymerase chain reaction (RT–PCR).

Gene	Forward Primer (5′-3′)	Reverse Primer (5′-3′)
Col [1]	GCTCCTCTTAGGGGCCACT	CCACGTCTCACCATTGGGG
Alp [2]	GGCTACATTGGTCTTGAGCTTTT	CCAACTCTTTTGTGCCAGAGA
Ocn [3]	CTGACAAAGCCTTCATGTCCAA	GCGCCGGAGTCTGTTCACTA

[1] Type I collagen; [2] Alkaline phosphatase; [3] Osteocalcin.

2.3. In Vivo Experiment

2.3.1. Animals

The rabbit tibia model was used. All the procedures were conducted with the approval of the Ethics Committee of Animal Experimentation of the Institutional Animal Care and Use Committee (CRONEX-IACUC 201803003; Cronex, Hwasung, Korea), according to the guidelines of Animal Research: Reporting In Vivo Experiments (ARRIVE).

Thereafter, four female New Zealand white rabbits (3–4 months old and 2.5–3.0 kg in weight) were anesthetized via a 1 mL intramuscular injection with a dose of 15 mg/kg of tiletamine/zolazepam (Zoletil 50, Vibrac Korea, Seoul, Korea) and 5 mg/kg of xylazine (Rompun, Bayer Korea, Seoul, Korea). Then the tibiae of the rabbits were shaved and disinfected with povidone iodine solution. Local anesthesia was administered in the surgical area with 2% lidocaine containing 1:100,000 epinephrine (Yuhan Co., Seoul, Korea).

2.3.2. Surgical Procedure

A full-thickness flap was made on the medial side of both tibiae, followed by exposure of the underlying bone. In each tibia, two holes for implant placement were drilled bicortically using implant surgical drills under copious sterile saline irrigation. The diameter of the drills was increased sequentially, with a final drill diameter of 2.8 mm. Then, the implant with a diameter of 3.3 mm was inserted into the hole and engaged bicortically with sufficient stability. The SLA and M + UV implants were allocated to each hole based on a 2 × 2 Latin square randomization. Following the implant placement, the periosteum and fascia were sutured with 4-0 resorbable polyglactin material (Vicryl, Ethicon, Somerville, MA, USA), and the skin was sutured with 4-0 monofilament nylon (Blue nylon, Ailee, Busan, Korea). Post-operatively, each rabbit was kept in a separate cage and administered with 5 mg/kg of enrofloxacin (Komibiotril, Komipharm International Co., Siheung, Korea) for seven days.

2.3.3. Sacrifice and Microcomputed Tomography (Micro-CT)

Two experimental animals were sacrificed at 10 days and the other two animals at 28 days after the surgery by an intravenous overdose of potassium chloride. The implants were surgically harvested en bloc with the surrounding bone. Then the implant–bone blocks were immediately immersed in a 10% neutral buffered formalin fixative. Micro-CT imaging was performed using a SkyScan 1275 (Bruker microCT, Kontich, Belgium). The X-ray source was set at an acceleration voltage of 100 kV and a pixel size of 10 μm. Each sample was scanned three times, using 360° spiral scanning on the SkyScan 1275 with a scanning time of 2 h. Reconstruction was performed using an NRecon (v. 1.7.3.2, Bruker microCT). The region-of-interest (ROI) was defined as the area within consecutive threads engaged in the upper cortical bone (Figure 1a). The analysis was performed using the CTAn software (v. 1.18.4.0, Bruker microCT; Figure 1b), and it also involved the visualization software DataViewer (v. 1.5.4.0, Bruker microCT) and CTVox (v. 3.3.0, Bruker microCT).

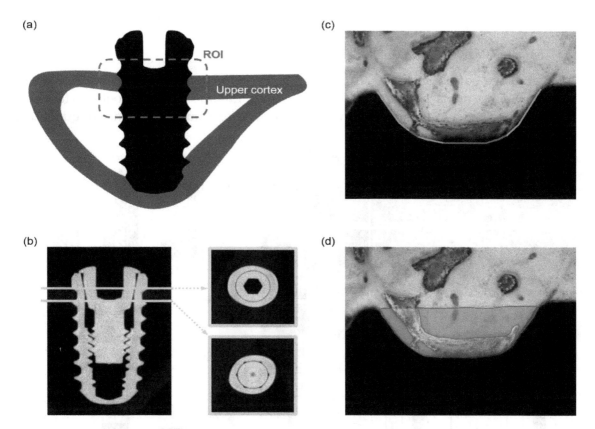

Figure 1. (**a**) The schematic drawing of the region-of-interest (ROI). The ROI was defined as an area within threads engaged in the upper cortical bone (red dot box); (**b**) microcomputed tomography (micro-CT) images for the measurement of the bone-to-implant contact ratio (BIC); (**c**) the bone-to-implant contact ratio (BIC) was calculated by the length of the green line divided by the total length of the well (green and red line); (**d**) the definition of the bone area (BA) was calculated by the area of red color divided by the total area of the well.

2.3.4. Histological Preparation and Histomorphometric Measurement

After μCT scanning, the implant–bone blocks were dehydrated in a series of ethanol with increasing concentrations and then embedded in light-curing resin (Technovit 7200 VLC, Hereaus Kulzer, Hanau, Germany). The embedded blocks were sectioned perpendicular to the longitudinal axis of the implant using the EXAKT system (EXAKT Apparatebau, Norderstedt, Germany), following the method described by Donath and Breuner [25]. The section was then ground to a thickness of 40 μm and stained with hematoxylin and eosin (H&E) for examination using a light microscope. These undecalcified, ground sections were observed under a light microscope (BX51, Olympus, Tokyo, Japan) to measure the BIC and bone area (BA; Figure 1c,d). The region-of-interest (ROI) was defined as the same area that was used in the micro-CT analysis. The measurement was performed under a ×100 magnification, using the SPOT software version 4.0 (Diagnostic Instruments, Sterling Heights, MI, USA) and Image-Pro Plus (Media Cybernetics, Rockville, MD, USA).

2.4. Statistical Analysis

The Kruskal–Wallis test was used to evaluate statistically significant differences amongst the three groups of discs. If there was a significant difference amongst the three groups, the post-hoc Tukey method was applied. To compare the two groups of implants, the Mann–Whitney U test was performed to determine the statistically significant differences. $p < 0.05$ was set as the statistical significance. All statistical analyses were performed using SPSS 20.0 (IBM Corp., Armonk, NY, USA).

3. Results

3.1. Surface Characteristics

In the overall evaluation of the Ti samples via the FE–SEM images, the M and M + UV surfaces showed similar evidence of machine turning (continuous straight traces) with smooth surfaces, although the SLA surface presented a rougher surface with a typical honeycomb appearance (Figures 2a and 3a).

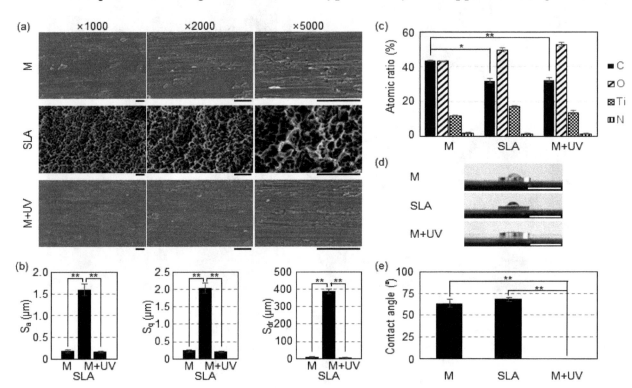

Figure 2. (**a**) Scanning electron microscopy (SEM) images of the Ti discs. M: Machined surface (top row); SLA: Sandblasted with large grit and acid etched surface (middle row); M + UV: machined surface treated with ultraviolet light (bottom row). Scale bars: 10 μm. (**b**) Surface roughness (Sa and Sq) and surface area ratio (Sdr) of the Ti discs evaluated by confocal laser scanning microscopy (CLSM) analysis. The values for the M and M + UV surfaces are similar and smaller than the SLA. (**c**) Element content of the surfaces of the Ti disc according to the energy dispersive x-ray spectrometer (XPS). M + UV shows a significantly lower carbon percentage than the M disc, but there is no significant difference between the SLA and M + UV. (**d**) The changes in wettability of the Ti discs. Superhydrophilicity after UV treatment for 48 h was observed. Scale bars: 10 mm. (**e**) The value of the contact angle of the Ti discs. Without UV treatment, the Ti disc was hydrophobic, but became superhydrophilic (zero degree angle) after UV treatment for 48 h. Error bars show the standard deviation. (*) and (**) represents significance compared with each pair, $p < 0.05$ and $p < 0.01$, respectively.

Surface roughness parameters for the samples are shown in Figures 2b and 3b. In the disc specimen, the SLA surface showed higher Sa, Sq, and Sdr values, and these were significantly different from the M and M + UV surfaces ($p < 0.01$). There was no statistical difference between the M and M + UV surfaces ($p > 0.05$). Similarly, for the implant specimen, the M + UV and SLA surfaces were statistically different across all the parameters ($p < 0.05$).

Chemical compositions from the x-ray spectrometer (XPS) revealed that, compared with the 43.42% ± 0.31% carbon in the M disc, the M + UV disc contained about 32.35% ± 1.50% carbon, which was statistically different ($p = 0.000$). The SLA showed 31.87% ± 1.42% carbon, with no significant difference from the M + UV disc ($p = 0.051$). On the other hand, the M + UV implant showed a significantly lower carbon percentage compared to the SLA implant ($p = 0.049$; Figures 2c and 3c).

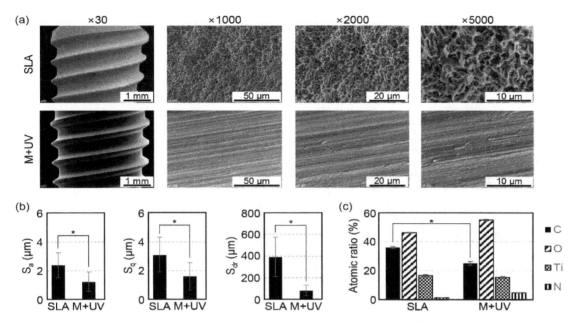

Figure 3. (**a**) Scanning electron microscopy (SEM) images of the Ti implants. SLA: Sandblasted with large grit and acid etched surface (top row); M + UV: Machined surface treated with ultraviolet light (bottom row). Magnification: ×30, ×1000, ×2000, and ×5000 from the left. (**b**) Surface roughness (Sa and Sq) and surface area ratio (Sdr) of the Ti discs according to the confocal laser scanning microscopy (CLSM) analysis. The values of the M + UV surfaces are smaller than the SLA, which means it is smoother than the SLA. (**c**) Element content of the surfaces of the Ti discs according to the energy dispersive x-ray spectrometer (XPS). The M + UV discs contain half of the carbon percentage of the SLA discs. Error bars show the standard deviation. (*) represents the significance compared with each pair, $p < 0.05$.

Contact angle measurement was performed for the disc-type specimens. The M and SLA discs showed a hydrophobic status with angles of 63.6 ± 4.7° and 68.3 ± 2.5°, respectively. On the other hand, 48 h after UV treatment, the M + UV discs showed superhydrophilicity at a 0° contact angle ($p = 0.000$; Figure 2d,e).

3.2. In Vitro Test

3.2.1. Cell Attachment

The CLSM images of the cells are shown in Figure 4a. A wider spread of cells was observed in the M + UV groups compared to the other groups. In the SLA discs, the cells were sharp and needle-like shaped, implying that the osteoblasts were not prone to attach to the SLA surfaces.

3.2.2. Cell Proliferation

The MTT assay showed that the amount of cells increased in a time-dependent way on all the surfaces. On the M + UV surface, the cells proliferated more significantly than the other surfaces at days 1, 3, and 7, with a p-value of less than 0.01, as shown in Figure 4b. On day 7, the amount of cells on the M + UV surface was two times greater than cells on the SLA surface (0.068 ± 0.0005 vs. 0.040 ± 0.001, $p = 0.000$). In particular, at day 3 and 7, the cells proliferated more on the M surface than on the SLA surface.

3.2.3. Quantitative Assessment of the Osteogenic Markers

Figure 4c shows the relative mRNA expression of Col, Alp, and Ocn. The RT–PCR analysis showed that Col was more significantly expressed on the M + UV and SLA surfaces at days 7, 10, and 14 compared to the M surface, although the M + UV and SLA surfaces were not significantly different.

The expression level of Alp on the SLA surface was not different from the M + UV surface at days 1 and 4, but it was significantly higher than the expression levels at days 7, 10, and 14. The M + UV surface expressed the Alp gene more than the M surface at days 4, 7, and 14. The expression level of Ocn on the M + UV surface was significantly higher at day 7, but it was lower at days 10 and 14.

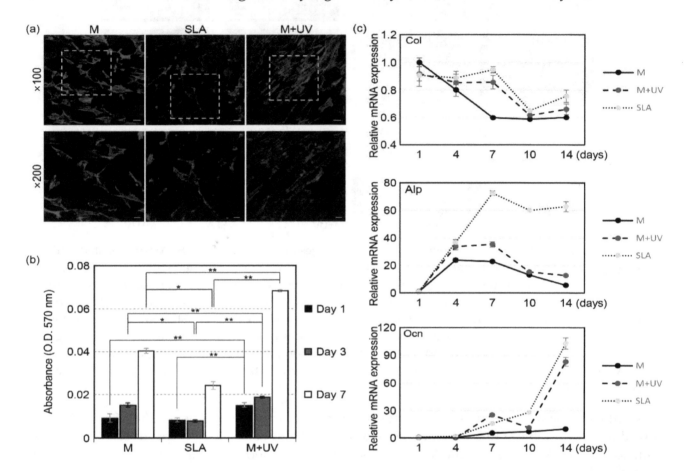

Figure 4. (**a**) Confocal microscopic images of the MC3T3-E1 cells, 24 h after being seeded on the Ti discs. The areas in the dotted box are magnified in the bottom row. Scale bars: 50 μm at ×100 and 20 μm at ×200 magnification. (**b**) Evaluation of cell proliferation of the MC3T3-E1 cells by an MTT assay at 1, 3, and 7 days after being seeded on the Ti discs. (**c**) Evaluation of the cell differentiation of MC3T3-E1 cells by real-time PCR at 1, 4, 7, 10, and 14 days after being seeded on the Ti discs. The relative mRNA expression levels were normalized to glyceraldehyde-3-phosphate dehydrogenase (GAPDH). The osteogenic markers are type I collagen (top), alkaline phosphatase (ALP, middle), and osteocalcin (OCN, bottom). UV photofunctionalization enhanced the osteoblastic gene expression. Error bars show the standard deviation. (*) and (**) represent the significance compared with each pair, $p < 0.05$ and $p < 0.01$, respectively.

3.3. In Vivo Test

3.3.1. Histomorphometry

All the implants were successfully osseointegrated at days 10 and 28 (Figure 5a). At day 10, the BIC ratios of the M + UV implants (55.93% ± 6.19%) were significantly higher than that of the SLA implants (43.38% ± 3.20%, $p = 0.021$). However, at day 28, the BIC ratios of the M + UV implants (64.88% ± 5.35%) were not significantly different from that of the SLA implants (59.93% ± 6.44%, $p = 0.149$; Figure 5b).

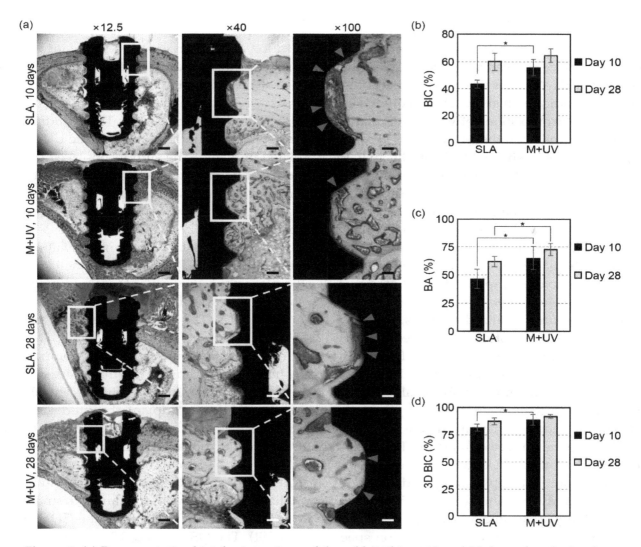

Figure 5. (a) Representative histologic sections of the rabbit tibia at 10 and 28 days after the implant placement. In the SLA implant, the osteoblast and organic matrix, which had not mineralized yet, was more observable on the interface between the bone and implant compared to the M + UV implant (red arrow head; magnification ×12.5, ×40, and ×100 from the left, hematoxylin and eosin staining). The scale bars: 1 mm at ×12.5, 200 μm at ×40, and 100 μm at ×100 magnification. (b) The bone-to-implant contact ratio (BIC) was evaluated histologically at days 10 and 28. The M + UV implant shows a significantly higher BIC than the SLA at day 10, but there is no significant difference at day 28. (c) The bone area ratio (BA) evaluated histologically at 10 and 28 days. The M + UV implants show significantly more BA than the SLA at days 10 and 28. (d) The bone-to-implant contact ratio evaluated by micro-CT (3D BIC) at days 10 and 28. The M + UV implants show a significantly higher 3D BIC than the SLA at day 10, but there is no significant difference at day 28. Error bars show the standard deviation. (*) represents the significance compared with each pair, $p < 0.05$.

In terms of the BA, the M + UV implants were significantly higher compared to the SLA implants (46.55% ± 8.59%) at day 10 (65.09% ± 10.42% vs. 46.55% ± 8.59%, $p = 0.042$) and at day 28 (72.70% ± 5.52% vs. 61.83% ± 4.89%, $p = 0.043$; Figure 5c).

3.3.2. Micro-CT

The three-dimensional BIC was evaluated using micro-CT. The micro-CT analysis revealed that the three-dimensional BIC of the M + UV implants was significantly higher than that of the SLA implants at day 10 (88.87% ± 5.1% vs. 81.6% ± 3.28%, $p = 0.046$), but it was not statistically different at day 28 (91.91% ± 1.55% vs. 87.47% ± 2.93%, $p = 0.201$; Figure 5d).

4. Discussion

In this study, we found that UV photofunctionalization on a Ti screw-shaped implant with an M + UV surface showed a higher BIC than the SLA surface at day 10, and there was no significant difference at day 28. This was confirmed in both two-dimensional and three-dimensional measurements. The results indicated that the UV photofunctionalization could accelerate the osseointegration process, and achieve firm fixation between the implant and the surrounding bone earlier. These findings are supported by other studies, where Park et al. found that after four months of healing, the UV-treated implants in rabbits showed a higher BIC than the untreated implants. The authors observed that UV treatment decreased both carbon impurities on the surface and water contact angles [26]. Similarly, Aita et al. showed that the UV-treated acid-etched implants at week two had a push-in value equivalent to the untreated acid-etched implant [18]. Pyo et al. measured the removal torque test in UV-treated implants and showed that it was 50% higher than in untreated implants [27]. Hirota et al. retrospectively studied and found that the use of photofunctionalization reduced the risk of early implant failure with an odds ratio of 0.30 ($p < 0.05$) [28]. Soltanzadeh studied the effect of UV photofunctionalization on immediately loaded implants in a rat model. After the placement, the implants were immediately loaded with 0.46 N of static lateral force. The results showed that osseointegration was successful in 100% of photofunctionalized implants, but 28.6% of untreated ones. The value of the push-in test was 2.4 times higher in photofunctionalized implants [29].

Histologically, the BA was significantly higher at days 10 and 28 in the M + UV compared to the SLA implants, meaning that the M + UV implant had a higher amount of mineralized bones between threads of implants. Pyo et al. evaluated the osteogenic dynamics using fluorescent labeling at four weeks after implant placement; and found that in the UV-treated implant, the interfacial areas between the bone and implant and the areas within the threads were filled with calcein-positive tissues compared to the untreated implants. This meant that UV photofunctionalization could lead to earlier bone deposition [27]. Ueno et al. showed that the UV-treated acid-etched implant had a marked bone formation in a gap healing model without cortical support [20]. Kitajima et al. measured the implant stability quotients (ISQ) for 55 photofunctionalized implants with low and extremely low initial stability at the time of placement and stage-two surgery. Then they calculated the ISQ increase per month, defining the osseointegration speed index (OSI). The OSI ranged 3.9–4.7 substantially higher than the OSIs for untreated implants reported in other literatures (0.36–2.8) [30]. Ijishima et al. evaluated the effect of photofunctionalization on aged rats. The aged rats showed considerably lower biological capabilities (cell attachment, proliferation, and ALP activity) than the young. However, the enhancement of cell attachment and differentiation were observed on the photofunctionalized Ti discs compared with untreated one. Moreover, in the femurs of aged rats, the photofunctionalized mini-implant showed the higher push-in value than untreated one after two weeks of healing. These findings supported that UV photofunctionalization could be also valuable in the compromised sites [31].

Generally, the surface roughness is considered as a main factor for the improvement of osseointegration. However, in this study, UV treatment did not physically change any surface roughness as shown in the SEM and CLSM. Rather, it induced superhydrophilicity (0° angle), reduced the percentage of hydrocarbons, and increased the osteoblast proliferation, attachment, and differentiation, as shown in the in vitro study. This indicated that the only physico-chemical changes in the Ti surface could enhance the biological activities. In the XPS analysis, Roy et al. found that UVC photon energy decreased carbon deposition and the amount of H_2O on Ti surface, and produced many –OH groups (TiOH) without any changes in surface topography. They explained that, through these chemical changes, the UV photofunctionalization could create the superhydrophilicity of Ti. The improvement of biological capabilities by UV photofunctionalization was supported by other studies [32]. Aita et al. showed that Col and osteopontin (Opn) were more expressed in the UV-treated discs [18]. The RT–PCR analysis performed by Zhang et al. showed that the expression of genes encoding Col, Runx2, BMP, and Opn increased in the UV-treated surface [33]. In contrast, Att et al. assessed the RT–PCR of genes for Opn and Ocn in bone marrow cells derived from the femur of eight-week-old male Sprague-Dawley rats, and found that there was no significant difference at days 10 and 20. The differences may have been caused by the kinds of cells, time points, and intensity and wavelength of the UV generator. Further research is required to elucidate this aspect.

With regard to plaque accumulation and peri-implant disease, the implant with a smooth surface is considered to be superior to an implant with a rough surface. Berglundh et al. observed that, at five months after the removal of ligature, bone loss accelerated in the SLA implant but not in the polished implant. Histologically, the size of the inflammatory lesion and the area of plaque were larger in the SLA surface [12]. Additionally, Albouy et al. compared the turned and the roughened implant (Ti-Unite), at six months after the ligature removal, and observed a larger amount of bone loss in the Ti-Unite implant compared to the turned implant (1.47 mm vs. 0.3 mm). This meant that spontaneous progression of peri-implantitis had occurred in the implant with a rough surface [17]. However, the machined implant had a definite drawback in that it had a low BIC level, because the osteoblastic differentiation was lower compared to the smooth surface [34,35]. Therefore, the enhancement of osteoblastic differentiation on the Ti with an M surface by UV photofunctionalization is considered to be inspired. Additionally, UV photofunctionalization itself could decrease plaque formation on Ti surface. De Avila et al. found that after 16 h incubation, there were significantly lower oral bacterial attachment on the UV-treated Ti disc compared to the untreated one [36].

The hydrophilicity of the implant surface can be induced by UV photofunctionalization [18–20,27,37] or preservation in a storage medium [38–40]. Both methods are effective and can improve the bone healing process and attain early osseointegration. However, the latter method has been reported to lead to foreign deposition and little elimination of hydrocarbons on the Ti surface. Moreover, the saline storage method is inferior to UV photofunctionalization in osteoblast spreading and adhesion [41]. Considering this point, UV treatment is considered a safer method to modify the implant surface to make it hydrophilic. On the other hand, Att et al. mentioned that, in UV photofunctionalization, the superhydrophilicity is not a significant factor in explaining the higher BIC in the UV-treated Ti discs compared to the acid-etched ones. The elimination of hydrocarbon on the surface was considered to be a significant factor [19]. The aging of the Ti is related to the contamination and accumulation of the hydrocarbon on the Ti surface, and it can suppress cell recruitment and biologic activity [42,43].

The combination of variables such as duration, intensity, and wavelength can create various modes of UV photofunctionalization, noting that the optimal combination is a controversial issue. The exposure time has been used from 12 min to 48 h [44,45]. However, Aita et al. and Att et al. have shown that, between 24 and 48 h, there was an increase in hydrophilicity and biological effects [18,19]. Additionally, treatment with UVC ($\lambda = 240 \pm 40$ nm) has shown more biological improvements compared to UVA ($\lambda = 360 \pm 40$ nm). Consequently, in our experiment, to maximize the effects of UV, the mode of UV photofunctionalization was determined as UVC treatment for 48 h.

There are still several questions regarding UV photofunctionalization. Strictly, the UV light treatment used in this study may be called physical photo-activation, rather than functionalization, because no chemical application to the surface, which have been shown in the previous studies, were used for enhanced bone response [11,46]. More obvious concept of the UV surface treatment needs to be established in the physical and chemical aspects. Amongst several factors following UV photofunctionalization, we also still need to identify the main factors for the enhancement of biological activity, superhydrophilicity, and removal of hydrocarbon. If they contribute to the improvement, there is a need to understand the mechanism through which they are inter-connected. Therefore, further studies are needed to fully appreciate the effects of UV photofunctionalization.

5. Conclusions

Within the limitations of the present study, UV photofunctionalization of a Ti dental implant with an M surface attained an earlier osseointegration compared to an implant with an SLA surface. The enhancement was considered to result from the superhydrophilicity, the elimination of hydrocarbon on the surface, and the improvement of osteoblastic activities.

Author Contributions: Conceptualization, J.-B.L., I.-C.R., I.-S.L.Y.; methodology, J.-B.L., Y.-H.C., J.-Y.C., I.-S.L.Y.; software, J.-B.L., Y.-H.C.; validation, I.-C.R., I.-S.L.Y.; formal analysis, J.-B.L., I.-S.L.Y.; investigation, J.-B.L., Y.-H.C., J.-Y.C.; resources, J.-Y.C., Y.-J.S., I.-C.R., I.-S.L.Y.; data curation, J.-B.L., J.-Y.C.; writing—original draft preparation, J.-B.L.; writing—review and editing, Y.-H.C., J.-Y.C., Y.-J.S., Y.-M.L., Y.K., I.-C.R., I.-S.L.Y.; visualization, J.-B.L., J.-Y.C.; supervision, I.-C.R., I.-S.L.Y.; project administration, I.-S.L.Y.; funding acquisition, I.-S.L.Y.

Acknowledgments: The authors greatly thank Kyoung-Hwa Kim and Young-Dan Cho for the material preparation and support.

References

1.   Henry, P.J. Oral implant restoration for enhanced oral function. *Clin. Exp. Pharmacol. Physiol.* **2005**, *32*, 123–127. [CrossRef] [PubMed]
2.   Srinivasan, M.; Meyer, S.; Mombelli, A.; Müller, F. Dental implants in the elderly population: A systematic review and meta-analysis. *Clin. Oral Implant. Res.* **2017**, *28*, 920–930. [CrossRef] [PubMed]
3.   De Angelis, F.; Papi, P.; Mencio, F.; Rosella, D.; Di Carlo, S.; Pompa, G. Implant survival and success rates in patients with risk factors: Results from a long-term retrospective study with a 10 to 18 years follow-up. *Eur. Rev. Med. Pharmacol. Sci.* **2017**, *21*, 433–437. [PubMed]
4.   Albrektsson, T.; Branemark, P.I.; Hansson, H.A.; Lindstrom, J. Osseointegrated titanium implants. Requirements for ensuring a long-lasting, direct bone-to-implant anchorage in man. *Acta Orthop. Scand.* **1981**, *52*, 155–170. [CrossRef]
5.   Gallucci, G.O.; Hamilton, A.; Zhou, W.; Buser, D.; Chen, S. Implant placement and loading protocols in partially edentulous patients: A systematic review. *Clin. Oral Implant. Res.* **2018**, *29*, 106–134. [CrossRef]
6.   Chrcanovic, B.R.; Kisch, J.; Albrektsson, T.; Wennerberg, A. Factors Influencing Early Dental Implant Failures. *J. Dent. Res.* **2016**, *95*, 995–1002. [CrossRef] [PubMed]
7.   Manzano, G.; Montero, J.; Martin-Vallejo, J.; Del Fabbro, M.; Bravo, M.; Testori, T. Risk Factors in Early Implant Failure: A Meta-Analysis. *Implant Dent.* **2016**, *25*, 272–280. [CrossRef] [PubMed]
8.   Diz, P.; Scully, C.; Sanz, M. Dental implants in the medically compromised patient. *J. Dent.* **2013**, *41*, 195–206. [CrossRef]
9.   Chrcanovic, B.R.; Albrektsson, T.; Wennerberg, A. Bone Quality and Quantity and Dental Implant Failure: A Systematic Review and Meta-analysis. *Int. J. Prosthodont.* **2017**, *30*, 219–237. [CrossRef]
10.   Neves, J.; de Araujo Nobre, M.; Oliveira, P.; Martins Dos Santos, J.; Malo, P. Risk Factors for Implant Failure and Peri-Implant Pathology in Systemic Compromised Patients. *J. Prosthodont.* **2018**, *27*, 409–415. [CrossRef]
11.   Albrektsson, T.; Wennerberg, A. Oral implant surfaces: Part 1—Review focusing on topographic and chemical properties of different surfaces and in vivo responses to them. *Int. J. Prosthodont.* **2004**, *17*, 536–543. [PubMed]
12.   Berglundh, T.; Gotfredsen, K.; Zitzmann, N.U.; Lang, N.P.; Lindhe, J. Spontaneous progression of ligature induced peri-implantitis at implants with different surface roughness: An experimental study in dogs. *Clin. Oral Implant. Res.* **2007**, *18*, 655–661. [CrossRef] [PubMed]
13.   Albouy, J.P.; Abrahamsson, I.; Persson, L.G.; Berglundh, T. Spontaneous progression of peri-implantitis at different types of implants. An experimental study in dogs. I: Clinical and radiographic observations. *Clin. Oral Implant. Res.* **2008**, *19*, 997–1002. [CrossRef] [PubMed]
14.   Rasmusson, L.; Kahnberg, K.E.; Tan, A. Effects of implant design and surface on bone regeneration and implant stability: An experimental study in the dog mandible. *Clin. Implant Dent. Relat. Res.* **2001**, *3*, 2–8. [CrossRef] [PubMed]
15.   Wennerberg, A.; Albrektsson, T. Effects of titanium surface topography on bone integration: A systematic review. *Clin. Oral Implant. Res.* **2009**, *20*, 172–184. [CrossRef] [PubMed]
16.   Feller, L.; Jadwat, Y.; Khammissa, R.A.; Meyerov, R.; Schechter, I.; Lemmer, J. Cellular responses evoked by different surface characteristics of intraosseous titanium implants. *Biomed. Res. Int.* **2015**, *2015*, 171945. [CrossRef]
17.   Albouy, J.P.; Abrahamsson, I.; Berglundh, T. Spontaneous progression of experimental peri-implantitis at implants with different surface characteristics: An experimental study in dogs. *J. Clin. Periodontol.* **2012**, *39*, 182–187. [CrossRef]
18.   Aita, H.; Hori, N.; Takeuchi, M.; Suzuki, T.; Yamada, M.; Anpo, M.; Ogawa, T. The effect of ultraviolet functionalization of titanium on integration with bone. *Biomaterials* **2009**, *30*, 1015–1025. [CrossRef]

19. Att, W.; Hori, N.; Iwasa, F.; Yamada, M.; Ueno, T.; Ogawa, T. The effect of UV-photofunctionalization on the time-related bioactivity of titanium and chromium-cobalt alloys. *Biomaterials* **2009**, *30*, 4268–4276. [CrossRef]

20. Ueno, T.; Yamada, M.; Suzuki, T.; Minamikawa, H.; Sato, N.; Hori, N.; Takeuchi, K.; Hattori, M.; Ogawa, T. Enhancement of bone-titanium integration profile with UV-photofunctionalized titanium in a gap healing model. *Biomaterials* **2010**, *31*, 1546–1557. [CrossRef]

21. Keleher, J.; Bashant, J.; Heldt, N.; Johnson, L.; Li, Y. Photo-catalytic preparation of silver-coated TiO_2 particles for antibacterial applications. *World J. Microbiol. Biotechnol.* **2002**, *18*, 133–139. [CrossRef]

22. Nakashima, T.; Ohko, Y.; Kubota, Y.; Fujishima, A. Photocatalytic decomposition of estrogens in aquatic environment by reciprocating immersion of TiO_2-modified polytetrafluoroethylene mesh sheets. *J. Photochem. Photobiol. A Chem.* **2003**, *160*, 115–120. [CrossRef]

23. Wang, R.; Hashimoto, K.; Fujishima, A.; Chikuni, M.; Kojima, E.; Kitamura, A.; Shimohigoshi, M.; Watanabe, T. Light-induced amphiphilic surfaces. *Nature* **1997**, *388*, 431. [CrossRef]

24. Chomczynski, P.; Mackey, K. Short technical reports. Modification of the TRI reagent procedure for isolation of RNA from polysaccharide-and proteoglycan-rich sources. *Biotechniques* **1995**, *19*, 942–945. [PubMed]

25. Donath, K.; Breuner, G. A method for the study of undecalcified bones and teeth with attached soft tissues * The Säge-Schliff (sawing and grinding) Technique. *J. Oral Pathol.* **1982**, *11*, 318–326. [CrossRef]

26. Park, K.H.; Koak, J.Y.; Kim, S.K.; Han, C.H.; Heo, S.J. The effect of ultraviolet-C irradiation via a bactericidal ultraviolet sterilizer on an anodized titanium implant: A study in rabbits. *Int. J. Oral Maxillofac. Implant.* **2013**, *28*, 57–66. [CrossRef] [PubMed]

27. Pyo, S.W.; Park, Y.B.; Moon, H.S.; Lee, J.H.; Ogawa, T. Photofunctionalization enhances bone-implant contact, dynamics of interfacial osteogenesis, marginal bone seal, and removal torque value of implants: A dog jawbone study. *Implant Dent.* **2013**, *22*, 666–675. [CrossRef] [PubMed]

28. Hirota, M.; Ozawa, T.; Iwai, T.; Ogawa, T.; Tohnai, I. Effect of Photofunctionalization on Early Implant Failure. *Int. J. Oral Maxillofac. Implant.* **2018**, *33*, 1098–1102. [CrossRef]

29. Soltanzadeh, P.; Ghassemi, A.; Ishijima, M.; Tanaka, M.; Park, W.; Iwasaki, C.; Hirota, M.; Ogawa, T. Success rate and strength of osseointegration of immediately loaded UV-photofunctionalized implants in a rat model. *J. Prosthet. Dent.* **2017**, *118*, 357–362. [CrossRef]

30. Kitajima, H.; Ogawa, T. The Use of Photofunctionalized Implants for Low or Extremely Low Primary Stability Cases. . *Int. J. Oral Maxillofac. Implant.* **2016**, *31*, 439–447. [CrossRef]

31. Ishijima, M.; Ghassemi, A.; Soltanzadeh, P.; Tanaka, M.; Nakhaei, K.; Park, W.; Hirota, M.; Tsukimura, N.; Ogawa, T. Effect of UV Photofunctionalization on Osseointegration in Aged Rats. *Implant Dent.* **2016**, *25*, 744–750. [CrossRef] [PubMed]

32. Roy, M.; Pompella, A.; Kubacki, J.; Szade, J.; Roy, R.A.; Hedzelek, W. Photofunctionalization of Titanium: An Alternative Explanation of Its Chemical-Physical Mechanism. *PLoS ONE* **2016**, *11*, e0157481. [CrossRef] [PubMed]

33. Zhang, H.; Komasa, S.; Mashimo, C.; Sekino, T.; Okazaki, J. Effect of ultraviolet treatment on bacterial attachment and osteogenic activity to alkali-treated titanium with nanonetwork structures. *Int. J. Nanomed.* **2017**, *12*, 4633–4646. [CrossRef] [PubMed]

34. Bowers, K.T.; Keller, J.C.; Randolph, B.A.; Wick, D.G.; Michaels, C.M. Optimization of surface micromorphology for enhanced osteoblast responses in vitro. *Int. J. Oral Maxillofac. Implant.* **1992**, *7*, 302–310. [CrossRef]

35. Keller, J.C.; Schneider, G.B.; Stanford, C.M.; Kellogg, B. Effects of implant microtopography on osteoblast cell attachment. *Implant Dent.* **2003**, *12*, 175–181. [CrossRef] [PubMed]

36. De Avila, E.D.; Lima, B.P.; Sekiya, T.; Torii, Y.; Ogawa, T.; Shi, W.; Lux, R. Effect of UV-photofunctionalization on oral bacterial attachment and biofilm formation to titanium implant material. *Biomaterials* **2015**, *67*, 84–92. [CrossRef] [PubMed]

37. Sawase, T.; Jimbo, R.; Baba, K.; Shibata, Y.; Ikeda, T.; Atsuta, M. Photo-induced hydrophilicity enhances initial cell behavior and early bone apposition. *Clin. Oral Implant. Res.* **2008**, *19*, 491–496. [CrossRef] [PubMed]

38. Buser, D.; Broggini, N.; Wieland, M.; Schenk, R.; Denzer, A.; Cochran, D.L.; Hoffmann, B.; Lussi, A.; Steinemann, S. Enhanced bone apposition to a chemically modified SLA titanium surface. *J. Dent. Res.* **2004**, *83*, 529–533. [CrossRef] [PubMed]

39. Ehlers, H.; Jacobs, F.; Kloppers, H.; Postma, T. The influence of storage media on early osseointegration of titanium implants. *J. Dent. Implant* **2016**, *6*, 3–12. [CrossRef]

40. Wennerberg, A.; Galli, S.; Albrektsson, T. Current knowledge about the hydrophilic and nanostructured SLActive surface. *Clin. Cosmet. Investig. Dent.* **2011**, *3*, 59–67. [CrossRef]

41. Ghassemi, A.; Ishijima, M.; Hasegawa, M.; Mohammadzadeh Rezaei, N.; Nakhaei, K.; Sekiya, T.; Torii, Y.; Hirota, M.; Park, W.; Miley, D.D.; et al. Biological and Physicochemical Characteristics of 2 Different Hydrophilic Surfaces Created by Saline-Storage and Ultraviolet Treatment. *Implant Dent.* **2018**, *27*, 405–414. [CrossRef] [PubMed]

42. Kasemo, B.; Lausmaa, J. Biomaterial and implant surfaces: On the role of cleanliness, contamination, and preparation procedures. *J. Biomed. Mater. Res.* **1988**, *22*, 145–158. [CrossRef] [PubMed]

43. Serro, A.; Saramago, B. Influence of sterilization on the mineralization of titanium implants induced by incubation in various biological model fluids. *Biomaterials* **2003**, *24*, 4749–4760. [CrossRef]

44. Choi, S.H.; Jeong, W.S.; Cha, J.Y.; Lee, J.H.; Lee, K.J.; Yu, H.S.; Choi, E.H.; Kim, K.M.; Hwang, C.J. Overcoming the biological aging of titanium using a wet storage method after ultraviolet treatment. *Sci. Rep.* **2017**, *7*, 3833. [CrossRef] [PubMed]

45. Flanagan, D. Photofunctionalization of Dental Implant. *J. Oral Implantol.* **2016**, *42*, 445–450. [CrossRef] [PubMed]

46. Shayganpour, A.; Rebaudi, A.; Cortella, P.; Diaspro, A.; Salerno, M. Electrochemical coating of dental implants with anodic porous titania for enhanced osteointegration. *Beilstein J. Nanotechnol.* **2015**, *6*, 2183–2192. [CrossRef] [PubMed]

10

Etiology and Measurement of Peri-Implant Crestal Bone Loss (CBL)

Adrien Naveau [1,2], Kouhei Shinmyouzu [3,4], Colman Moore [5], Limor Avivi-Arber [6], Jesse Jokerst [5,7,8] and Sreenivas Koka [9,10,11,*]

[1] Department of Prosthodontics, Dental Science Faculty, University of Bordeaux, 33000 Bordeaux, France; Adrien.naveau@laposte.net

[2] Dental and Periodontal Rehabilitation Unit, Saint Andre Hospital, Bordeaux University Hospital, 33000 Bordeaux, France

[3] Department of Oral Implants, Kyushu Dental University, Kitakyushu, Fukuoka 803-8580, Japan; k.shinmyouzu@spice.ocn.ne.jp

[4] Tanpopo Dental Clinic, Nerima ward, Tokyo 178-0062, Japan

[5] Department of NanoEngineering, University of California San Diego, La Jolla, CA 92093, USA; cam081@eng.ucsd.edu (C.M.); jjokerst@eng.ucsd.edu (J.J.)

[6] Faculty of Dentistry, University of Toronto, Toronto M5G1G6, ON M5G 1G6, Canada; Limor.Avivi-Arber@dentistry.utoronto.ca

[7] Materials Science Program, University of California San Diego, La Jolla, CA 92093, USA

[8] Department of Radiology, University of California San Diego, La Jolla, CA 92093, USA

[9] Private practice, Koka Dental Clinic, San Diego, CA 92111, USA

[10] Advanced Prosthodontics, Loma Linda University School of Dentistry, Loma Linda, CA 92350, USA

[11] Advanced Prosthodontics, University of California Los Angeles School of Dentistry, Los Angeles, CA 90095, USA

* Correspondence: skoka66@gmail.com

Abstract: The etiology of peri-implant crestal bone loss is today better understood and certain factors proposed in the past have turned out to not be of concern. Regardless, the incidence of crestal bone loss remains higher than necessary and this paper reviews current theory on the etiology with a special emphasis on traditional and innovative methods to assess the level of crestal bone around dental implants that will enable greater sensitivity and specificity and significantly reduce variability in bone loss measurement.

Keywords: Crestal bone loss; osseosufficiency; osseoseparation; peri-implantitis; photoacoustic ultrasound; brain–bone axis; foreign body reaction; overloading; radiography; CBCT (cone beam computerized tomography)

1. Introduction

Crestal bone loss (CBL) was relatively uncommon and non-progressing with the commercially pure titanium implants with a machined surface introduced by Per-Ingvar Branemark. It was accepted in the late 1980s and 1990s that 1 mm of CBL could be expected in the first year after implant placement and then 0.2 mm of CBL on average might occur after that. In fact, an adage took hold that with these implants, CBL to between the first and second thread is common after which time bone levels remained remarkably stable for years.

Predictably, as the application of the initial wave of implants was so successful, an expansion of clinical scenarios amenable to dental implant therapy took place. Following on, an expansion of the clinical provider pool considered appropriate to place and restore implants took place. Finally, "innovations" to the dental implant systems with the goal of fostering the expansion of clinical scenarios and provider pool also took place. Unfortunately, despite the noblest of intentions, and indeed some not so noble, the number of complications associated with dental implant therapy reported today is high. Indeed, it is far higher than necessary, and puts patients at unnecessary, and hence unjustifiable, risk for suboptimal clinical outcomes including implant loss, biological tissue loss, financial loss, and psychological trauma.

Koka and Zarb first proposed the concept of osseosufficiency to describe the role of the interplay between clinician, patient, and implant system inasmuch as promoting and perpetuating osseointegration [1]. In this model, if the combination of the ingredients that clinician (skill, knowledge, experience), patient (genetic, environmental, behavioral), and implant system (design, material) are "enough" to promote and perpetuate osseointegration, a state of osseosufficiency is attained. If the combination of ingredients is "not enough", a state of osseoinsufficiency results. Although it is commonplace to attribute implant loss as representing "implant failure", this is clearly not the case in most instances where implants are retrieved from jawbones, the main exception being when an implant body fractures. To state that an implant failed implies that the implant was at fault for its retrieval and assigns blame for the undesirable outcome to the one ingredient in the osseointegration recipe that is the most predictable and by far, compared to patient and clinician, the least variable. Conveniently, it is also the one element that is unable to defend itself in conversations about why an implant was retrieved. Clearly, albeit an uncomfortable state of affairs, most complications in implant therapy are clinician-dependent (inexperience, incompetence, or ignorance) and the remainder are patient-dependent or a combination of clinician and patient factors. Therefore, throughout this manuscript, the term "implant failure" will not be used. In the place of "implant failure", terms like "implant retrieval", "implant removal", or "implant loss" will be used to more accurately describe the clinical outcome and to avoid inaccurate assignment of blame.

One manifestation of osseoinsufficiency that has significant clinical ramifications is peri-implant CBL because it can lead to implant retrieval, osseous deformation, soft tissue deformation, esthetic compromise, and a dissatisfied/upset patient who loses confidence in their clinical provider. Clearly, prevention is better than cure when it comes to peri-implant CBL as effective and predictable methods to restore lost bone remain elusive.

Crestal bone loss has been postulated to have a multi-factorial etiology [2] and can be considered to occur early or late in the lifetime of a dental implant. Here, early means within the first year after placement and CBL observed is a consequence of bone remodeling subsequent to surgical and restorative procedures and early loading challenges undertaken by an implant and its associated prosthesis [2,3]. Given the role of adaptive bone remodeling, early CBL is not necessarily influenced by infection from oral microflora. Over the longer term, the cumulative effect of chronic etiological factors that are immunological (foreign body reaction), environmental, including patient factors such as motivation, smoking, bruxism, and infection/inflammation, and the influence of clinician (surgeon/prosthodontist) may influence late CBL [2–5]. Given that other manuscripts in this volume will address different etiological factors of CBL, in Section A, this manuscript will provide a summary of current knowledge related to two common etiological factors, mechanical overloading and periodontopathogens/perimplantopathogens/bacteria. It will also discuss the role of the immune system through the foreign body reaction mechanisms that lie at the heart of osseointegration, and describe how adverse immune reactions and a tantalizing new potential mechanism involving the brain–bone axis may lead to CBL. In Section B, it will focus on a key and related issue of how CBL is currently measured and how it can be improved in the future.

2. Section A. Selected Etiological Factors in Crestal Bone Loss

2.1. Overloading

After an implant body osseointegrates and is exposed to functional loading, Esposito et al. reported that overload of the implant prosthesis may lead to implant loss. Furthermore, the report suggests that overload contributes to peri-implantitis and is one of the major determinants of late implant retrieval [6].

There are a wide variety of experimental reports about overloading and implant therapy including computer simulations, such as finite element analysis, and in vivo and in vitro experiment. However, the results are inconclusive regarding the strength and validity of the evidence clearly linking overloading to CBL. Here, we consider the clinical significance of overloading in peri-implant CBL.

What is 'overloading'? 'Overloading' is difficult to describe but could be considered to be the force level and/or nature of force application that exceeds the permissible or tolerable range of the prosthetic and biological resistance to CBL. Each patient presents with a unique prosthetic and biological resistance profile and reference ranges of permissibility are, as yet, unknown. Hence, predicting who will be more or less susceptible to the effects of overloading is difficult. Most reports draw a conclusion of overloading based on the findings of a complication (fracture of the prosthesis, marginal bone loss etc.) as a post hoc event. Nevertheless, the complication is a result of distortion between implant and marginal bone interface caused by stress applied to the structural components of the implant prosthesis instead of the occlusal bite force itself.

Notationally, 0.1% deformation in volume is transcribed to 1000 με (microstrain). Frost et al. divided the reaction of bone as a result of strain application into four phases or "windows" according to the amount of distortion between bone and implant (Figure 1). (i) Disuse atrophy window (50–100 με). Bone resorption may result in this phase where the net effect of bone formation and resorption is negative; (ii) Steady state window (100–1500 με). Here, the net volume of the bone remains steady; (iii) Mild overload window (1500–3000 με). Here, the net effect of bone formation and resorption is positive and bone volume increases; (iv) Fatigue failure window (>3000 με). Here, bone resorption and destruction occur [6].

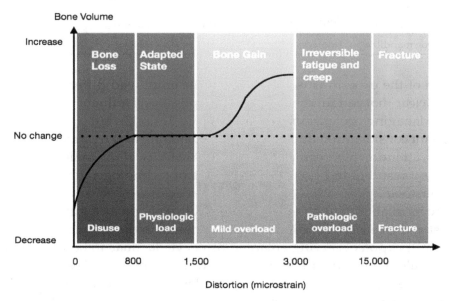

Figure 1. Diagram showing clinical effect on bone relative to strain level applied.

Theoretically, when we classify the reaction of bone to force application/distortion at the implant–bone interface, we can use Frost's definition of overload, the fatigue failure window. However, Naert et al. noted that the definition of overload in implant dentistry is more complex, open to interpretation and they suggested the range of distortion represented by Frost's fatigue failure window does not accurately represent the over load in the clinical situation [7].

Past reports focused on overload and CBL are presented in Table 1. Isidor et al. reported on crestal bone reaction following excessive occlusal load or plaque accumulation in monkeys. In this report, 6 months after insertion of implants, a fixed partial prosthesis was mounted and there were two experimental groups: Excessive occlusal over load and plaque accumulation. A loss of osseointegration and/or CBL was observed 4.5 months to 15.5 months after overloading was initiated. None of the implants with plaque accumulation experienced CBL [8]. Miyata et al. reported the influence of controlled occlusal overload on peri-implant tissue, again in monkeys and in this model, supra-occlusal contact was applied for four weeks to implants starting fourteen weeks after insertion. Neither inflammation nor CBL was observed when supra-occlusal contact was of approximately 100 microns. In contrast, CBL was observed in the group with supra-occlusal contact was over 180 microns. The authors concluded that peri-implant CBL occurred with 180 microns or more of supra-occlusion [9]. Esaki et al. reported the relationship between the magnitude of immediate loading and peri-implant osteogenesis in a canine model [10]. In this report, immediate load (0 N, 10 N, 50 N) using a cyclic loading device was applied to implants placed in healed sites. In the 10 N group, newly formed bone was observed over a wide area from the implant neck toward the tip. In contrast, in the 50 N group, newly formed bone was rarely observed around the neck and signs of infection were seen. The authors suggested there is a certain load that is beneficial and promotes osteogenesis and an overload threshold that is detrimental. Heitz-Mayfield et al. evaluated the effect of excessive occlusal load following placement of implants in dog [11]. After six months of healing after implant insertion, supra-occlusal crowns were placed. At eight months, all implants were osseointegrated with no statistically difference between test and control implants observed with regard to osseous response.

Table 1. Animal experiments about biological complications related to implant loading.

Year	Animal Model	Loading Pattern	Bone Resorption	Healing Period	Loading Period	Implant System
Isidor [9]	Monkey mandible	10–300 N330 N/s for 5 days	Yes	6 months	4–15 months	Astra
Miyata et al. [10]	Monkey mandible	Supra-occlusal contact	Yes	3.5 months	4 weeks	Intra-mobile element (IMZ)
Heitz-Mayfield et al. [12]	Dog mandible	Supra-occlusal contact	No	6 months	8 months	Straumann
Esaki et al. [11]	Dog mandible	Immediate load	Yes	None	3 weeks	Branemark

Although each of the experiments described above employed different experimental models, taken together, it is clear that certain dynamic force applications influence CBL and bone formation around implants. Managing occlusal loading to achieve desirable effects and prevent undesirable effects is an important consideration during treatment planning and treatment.

In recent years, attention has been paid to osseous activity at the molecular level when force is applied to bone. As a result of technological advances of technology, the role of the osteocyte has become better understood.

Osteocytes are most abundant bone cell in the adult skeleton and function as mechanosensors directing osteoblast and osteoclast function in order to maintain the optimal integrity of load bearing bone. Early histologists upon observing enlarged osteocyte lacunae in bone sections proposed that mature osteocytes could remove their perilacunar matrix, a term called "osteocytic osteolysis". New insights into this process have occurred during the last decade using novel technology thereby providing a means to identify molecular mechanisms responsible for osteocytic osteolysis [12].

Dendritic osteocytes connect to the vasculature, to each other and to periosteal bone surface cells creating a broad communication network within bone tissue. Osteocytes lie in a fluid-filled interstitium of lacunae and canaliculi and are capable of sensing when mechanical load that applied to the skeleton [13]. In response to force application, osteocytes react to and transmit information via secretion of molecules with a signaling function such as sclerostin and receptor activator of nuclear factor kappa-B ligand (RANKL) which then regulate bone matrix turnover by osteoblasts and osteoclasts [14,15]. Due to the recently discovered multi-functionality of osteocytes, ranging from phosphate homeostasis to interaction with distant organs, the regulation of the osteoblast–osteoclast axis is one mechanism by which the osteocyte network contributes to mechanosensory response to loading and may lead to osteocyte apoptosis and targeted bone resorption by osteoclasts [16]. As a result of this mechanosensing communication stream, bone resorption and targeted bone remodeling, in the absence of bacterial inflammation, may change peri-implant crestal bone contours.

2.2. Peri-Implant CBL and Periodontal Pathogens

The success of implant therapy ad modum Branemark in experiencing minimal CBL led to the proposal of optimistic criteria for success of implant therapy by Albrektsson et al. in 1986 [1]. These criteria were quickly accepted as clinicians and scholars worldwide were able to achieve the criteria proposed based on $\leq$1–2 mm of CBL in the first year after placement and $\leq$0.2 mm mean CBL bone loss in subsequent years. The fact that these criteria were based on clinical outcomes from implant therapy in edentulous patients/subjects was appreciated and concern remained that implants placed in partially edentulous patients with their dental reservoirs of periodontopathogens would not be able to duplicate the excellent crestal bone response seen in edentulous patients. These concerns were laid to rest by Van Steenberghe et al. who, from multi-center study findings published in 1993, clearly demonstrated that implant therapy ad modum Branemark in partially edentulous patients also exhibited the same excellent resistance to CBL as observed in edentulous patients [17].

Nevertheless, in the relatively uncommon cases of CBL seen, the concurrent peri-implant mucosal inflammation and bacterial cultures yielding traditional periodontopathogens spawned an erroneous belief system that peri-implant CBL was fashioned after the same etiology as periodontitis. This despite that nowhere else in the human body is an artificial substitute considered to be the same as the original biological tissue: A man-made substance is yet to be fabricated that is identical to natural tissue (see next section). Today, one comes across people who simultaneously claim that bone created from an allograft is different to native bone and yet who argue that periodontal bone loss is the same as peri-implant CBL and should be prevented, diagnosed, and treated similarly. The use of the term peri-implantitis has merely cemented the error of association in the minds of clinicians and scholars despite the fact that, to date, there is no clear and compelling evidence that peri-implant CBL is primarily a consequence of bacterial insult. Of course, many of the same bacteria are found in diseased periodontal and peri-implant sites, more a consequence of anaerobic environments that lend themselves to colonization and propagation of these bacteria [18]. The osseosufficiency model presents the patient as an important element of the path towards successful implant therapy. Yet, it is critical to recognize that is the host response of the patient that is important, not the presence or absence or site concentration of specific bacterial species that prevails and the host response to an artificial implant substitute is markedly different than the host response to a natural tooth. Once peri-implant CBL or inflammation is observed, addressing the bacterial component may alleviate the symptoms and signs, but it will not address the root cause of the problem which is more likely to be improper diagnosis, treatment planning and treatment by the unaware clinician that then leads to peri-implant CBL.

Further erroneous implications are engendered when research models used to study periodontitis are applied to the dental implant ecosystem, most notably, the use of ligature-induced peri-implantitis canine model that creates an artificial scenario by which bacterial inflammation is induced around implants in order to study the degree of CBL. Clinically irrelevant periods of oral hygiene cessation, sometimes 4 months in duration, are combined with the introduction of plaque-attracting sulcular ligatures in order to create a scenario that bears no resemblance to clinical practice and which, therefore, have no clinical meaning [19,20].

2.3. Bone and the Immune System—Foreign Body Reaction

Any foreign-body implant that is placed in contact with vital tissues can activate the immune/inflammatory systems whereby under normal conditions the defense cells, including neutrophils, lymphocytes, reactive pro-inflammatory macrophages (i.e., M1 and OsteoMac), and osteoclasts are activated and engulf and then digest the foreign body. The repair cells, such as fibroblasts, osteoblasts as well as macrophages (M2 and OsteoMacs) are also activated and assist in tissue repair and remodeling, and protection of the tissues from further destruction. However, when a foreign body is too large to be engulfed or digested by the immune cells, a fibrous (granuloma) or osseous encapsulation of the foreign body is formed around the foreign body. This encapsulation isolates the foreign body from the surrounding tissue and is characterized by a chronic presence of macrophages and multinucleated foreign body giant cells (i.e., Langerhan's cells) at the foreign-body surface. These foreign-body giant cells are the result of fusion of monocytes and macrophages activated upon adherence to the foreign-body surface during the earlier inflammation and tissue-repair stages. While these giant cells may present throughout the foreign-body life-time, it is unclear whether they remain active or become inactive with time. Another possible immune reaction to a foreign-body occurs when the immune response is too vigorous or too prolonged, or its function is disrupted. In such situations, the defense/repair balance may shift towards chronic inflammation and chronic tissue destruction [21–24].

In the case of dental implants (see above), it is well established that when titanium implants are placed in the jaw-bone, an evoked inflammatory reaction is followed by formation of new bone in close approximation around the implant. Subsequently, a long-lasting (i.e., implant lifetime) steady state bone remodeling activity is established which maintains the bone around the implant including the marginal bone level height. This process has been named by Branemark 'osseointegration', whereby titanium has been considered an immunologically inert material that supports the bone healing process. It was Donath et al [25] who first suggested that in fact, this reaction of bone-tissue engulfing a dental implant is consistent with a protective foreign body immune response whereby the bone formed around the implant isolates it and thus protects the surrounding bone marrow tissue (Figure 2). This hypothesis has been further investigated and subsequently supported by the Wennerberg and Albrektsson group and others who have further suggested that once new bone is formed around the implant, maintenance of a balance between bone resorption and bone formation (i.e., 'foreign-body equilibrium') can maintain the osseointegration and the marginal bone height around the implants [4,21,22,26–33]. Albrektsson and colleagues have proposed a revised definition of osseointegration to state that "osseointegration is a foreign body reaction where interfacial bone is formed as a defense reaction to shield off the implant from the tissues [34] and further elucidated the importance of host response in long-term osseointegration outcomes [35]. However, the majority of the studies on foreign-body response are in vitro studies or studies that have utilized titanium or other biomaterial implants placed in limb bones or other body tissues. In vitro studies have shown that titanium can activate macrophages [30], and that complement factors in blood plasma binds to titanium implant surface which suggests that during the early stage of inflammation following titanium implant placement, the implant surfaces can be recognized by the immune cells through complement factors in the blood [36]. In the recent study in rabbits, it has been shown that the formation and subsequent maintenance of new bone around titanium implants placed in a femur bone are associated with time-dependent immune responses. These responses were manifested first (10 days) as up-regulation of immune defense cells (i.e., macrophages), and subsequently (at 28 days) by up-regulation of immune repair cells (macrophages, lymphocytes, neutrophils, and the complement system), plus down-regulation of bone-resorbing cells (osteoclasts) around the implants [33]. In addition, similar to foreign-body host response in other body parts, multinucleated giant cells are present at the dental implant–bone interface [25,37], and while these giant cells can be present throughout the implant life-time, it is unclear whether they become inactive with time, or remain active, or become active under certain conditions leading to marginal bone resorption.

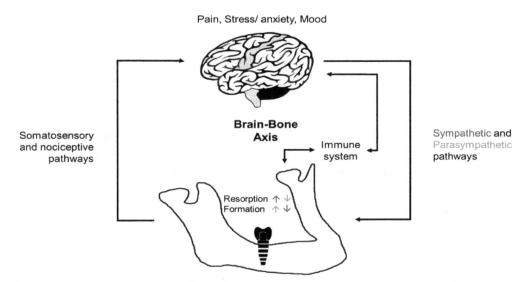

Pain, Stress/ anxiety, Mood

Brain-Bone Axis

Somatosensory and nociceptive pathways

Immune system

Sympathetic and Parasympathetic pathways

Resorption ↑ ↓
Formation ↑ ↓

Figure 2. A diagram illustrating brain–bone axis involving the sympathetic and parasympathetic nervous systems that act through direct and direct neuronal innervation of bone tissue (black arrows). Centrally modulated sympathetic activity inhibits osteoblasts and bone formation and enhances osteoclast activity and bone resorption (red), while centrally modulated parasympathetic activity enhances osteoblast activity and bone formation and inhibits osteoclasts and bone resorption (green). Somatosensory and nociceptive inputs from the bone to the brain as well as pain, stress, and mood responses can impact bone formation and resorption either directly through the autonomic nervous system or indirectly through activation of the immune system that can also be activated directly by bone injury.

Considering the intimate relations between the immune system and bone healing and remodeling, when the immune response to titanium implants is coupled with certain factors or health conditions that impact the immune system or the immune response, the balance between osteoblast and osteoclast activity can shift during the healing phase from a net bone apposition to a net bone resorption resulting in osseointegration failure or unwarranted CBL. Moreover, since osseointegration is a dynamic state of bone remodeling, these factors or health conditions may also impact the osseointegration after it had already been established. These factors or conditions include genetic factors, immunosuppressed diseases, smoking, poorly controlled surgery, excess cement, and medications [26,38–42]. Therefore, patient examination and medical history taking should be evaluated not only prior to implant placement, but also on a regular basis as part of the postoperative follow-up appointments. Other possible causes for impaired bone healing or marginal bone loss could be titanium ion leakage, titanium particles detachment and implant surface contamination with metal or organic particles that are residues of the implant manufacturing, implant cleaning and handling, surgical placement or prosthetic installation processes, as well as prosthetic materials [43,44]. Such particles in the bone surrounding the dental implants can induce chronic inflammatory reaction and immune response which include activation of immune cell mediators such as cytokines (e.g., tumor necrosis factor-alpha (TNF-α)) that can influence the activities of osteoblasts and osteoclasts and thereby impact on bone healing and bone turnover around the implants [29,45–47]. On the other hand, if osseointegration had already occurred, considering osseointegration is dynamic, the above-mentioned factors can also impact bone homeostasis and shift bone turnover into a net bone resorption manifested as aseptic osseoseparation and/or marginal bone resorption (see above). This condition is considered aseptic since its initiation does not involve the oral microbiota however, this does not rule out the possibility of a secondary bacterial infection or a bacterial-derived marginal bone resorption in individual cases [4,22,26,27,29,34,35,47,48].

2.4. The Role of the Brain in Modulating Osseointegration: Brain–Bone Axis

Novel evidence suggests that the brain and the nervous system in general play vital roles in long-bone healing and remodeling processes [49–51]. Complex neural networks exist between the central nervous system and the bones, and nerve fibers of sympathetic, parasympathetic, and somatic origin innervate long bones [52,53]. Furthermore, nerve-derived neuropeptides [e.g., neuropeptide Y, endocannabinoids (CB)], and neurotransmitters (e.g., norepinephrine, dopamine, serotonin, and calcitonin gene-related peptide) were found in the vicinity of long-bone cells that express receptors for these neuropeptides (e.g., β2-adrenergic, Y1 (the name of the receptor) and Y2 (the name of the receptor), CB1 and CB2) and neurotransmitters (e.g., dopamine, and serotonin). These neuropeptides, neurotransmitters and receptors can in turn contribute to the regulatory mechanisms underlying bone remodeling [49,54]. In addition, the central nervous system can integrate internal (e.g., glycemia, menstruation hormones) and external signals that can impact brain control of bone formation and remodeling [51]. For example, experimental denervation of sensory and sympathetic nerve fibers can impact bone development and remodeling [55,56]. While nerve fibers of sympathetic, parasympathetic, and somatic origin also innervate jaw-bones including extraction sockets and peri-implant tissues [53,57–61], no information is available on the role of the nervous system in the healing and remodeling of jaw bones.

Recent studies have also shown important functional links between the central nervous system and the immune system that as we have discussed above plays a key role in peri-implant bone healing. Immune organs, such as lymphoid organs (e.g., lymph nodes, spleen) are innervated by sympathetic and parasympathetic nerve fibers of the autonomic nervous system which can in turn control bone remodeling [52,62]. The notion that the brain can modulate the immune response is also supported by studies showing the effects of mental and physical stress on the general health and immunity [63]. Moreover, usage of central nervous system medications (e.g., opioids, antidepressants, anticonvulsants) as well as depression conditions are associated with low bone mass and increased risk of osteoporosis and fractures [64]. It is interesting to note that recent studies have shown that impaired osseointegration and failures of dental implants are higher in patients treated with antidepressant drugs (selective serotonin reuptake inhibitors) [65–67]. However, it is unclear if the increased loss of osseointegration is produced by the drug or by the mental health condition itself and the impaired communication between the nervous system, immune system and bone healing and remodeling and thus, more robust research is required to identify the exact cause of osseointegration loss.

Another evidence for the role of the brain in bone growth in general comes from the effects of growth hormones in regulating bones growth during development, and bone remodeling throughout life. Growth hormones are secreted from the cerebral pituitary gland under the control of the cerebral hypothalamus. In fact, growth hormones can induce proliferation and activation of both osteoblasts and osteoclasts with an overall net effect of either bone growth, bone resorption or homeostasis [68]. Furthermore, growth hormones play a crucial role in fracture healing, and novel therapeutic approaches utilizing growth hormones (and other growth factors) to improve long bone healing are currently under investigation and development [69].

Altogether, the clinical significance of these studies on brain–bone axis (Figure 2) lies in them providing novel potential therapeutic targets for modulating bone remodeling. Thus, research is needed to gain a better understanding of the possible role of brain–immune system interaction also on jaw-bone remodeling and peri-implant bone healing and CBL.

3. Section B. Methods of Measuring Crestal Bone Loss

3.1. Current Methods

The need for measuring CBL has come with the spectrum of osseoseparation and peri-implantitis. A "lifetime" treatment for a patient requires osseosufficiency, i.e., the harmonious relationship between the host, the implant, and the clinician [3]. The rise of osseointegration science (and related expectations) led to the preservation of crestal bone height after implant placement in the context of quantitative success criteria for implant osseointegration. Monitoring changes in the bony anchorage routinely, at regular intervals, was advocated [1]. In this context, X-ray imaging techniques naturally emerged as a convenient tool for characterizing the marginal bone loss.

Change in bone height (loss or gain) represents the difference in bone levels at the same site at separate time-points. The initial reference bone level value is subtracted from each of the later values, usually but not always, resulting in a negative measurement representing loss of crestal bone. The initial reference is often recorded either right after implant placement (post-operative value) or once the implant becomes functionally loaded (prosthetic loading). These calculations compare the vertical distance between the crestal bone level at the implant contact and a reference point on the implant (implant platform for example), and as a consequence, should be referred as "distance to bone" values than to "bone level" values. Clinical routine measurements are often reported at the tenth of millimeter, while experimental ones may exhibit more accuracy.

To be consistent, the use of a single technique for both measurements is recommended (same imaging materials, same settings and same measure method). Then the known implant diameter, platform diameter, implant length or distance between two threads of screw-type implants may be used for calibration [70].

In the scientific literature, various imaging techniques have been used for measuring CBL, such as standardized intraoral radiographs (SIR), panoramic radiographs, computerized tomography scans, and cone beam computerized tomography (CBCT) scans [71]. The accuracy of the measurements have usually been assessed on jaws from animals or human cadavers, and those studies have repeatedly showed that panoramic radiographs lack reproducibility and resolution due to structure distortions and superimpositions, while computed tomography scans are affected by metal artifacts combined with an excessive exposure dose [71]. Today, SIR and CBCT appear to be the appropriate methods for routine assessment of crestal bone levels on living patients.

3.1.1. Standardized Intraoral Radiographs (SIR)

Standardized intraoral (or periapical) radiographs have historically been, and remain to be, the most commonly used method for longitudinal assessment of peri-implant bone loss. For limiting distortion, the long cone paralleling technique is preferred to the intra-oral bisecting angle technique [72,73]. This technique, routinely used in periodontology, consists in holding the radiographic film parallel to the long axis of the implant and placing the X-ray beam perpendicularly to the receptor [74]. This paralleling technique requires the use of a film holder for routine clinical care, but for research purpose, a customized occlusal bite jig may be also fabricated to standardize the procurement of the implant image at different time points. The bite jig improves comparative measurements by limiting the parallax effect (apparent displacement of bony structures when radiographs are taken from different angles). The bite jig, typically fabricated from silicone, wax, or resin, is a repositioning key that fits to the film holder and can be stored by the dentist until next use. In some clinical studies, the bite jig is clipped on the attachment (locator, ball) or screwed into the implant. However, bone level interventions are not advocated as they may predispose to the bone loss. Some interesting devices have been described for the assessment of functional implants, such as a bite jig designed to be perpendicular to the initial implant placement driver [75].

Periapical radiographs used to be obtained on conventional films; however, the use of digital radiography is expanding in dental practice. When routine measurements are performed on conventional films, a magnifying lens can be used. Nowadays however, most research protocols incorporate high-resolution digitalization of a conventionally-obtained radiograph film. When routine measurements are performed directly with digital radiography, a sliding gauge tool can be used with most of the currently-available radiograph-related software to assess the distance between the crestal bone and the implant reference-point chosen. For research purposes, a method called the digital subtraction technique has been developed to directly measure bone loss by superimposing two serial radiographic images before subtracting them to isolate/quantify bone changes using specially-designed software [72].

Accuracy

Measurement accuracy is the closeness of agreement between measured and the true bone level. The accuracy relies not only on the resolution and sharpness of the radiographic material, but also on many clinical parameters, such as the degree of CBL, the jaw anatomy and configuration, the delay between placement and function, and the quantity of serial radiographs on the same implant [76].

When using a magnifying lens, e.g. ×10, with conventional SIR, inter- and intra-observer variability were shown to be approximately 0.14 mm and 0.08 mm respectively [76]. Conventional film and digital radiography exhibit the same accuracy [77]. Digitized conventional films may exhibit more noise artifacts and may lose density range but still provide comparable measurements [77,78].

Sensitivity and Specificity

In our context, the sensitivity of a radiographic technique consists in detecting the presence of crestal bone, while its specificity is about correctly detecting the bone (or defect) absence. These parameters have been tested in animals or in cadaver studies, when bone level estimations can be compared to the physical measurements. In a recent meta-analysis pooling the results of 5 studies, the SIR exhibited clinically acceptable sensitivity (60% when pooled; 56–100%) and specificity (59% when pooled; 51–98%) [71]. SIR detected more precisely large defects (around 3 mm) than small ones (1–2 mm) [71,79,80]. As a consequence, many authors reported the proximal bone loss to be underestimated by SIR measurements [81–83].

Pros and Cons

The primary advantages of SIR are the low exposure dose and being the least invasive of all the radiographic techniques. Combined with its low cost, the reliability of linear distance measurements, easy access and easy handling for dentists, this technique remains the gold standard for routine clinical measurements.

However, only the mesial and distal CBL can be assessed with this technique. Furthermore, in the context of peri-implantitis, proximal bone levels were often shown to be more apical than the radiographically measured ones [81–83]. The tangential measurements can be affected by geometric distortions and anatomical superimpositions, especially since a strict parallel projection is difficult to obtain in some clinical situations [84]. In addition, SIR do not allow identification of the 3D morphology of a bone defect (intra-bony and supracrestal components) that influences diagnosis, prognosis and treatment planning [83,85,86].

3.1.2. Cone Beam Computerized Tomography (CBCT)

The use of CBCT, also called digital volume tomography, to assess peri-implant bone level is more recent as this technology emerged in dentistry only 20 years ago. Compared with traditional CT, the lower irradiation dose and less severe metallic artifacts raised opportunities for new dental applications.

In comparison with SIRs, CBCT image quality relies mainly on the technological performance of the material. Some of the most influencing parameters are the voxel size and the field of view. Indeed, image resolution is related to the size of volume elements, called voxels, which are often cubes (with edge ranging from 0.08–0.3 mm in research studies on peri-implant defects). However, small voxels come with additional noise [87]. Also, the field of view defines the volume of interest undergoing examination (cube ranging from 4 × 4 to 8 × 8 cm) and influences accuracy. This technological parameter is determined by the available detector, beam projection geometry and beam collimation. Small voxels and small fields of view improve measurements; but seeking the most precise peri-implant morphology when combining these two parameters will still deliver high radiation levels [80,88]. Image reconstruction parameters and filter software (used to lower metal artifacts) also influence the performance quality of the peri-implant measurements [89,90].

Accuracy

As previously mentioned, CBCT accuracy is defined by the field of view size, but also by the device scan mode and arc of rotation [91–93]. Indeed, the full-scan mode (360°) provides a higher diagnostic accuracy for peri-implant defects [90]. A recent systematic review concluded that large defects are more accurately detected than small ones, and that circumferential and fenestration peri-implant defects are more accurately detected than dehiscence defects [94].

Experimental measurements of peri-implant defects showed very low deviation when compared with direct measurement (0.18 ± 0.12 mm) and the proximal values were comparable to those obtained with periapical radiographs [95,96]. The spatial resolution can reach around 150–200 μm [72,97].

Sensitivity and Specificity

In a recent meta-analysis pooling the results of 9 studies, the CBCT exhibited clinically acceptable sensitivity (59% when pooled; 28–97%) and specificity (67% when pooled; 25–97%) [71]. Sensitivity globally increases with small voxels but remains challenged by small defects [90]. On the other hand, some authors suggested that specificity may increase with bigger voxels [80]. Filters can improve the detection of true positive or negative values [90].

Pros & Cons

When compared with SIR, CBCT delivers more radiation to patients, is more expensive for the patient and for the medical team, and has relatively limited availability. Metal artifacts (streaking, beam hardening, or scatter) increase with CBCT low energy settings and may add some false-positive bone on the vestibular side and false-negative bone on the other sides [96].

Both SIR and CBCT are interesting and validated imaging techniques for measuring peri-implant CBL. Their accuracy, sensitivity, and specificity are clinically acceptable [71,98]. On one hand, SIR provides only proximal values, but the data obtained often are sufficient to confirm changes in peri-implant CBL. On the other hand, CBCT exposes the patient to higher cost and radiation dose but offers a 3D characterization of the peri-implant defect. For these reasons, SIR remains the gold standard for routine assessment of bone level changes and for helping in peri-implantitis diagnosis, while CBCT is still confined to providing clear 3D images of diagnosed peri-implantitis that require a treatment plan [71,94,99]. In the future, CBL assessment may not be in X-ray imaging but rather in non-invasive 3D procedures such as ultrasound [100].

3.2. Novel Method: Photoacoustic Ultrasound as an Innovative Method to Measure Peri-Implant Pocket Depths and Bone Loss over Time

Ultrasound is the most widely used clinical imaging modality in medicine but has limited deployment in dental and periodontal practices [101]. In recent years, however, the number of preclinical dental applications of ultrasound has been increasing [102]. The advantages of ultrasound include the ability to image soft tissues in real-time without ionizing radiation at a relatively low cost.

One of the drawbacks of ultrasound is its limited contrast (signal from target versus signal from background). Contrast in conventional ultrasound is a function in differences in the acoustic impedance of different tissue types. Photoacoustic imaging is a hybrid form of ultrasound that can overcome this limitation and increase the contrast of ultrasound (Figure 3) [103]. It has a rapidly growing number of applications and uses optical—rather than acoustic—excitation to harness the photoacoustic effect. Photoacoustic imaging converts the incident light into sound following absorption and thermoelastic expansion of a target material [104]. It combines the good spatial and temporal resolution of ultrasound with the contrast and spectral imaging capabilities of optics. Typically, the optical excitation source (5–50 ns pulses at ~ 5 Hz) is a pulsed near-infrared laser (Nd:YAG/OPO) but low-power LED sources can also be used [105]. These pulses are absorbed by tissue, and the energy is released acoustically and detected by ultrasound transducers with center frequencies in the MHz range. The coupling of fiber optics with ultrasound transducers allows simultaneous ultrasound and photoacoustic imaging [106]. A variety of algorithms can be used for image reconstruction to maximize contrast, resolution, and signal-to-noise [107–110].

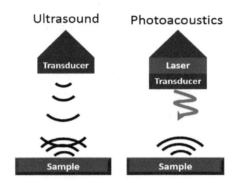

Figure 3. Acoustic Modalities. Ultrasound uses echoes to create contrast ("sound in/sound out"). Photoacoustics is "light in/sound out" and is based on thermal expansion of the target tissue or contrast agent.

The most common uses of photoacoustic imaging are image-guided therapies [111], diagnosis of disease states [112,113], surgeries [114,115], and drug delivery [116,117]. These applications can be achieved through either endogenous or exogenous contrast. Endogenous contrast is based on the optical absorption of naturally occurring targets such as oxygenated/deoxygenated hemoglobin, melanin, lipids, and water [118]. Exogenous contrast mechanisms leverage the absorption of materials such as small-molecule dyes, fluorophores, and nanoparticles that originate from outside of the body [119]. In both cases, because photoacoustic intensity is proportional to optical absorption, light sources with specific wavelengths can be used for spectral differentiation between materials according to their absorption spectra.

Imaging the Periodontal Pocket with Photoacoustic Ultrasound

Assessment of periodontal disease uses physical measurements (e.g., attachment level, probing depth, bone loss, mobility, recession, and degree of inflammation) [120]. Periodontal probing offers a numerical metric that reflects the extent of apical epithelial attachment relative to the gingival margin [121] but suffers from poor reproducibility due to variation in probing force [122]. Indeed, a recent meta-analysis showed a wide range of probing forces (51 to 995 N/cm^2)—a variation of ~20-fold [123]. Other error sources include variation in the insertion point, probe angulation, the patient's overall gingival health (weakly inflamed tissue), and the presence of calculus [121,124]. Thus, the exam is subject to large errors with inter-operator variation as high as 40% with r values between technicians <0.80 [125]. These errors can hamper clinical decision-making and epidemiological studies ultimately resulting in poor patient outcomes [126]. Furthermore, many patients find probing to be uncomfortable or painful—this can prevent patients from seeking care [127,128]. Moreover, the periodontal probing is time consuming for the practitioners. It is perhaps not surprising that periodontal examination was not performed in 50–90% of the audited dental records offices [129–131]. Finally, the benefit of traditional periodontal probing around implants is abrogated due to implant threads that impede probe penetration along the implant surface [132,133]. This limits the clinical assessment of these tissues, potentially leading to peri-implantitis [134,135].

The first study to use photoacoustic imaging for visualizing pocket depths was conducted by Lin et al. in 2017 [136]. A commercially available tomographic system (Visualsonics Vevo LAZR) was used for imaging porcine jaws extracted from frozen cadavers. A food-grade contrast agent containing melanin nanoparticles derived from cuttlefish ink was used to increase the photoacoustic signal of the pockets. This material acted as a safe, highly absorbing material capable of filling the gingival sulcus following oral irrigation. It had broad absorbance and photoacoustic signal.

This technique was recently expanded to a healthy young adult case [137]. The same imaging system was adapted so that a subject could be scanned while seated (Figure 4A). Here, ultrasound gel was used for coupling and a medical head immobilizer and cheek retractors were used to minimize movements from the subject; 40 MHz ultrasound was used throughout. Again, the procedure began with irrigation of the pocket followed by laser pulsing and imaging, removal of the contrast agent, and image processing. The pocket depth could be visualized for a given sagittal plane (Figure 4B–D) after administration of the agent. Because these experiments used ultrasound gel for coupling, it was common during scanning for the agent to nonspecifically coat the surface of tooth. However, this nonspecific signal could be removed in post-processing by using the ultrasound-only images to locate the gingival margin. Any signal originating from tooth surface occlusal to the margin was ignored allowing a final mapping of the pocket to be manually generated (Figure 4E). In the future, this processing step will be automated.

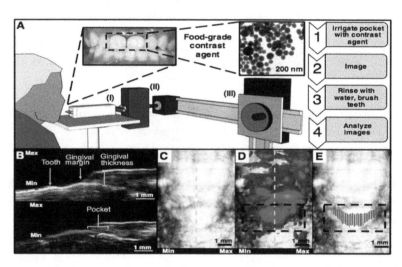

Figure 4. Representative human data of photoacoustic-ultrasound imaging for pocket depth measurements. (**A**) Overview of the imaging setup and methodology. The subject was seated in front of the transducer (I) and ultrasound gel was used for coupling. The stepper motor (II) was used for scanning the transducer and the sliding frame allowed positioning (III). First, the teeth of interest were irrigated with the contrast agent followed by imaging, removal of the agent, and image analysis. (**B**) A sagittal cross-section (dashed yellow line in Panel C) of a mandibular central incisor before (top) and after (before) irrigation with the contrast agent, revealing the pocket depth, measured from the gingival margin to the edge of photoacoustic signal. Nonspecific signal from the tooth, caused by the movement of coupling gel during scanning, did not contribute to the measurement. (**C**) A frontal view of the same tooth before (**D**) and after (**E**) irrigation. Nonspecific signal from contrast agent was removed during image processing by measuring the pocket from each sagittal plane as in Panel B and overlaying each measurement on the ultrasound-only image.

In the case of implants, physical probing is typically hindered by threads that impede probe penetration along the implant surface [132,133]. This limits the ability for clinical assessment of these tissues potentially leading to peri-implantitis [134,135]. We note that photoacoustic ultrasound has not been explicitly tested yet for imaging the pockets around implants. However, because it relies on the flow of contrast agent into the pocket rather than the physical penetration of a metal probe, the presence of implant threads should not affect measurements. For this reason, we believe photoacoustic imaging is promising for patients with implants that obstruct manual probing. Of course, additional work remains to improve the clinical feasibility of the technique including development of a mouthpiece transducer and the implementation of more affordable and stable excitation sources, such as LEDs or laser diodes.

4. Summary

New ways of appreciating CBL are blending traditional etiologies with novel mechanisms that better reconcile what was originally thought to be taking place during osseointegration with actual long-term clinical outcomes. Today, the ability to look back on osseointegration outcomes at the implant level, the prosthesis level, the patient level and even the clinician level allow us to recognize that osseointegration likely represents a form of foreign body reaction and focuses our attention on elements that, therefore, influence the immune response or the consequence of a patient's immune response. In this way, traditional etiologies such as inflammation from infection and overloading can be viewed as modulators of the immune response and the effect of immune response through neuroimmunomodulation opens up new and exciting avenues for future research.

Clinically, measuring crystal bone loss remains at the mercy of the constraints of radiographic imaging. Nevertheless, new methodologies and digital technologies portend the introduction of non-invasive methods that may be more sensitive and specific with regard to measurement of crestal bone position and changes in crestal bone position over time. Here too, innovations in imaging will allow us to better assess the effect of new techniques, products, protocols and materials.

Author Contributions: For this paper, individuals contributed to the following activities: Conceptualization, S.K.; writing—original draft preparation, A.N., K.S., C.M., L.A.-A., J.J., and S.K.; project administration, S.K.

References

1. Koka, S.; Zarb, G.A. On osseointegration: The healing adaptation principle in the context of osseosufficiency, osseoseparation, and dental implant failure. *Int. J. Prosthodont.* **2012**, *25*, 48–52. [PubMed]

2. Bryant, S.R. Oral Implant Outcomes Predicted by Age- and Site-Specific Aspects of Bone Condition. Ph.D. Thesis, University of Toronto, Toronto, ON, Canada, 2001.

3. Linkevicius, T.; Puisys, A.; Vindasuite, E.; Linkeviciene, L.; Apse, P. Does residual cement around implant-supported restorations cause peri-implant disease? A retrospective case analysis. *Clin. Oral Implants Res.* **2013**, *24*, 1179–1184. [CrossRef] [PubMed]

4. Roos-Jansaker, A.M. Long time follow up of implant therapy and treatment of peri-implantitis. *Swed. Dent. J. Suppl.* **2007**, *188*, 7–66.

5. Fransson, C.; Lekholm, U.; Jemt, T.; Berglundh, T. Prevalence of subjects with progressive bone loss. *Clin. Oral Implants Res.* **2005**, *16*, 440–446. [CrossRef] [PubMed]

6. Esposito, M.; Hirsch, J.M.; Lekholm, U.; Thomsen, P. Biological factors contributing to failures of osseointegrated oral implants. (I). Success criteria and epidemiology. *Eur. J. Oral Sci.* **1998**, *106*, 527–551. [CrossRef] [PubMed]

7. Frost, H.M. A 2003 update of bone physiology and Wolff's Law for clinicians. *Angle Orthod.* **2004**, *74*, 3–15. [PubMed]

8. Naert, I.; Duyck, J.; Vandamme, K. Occlusal overload and bone/implant loss. *Clin. Oral Implants Res.* **2012**, *23* (Suppl. 6), 95–107. [CrossRef]

9. Isidor, F. Loss of osseointegration caused by occlusal load of oral implants. *Clin. Oral Implants Res.* **1996**, *7*, 143–152. [CrossRef]

10. Miyata, T.; Kobayashi, Y.; Araki, H.; Ohto, T.; Shin, K. The influence of controlled occlusal overload on peri-implant tissue. Part 3: A histologic study in monkeys. *Int. J. Oral Maxillofac. Implants* **2000**, *15*, 425–431.

11. Esaki, D.; Matsushita, Y.; Ayukawa, Y.; Sakai, N.; Sawae, Y.; Koyano, K. Relationship between magnitude of immediate loading and peri-implant osteogenesis in dogs. *Clin. Oral Implants Res.* **2012**, *23*, 1290–1296. [CrossRef]

12. Heitz-Mayfield, L.J.; Schmid, B.; Weigel, C.; Gerber, S.; Bosshardt, D.D.; Jonsson, J.; Lang, N.P.; Jönsson, J. Does excessive occlusal load affect osseointegration? *Exp. Study Dog Clin. Oral Implants Res.* **2004**, *15*, 259–268. [CrossRef] [PubMed]

13. Tsourdi, E.; Jahn, K.; Rauner, M.; Busse, B.; Bonewald, L.F. Physiological and pathological osteocytic osteolysis. *J. Musculoskelet. Neuronal Interact.* **2018**, *18*, 292–303. [PubMed]

14. Klein-Nulend, J.; van der Plas, A.; Semeins, C.M.; Ajubi, N.E.; Frangos, J.A.; Nijweide, P.J.; Burger, E.H. Sensitivity of osteocytes to biomechanical stress in vitro. *FASEB J.* **1995**, *9*, 441–445. [CrossRef] [PubMed]

15. Van Bezooijen, R.L.; Roelen, B.A.; Visser, A.; van der Wee-Pals, L.; de Wilt, E.; Karperien, M.; Hamersma, H.; Papapoulos, S.E.; ten Dijke, P.; Löwik, C.W. Sclerostin is an osteocyte-expressed negative regulator of bone formation, but not a classical BMP antagonist. *J. Exp. Med.* **2004**, *199*, 805–814. [CrossRef] [PubMed]

16. Nakashima, T.; Hayashi, M.; Fukunaga, T.; Kurata, K.; Oh-Hora, M.; Feng, J.Q.; Bonewald, L.F.; Kodama, T.; Wutz, A.; Wagner, E.F.; et al. Evidence for osteocyte regulation of bone homeostasis through RANKL expression. *Nat. Med.* **2011**, *17*, 1231–1234. [CrossRef] [PubMed]

17. Dallas, S.L.; Prideaux, M.; Bonewald, L.F. The osteocyte: An endorine cell . . . and more. *Endocr. Rev.* **2013**, *34*, 658–690. [CrossRef] [PubMed]

18. Van Steenberghe, D.; Klinge, B.; Lindén, U.; Quirynen, M.; Herrmann, I.; Garpland, C. Periodontal indices around natural and titanium abutments: A longitudinal multicenter study. *J. Periodontol.* **1993**, *64*, 538–541. [CrossRef]

19. Charalampakis, G.; Abrahamsson, I.; Carcuac, O.; Dahlén, G.; Berglundh, T. Microbiota in experimental periodontitis and peri-implantitis in dogs. *Clin. Oral Implants Res.* **2014**, *25*, 1094–1098. [CrossRef]

20. Berglundh, T.; Gotfredsen, K.; Zitzmann, N.U.; Lang, N.P.; Lindhe, J. Spontaneous progression of ligature induced peri-implantitis at implants with different surface roughness: An experimental study in dogs. *Clin. Oral Implants Res.* **2007**, *18*, 655–661. [CrossRef]

21. Carcuac, O.; Abrahamsson, I.; Albouy, J.P.; Linder, E.; Larsson, L.; Berglundh, T. Experimental periodontitis and peri-implantitis in dogs. *Clin. Oral Implants Res.* **2013**, *24*, 363–371. [CrossRef]

22. Anderson, J.M. Inflammation, wound healing, and the foreign-body response. In *Biomaterials Science: An Introduction to Materials*, 3rd ed.; Academic Press: Cambridge, UK, 2013; pp. 503–512.

23. Anderson, J.M.; Rodriguez, A.; Chang, D.T. Foreign body reaction to biomaterials. *Semin. Immunol.* **2008**, *20*, 86–100. [CrossRef] [PubMed]

24. Miron, R.J.; Zohdi, H.; Fujioka-Kobayashi, M.; Bosshardt, D.D. Giant cells around bone biomaterials: Osteoclasts or multi-nucleated giant cells? *Acta Biomater.* **2016**, *46*, 15–28. [CrossRef] [PubMed]

25. Sheikh, Z.; Sima, C.; Glogauer, M. Bone replacement materials and techniques used for achieving vertical alveolar bone augmentation. *Materials* **2015**, *8*, 2953–2993. [CrossRef]

26. Donath, K.; Laass, M.; Gunzl, H.J. The histopathology of different foreign-body reactions in oral soft tissue and bone tissue. *Virchows Archiv. A* **1992**, *420*, 131–137. [CrossRef]

27. Albrektsson, T.; Chrcanovic, B.; Molne, J.; Wennerberg, A. Foreign body reactions, marginal bone loss and allergies in relation to titanium implants. *Eur. J. Oral Implantol.* **2018**, *11* (Suppl. 1), S37–S46.

28. Albrektsson, T.; Dahlin, C.; Jemt, T.; Sennerby, L.; Turri, A.; Wennerberg, A. Is marginal bone loss around oral implants the result of a provoked foreign body reaction? *Clin. Implant Dent. Relat. Res.* **2014**, *16*, 155–165. [CrossRef] [PubMed]

29. Bielemann, A.M.; Marcello-Machado, R.M.; Del Bel Cury, A.A.; Faot, F. Systematic review of wound healing biomarkers in peri-implant crevicular fluid during osseointegration. *Arch. Oral Biol.* **2018**, *89*, 107–128. [CrossRef]

30. Kzhyshkowska, J.; Gudima, A.; Riabov, V.; Dollinger, C.; Lavalle, P.; Vrana, N.E. Macrophage responses to implants: Prospects for personalized medicine. *J. Leukoc. Biol.* **2015**, *98*, 953–962. [CrossRef]

31. Takayanagi, H. Osteoimmunology: Shared mechanisms and crosstalk between the immune and bone systems. *Nat. Rev. Immunol.* **2007**, *7*, 292–304. [CrossRef]

32. Takayanagi, H. New developments in osteoimmunology. *Nat. Rev. Rheumatol.* **2012**, *8*, 684–689. [CrossRef]

33. Trindade, R.; Albrektsson, T.; Galli, S.; Prgomet, Z.; Tengvall, P.; Wennerberg, A. Osseointegration and foreign body reaction: Titanium implants activate the immune system and suppress bone resorption during the first 4 weeks after implantation. *Clin. Implants Dent. Relat Res.* **2018**, *20*, 82–91. [CrossRef] [PubMed]

34. Trindade, R.; Albrektsson, T.; Tengvall, P.; Wennerberg, A. Foreign body reaction to biomaterials: On mechanisms for buildup and breakdown of osseointegration. *Clin. Implants Dent. Relat. Res.* **2016**, *18*, 192–203. [CrossRef] [PubMed]

35. Albrektsson, T.; Chrcanovic, B.; Jacobsson, M.; Wennerberg, A. Osseointegration of implants—A biological and clinical overview. *JSM Dent. Surg* **2017**, *2*, 1022–1027.

36. Albrektsson, T.; Jämt, T.; Molne, J.; Tengvall, P.; Wennerberg, A. On inflammation-immunological balance theory—A critical apprehension of disease concepts around implants: Mucositis and marginal bone loss may represent normal conditions and not necessarily a state of disease. *J. Clin. Implant Dent. Relat. Res.* **2019**, in press. [CrossRef] [PubMed]

37. Chappuis, V.; Cavusoglu, Y.; Gruber, R.; Kuchler, U.; Buser, D.; Bosshardt, D.D. Osseointegration of zirconia in the presence of multinucleated giant cells. *Clin. Implants Dent. Relat. Res.* **2016**, *18*, 686–698. [CrossRef] [PubMed]

38. Avivi-Arber, L.; Avivi, D.; Perez, M.; Arber, N.; Shapira, S. Impaired bone healing at tooth extraction sites in cd24-deficient mice: A pilot study. *PLoS ONE* **2018**, *13*, e0191665. [CrossRef] [PubMed]

39. Berglundh, T.; Giannobile, W.V. Investigational clinical research in implant dentistry: Beyond observational and descriptive studies. *J. Dent. Res.* **2013**, *92* (Suppl. 12), 107s–108s. [CrossRef]

40. Brånemark, P.I.; Zarb, G.A.; Albrektsson, T. *Tissue-Integrated Prostheses. Osseointegration in Clinical Dentistry*; Quintessence: Chicago, IL, USA, 1985.

41. Nishimura, I. Genetic networks in osseointegration. *J. Dent. Res.* **2013**, *92* (Suppl. 12), 109s–118s. [CrossRef]

42. Wennerberg, A.; Ide-Ektessabi, A.; Hatkamata, S.; Sawase, T.; Johansson, C.; Albrektsson, T.; Martinelli, A.; Sodervall, U.; Odelius, H. Titanium release from implants prepared with different surface roughness. *Clin. Oral Implants Res.* **2004**, *15*, 505–512. [CrossRef]

43. Delgado-Ruiz, R.; Romanos, G. Potential causes of titanium particle and ion release in implant dentistry: A systematic review. *Int J. Mol. Sci.* **2018**, *19*, 3585. [CrossRef]

44. Franchi, M.; Bacchelli, B.; Martini, D.; Pasquale, V.D.; Orsini, E.; Ottani, V.; Fini, M.; Giavaresi, G.; Giardino, R.; Ruggeri, A. Early detachment of titanium particles from various different surfaces of endosseous dental implants. *Biomaterials* **2004**, *25*, 2239–2246. [CrossRef] [PubMed]

45. Trindade, R.; Albrektsson, T.; Galli, S.; Prgomet, Z.; Tengvall, P.; Wennerberg, A. Bone Immune Response to Materials, Part I: Titanium, PEEK and Copper in Comparison to Sham at 10 Days in Rabbit Tibia. *J. Clin. Med.* **2018**, *7*, 526. [CrossRef] [PubMed]

46. Lechner, J.; Noumbissi, S.; von Baehr, V. Titanium implants and silent inflammation in jawbone-a critical interplay of dissolved titanium particles and cytokines tnf-alpha and rantes/ccl5 on overall health? *EPMA J.* **2018**, *9*, 331–343. [CrossRef] [PubMed]

47. Noronha Oliveira, M.; Schunemann, W.V.H.; Mathew, M.T.; Henriques, B.; Magini, R.S.; Teughels, W.; Souza, J.C.M. Can degradation products released from dental implants affect peri-implant tissues? *J. Periodontal. Res.* **2018**, *53*, 1–11. [CrossRef] [PubMed]

48. Christiansen, R.J. Metal Release from Implants and Its Effect on the Immune System. Ph.D. Thesis, Technical University of Denmark, DTU Mechanical Engineering, Lyngby, Denmark, 2016.

49. Elefteriou, F. Regulation of bone remodeling by the central and peripheral nervous system. *Arch. Biochem. Biophys.* **2008**, *473*, 231–236. [CrossRef] [PubMed]

50. Kim, J.G.; Sun, B.H.; Dietrich, M.O.; Koch, M.; Yao, G.Q.; Diano, S.; Insogna, K.; Horvath, T.L. AGRP neurons regulate bone mass. *Cell Rep.* **2015**, *13*, 8–14. [CrossRef] [PubMed]

51. Takeda, S.; Ducy, P. Regulation of bone remodeling by central and peripheral nervous signals. In *Principles of Bone Biology*; Bilezekian, J., Raisz, L.G., Martin, T.J., Eds.; Academic Press: Cambridge, MA, USA, 2008; pp. 1059–1068.

52. Bajayo, A.; Bar, A.; Denes, A.; Bachar, M.; Kram, V.; Attar-Namdar, M.; Zallone, A.; Kovacs, K.J.; Yirmiya, R.; Bab, I. Skeletal parasympathetic innervation communicates central il-1 signals regulating bone mass accrual. *Proc. Natl. Acad. Sci. USA* **2012**, *109*, 15455–15460. [CrossRef]

53. Ysander, M.; Branemark, R.; Olmarker, K.; Myers, R.R. Intramedullary osseointegration: Development of a rodent model and study of histology and neuropeptide changes around titanium implants. *J. Rehabil. Res. Dev.* **2001**, *38*, 183–190.

54. Elefteriou, F. Neuronal signaling and the regulation of bone remodeling. *Cell. Mol. Life Sci.* **2005**, *62*, 2339–2349. [CrossRef]

55. Chenu, C. Role of innervation in the control of bone remodeling. *J. Musculoskelet. Neuronal Interact.* **2004**, *4*, 132–134.

56. Jiang, S.D.; Jiang, L.S.; Dai, L.Y. Mechanisms of osteoporosis in spinal cord injury. *Clin. Endocrinol.* **2006**, *65*, 555–565. [CrossRef] [PubMed]

57. Corpas Ldos, S.; Lambrichts, I.; Quirynen, M.; Collaert, B.; Politis, C.; Vrielinck, L.; Martens, W.; Struys, T.; Jacobs, R. Peri-implant bone innervation: Histological findings in humans. *Eur J. Oral Implants* **2014**, *7*, 283–292.

58. Fujii, N.; Ohnishi, H.; Shirakura, M.; Nomura, S.; Ohshima, H.; Maeda, T. Regeneration of nerve fibres in the peri-implant epithelium incident to implantation in the rat maxilla as demonstrated by immunocytochemistry for protein gene product 9.5 (pgp9.5) and calcitonin gene-related peptide (cgrp). *Clin. Oral Implants Res.* **2003**, *14*, 240–247. [CrossRef] [PubMed]

59. Mason, A.G.; Holland, G.R. The reinnervation of healing extraction sockets in the ferret. *J. Dent. Res.* **1993**, *72*, 1215–1221. [CrossRef] [PubMed]

60. Wada, S.; Kojo, T.; Wang, Y.H.; Ando, H.; Nakanishi, E.; Zhang, M.; Fukuyama, H.; Uchida, Y. Effect of loading on the development of nerve fibers around oral implants in the dog mandible. *Clin. Oral Implants Res.* **2001**, *12*, 219–224. [CrossRef] [PubMed]

61. Wang, Y.-H.; Kojo, T.; Ando, H.; Nakanishi, E.; Yoshizawa, H.; Zhang, M.; Fukuyama, H.; Wada, S.; Uchida, Y. Nerve regeneration after implantation in peri-implant area. A histological study on different implant materials in dogs. In *Osseoperception*; Jacobs, R., Ed.; Catholic University Leuven: Leuven, Belgium, 1998; pp. 3–11.

62. Elefteriou, F.; Campbell, P.; Ma, Y. Control of bone remodeling by the peripheral sympathetic nervous system. *Calcif. Tissue Int.* **2014**, *94*, 140–151. [CrossRef] [PubMed]

63. Schneiderman, N.; Ironson, G.; Siegel, S.D. Stress and health: Psychological, behavioral, and biological determinants. *Annu. Rev. Clin. Psychol.* **2005**, *1*, 607–628. [CrossRef] [PubMed]

64. Kinjo, M.; Setoguchi, S.; Schneeweiss, S.; Solomon, D.H. Bone mineral density in subjects using central nervous system-active medications. *Am. J. Med.* **2005**, *118*, 1414.e7–1414.e12. [CrossRef]

65. Chrcanovic, B.R.; Kisch, J.; Albrektsson, T.; Wennerberg, A. Factors influencing early dental implant failures. *J. Dent. Res.* **2016**, *95*, 995–1002. [CrossRef]

66. Gupta, B.; Acharya, A.; Pelekos, G.; Gopalakrishnan, D.; Kolokythas, A. Selective serotonin reuptake inhibitors and dental implant failure-a significant concern in elders? *Gerodontology* **2017**, *34*, 505–507. [CrossRef]

67. Wu, X.; Al-Abedalla, K.; Rastikerdar, E.; Abi Nader, S.; Daniel, N.G.; Nicolau, B.; Tamimi, F. Selective serotonin reuptake inhibitors and the risk of osseointegrated implant failure: A cohort study. *J. Dent. Res.* **2014**, *93*, 1054–1061. [CrossRef] [PubMed]

68. Olney, R.C. Regulation of bone mass by growth hormone. *Med. Pediatric Oncol.* **2003**, *41*, 228–234. [CrossRef] [PubMed]

69. Giannoudis, P.V. Bone healing the diamond concept. In *European Instructional Lectures: 15th EFORT Congress, London, United Kingdom*; Bentley, G., Ed.; Springer: Berlin/Heidelberg, Germany, 2014. [CrossRef]

70. Malloy, K.A.; Wadhwani, C.; McAllister, B.; Wang, M.; Katancik, J.A. Accuracy and reproducibility of radiographic images for assessing crestal bone height of implants using the precision implant X-ray locator (pixrl) device. *Int J. Oral Maxillofac. Implants* **2017**, *32*, 830–836. [CrossRef] [PubMed]

71. Bohner, L.O.L.; Mukai, E.; Oderich, E.; Porporatti, A.L.; Pacheco-Pereira, C.; Tortamano, P.; De Luca Canto, G. Comparative analysis of imaging techniques for diagnostic accuracy of peri-implant bone defects: A meta-analysis. *Oral Surg. Oral Med. Oral Pathol. Oral Radiol.* **2017**, *124*, 432.e5–440.e5. [CrossRef] [PubMed]

72. Wakoh, M.; Harada, T.; Otonari, T.; Otonari-Yamamoto, M.; Ohkubo, M.; Kousuge, Y.; Kobayashi, N.; Mizuta, S.; Kitagawa, H.; Sano, T. Reliability of linear distance measurement for dental implant length with standardized periapical radiographs. *Bull. Tokyo Dent. Coll.* **2006**, *47*, 105–115. [CrossRef] [PubMed]

73. Daros, P.; Carneiro, V.C.; Siqueira, A.P.; de-Azevedo-Vaz, S.L. Diagnostic accuracy of 4 intraoral radiographic techniques for misfit detection at the implant abutment joint. *J. Prosthet. Dent.* **2018**, *120*, 57–64. [CrossRef] [PubMed]

74. Duckworth, J.E.; Judy, P.F.; Goodson, J.M.; Socransky, S.S. A method for the geometric and densitometric standardization of intraoral radiographs. *J. Periodontol.* **1983**, *54*, 435–440. [CrossRef]

75. Lin, K.C.; Wadhwani, C.P.; Cheng, J.; Sharma, A.; Finzen, F. Assessing fit at the implant-abutment junction with a radiographic device that does not require access to the implant body. *J. Prosthet. Dent.* **2014**, *112*, 817–823. [CrossRef]

76. Grondahl, K.; Sunden, S.; Grondahl, H.G. Inter- and intraobserver variability in radiographic bone level assessment at Branemark fixtures. *Clin. Oral Implants Res.* **1998**, *9*, 243–250. [CrossRef]

77. Morner-Svalling, A.C.; Tronje, G.; Andersson, L.G.; Welander, U. Comparison of the diagnostic potential of direct digital and conventional intraoral radiography in the evaluation of peri-implant conditions. *Clin. Oral Implants Res.* **2003**, *14*, 714–719. [CrossRef]

78. Kamburoglu, K.; Gulsahi, A.; Genc, Y.; Paksoy, C.S. A comparison of peripheral marginal bone loss at dental implants measured with conventional intraoral film and digitized radiographs. *J. Oral Implants* **2012**, *38*, 211–219. [CrossRef] [PubMed]

79. Sewerin, I.P.; Gotfredsen, K.; Stoltze, K. Accuracy of radiographic diagnosis of peri-implant radiolucencies–an in vitro experiment. *Clin. Oral Implants Res.* **1997**, *8*, 299–304. [CrossRef] [PubMed]

80. Dave, M.; Davies, J.; Wilson, R.; Palmer, R. A comparison of cone beam computed tomography and conventional periapical radiography at detecting peri-implant bone defects. *Clin. Oral Implants Res.* **2013**, *24*, 671–678. [CrossRef] [PubMed]

81. Tonetti, M.S.; Pini Prato, G.; Williams, R.C.; Cortellini, P. Periodontal regeneration of human infrabony defects. Iii. Diagnostic strategies to detect bone gain. *J. Periodontol.* **1993**, *64*, 269–277. [CrossRef] [PubMed]

82. Eickholz, P.; Hausmann, E. Accuracy of radiographic assessment of interproximal bone loss in intrabony defects using linear measurements. *Eur. J. Oral Sci.* **2000**, *108*, 70–73. [CrossRef] [PubMed]

83. Garcia-Garcia, M.; Mir-Mari, J.; Benic, G.I.; Figueiredo, R.; Valmaseda-Castellon, E. Accuracy of periapical radiography in assessing bone level in implants affected by peri-implantitis: A cross-sectional study. *J. Clin. Periodontol.* **2016**, *43*, 85–91. [CrossRef]

84. Hermann, J.S.; Schoolfield, J.D.; Nummikoski, P.V.; Buser, D.; Schenk, R.K.; Cochran, D.L. Crestal bone changes around titanium implants: A methodologic study comparing linear radiographic with histometric measurements. *Int. J. Oral Maxillofac. Implants* **2001**, *16*, 475–485.

85. Schwarz, F.; Herten, M.; Sager, M.; Bieling, K.; Sculean, A.; Becker, J. Comparison of naturally occurring and ligature-induced peri-implantitis bone defects in humans and dogs. *Clin. Oral Implants Res.* **2007**, *18*, 161–170. [CrossRef]

86. Schwarz, F.; Sahm, N.; Schwarz, K.; Becker, J. Impact of defect configuration on the clinical outcome following surgical regenerative therapy of peri-implantitis. *J. Clin. Periodontol.* **2010**, *37*, 449–455. [CrossRef]

87. Demirturk Kocasarac, H.; Helvacioglu Yigit, D.; Bechara, B.; Sinanoglu, A.; Noujeim, M. Contrast-to-noise ratio with different settings in a cbct machine in presence of different root-end filling materials: An in vitro study. *Dentomaxillofac. Radiol.* **2016**, *45*, 20160012. [CrossRef]

88. Sirin, Y.; Horasan, S.; Yaman, D.; Basegmez, C.; Tanyel, C.; Aral, A.; Guven, K. Detection of crestal radiolucencies around dental implants: An in vitro experimental study. *J. Oral Maxillofac. Surg.* **2012**, *70*, 1540–1550. [CrossRef] [PubMed]

89. Fienitz, T.; Schwarz, F.; Ritter, L.; Dreiseidler, T.; Becker, J.; Rothamel, D. Accuracy of cone beam computed tomography in assessing peri-implant bone defect regeneration: A histologically controlled study in dogs. *Clin. Oral Implants Res.* **2012**, *23*, 882–887. [CrossRef] [PubMed]

90. De-Azevedo-Vaz, S.L.; Alencar, P.N.; Rovaris, K.; Campos, P.S.; Haiter-Neto, F. Enhancement cone beam computed tomography filters improve in vitro periimplant dehiscence detection. *Oral Surg. Oral Med. Oral Pathol. Oral Radiol.* **2013**, *116*, 633–639. [CrossRef] [PubMed]

91. Neves, F.S.; Vasconcelos, T.V.; Campos, P.S.; Haiter-Neto, F.; Freitas, D.Q. Influence of scan mode (180 degrees/360 degrees) of the cone beam computed tomography for preoperative dental implant measurements. *Clin. Oral Implants Res.* **2014**, *25*, e155–e158. [CrossRef] [PubMed]

92. Pinheiro, L.R.; Scarfe, W.C.; Augusto de Oliveira Sales, M.; Gaia, B.F.; Cortes, A.R.; Cavalcanti, M.G. Effect of cone-beam computed tomography field of view and acquisition frame on the detection of chemically simulated peri-implant bone loss in vitro. *J. Periodontol.* **2015**, *86*, 1159–1165. [CrossRef] [PubMed]

93. Al-Nuaimi, N.; Patel, S.; Foschi, F.; Mannocci, F. The detection of simulated periapical lesions in human dry mandibles with cone-beam computed tomography: A dose reduction study. *Int. Endod. J.* **2016**, *49*, 1095–1104. [CrossRef] [PubMed]

94. Pelekos, G.; Acharya, A.; Tonetti, M.S.; Bornstein, M.M. Diagnostic performance of cone beam computed tomography in assessing peri-implant bone loss: A systematic review. *Clin. Oral Implants Res.* **2018**, *29*, 443–464. [CrossRef]

95. Mengel, R. Kruse, B. Flores-de-Jacoby, L. Digital volume tomography in the diagnosis of peri-implant defects: An in vitro study on native pig mandibles. *J. Periodontol.* **2006**, *77*, 1234–1241. [CrossRef]

96. Ritter, L.; Elger, M.C.; Rothamel, D.; Fienitz, T.; Zinser, M.; Schwarz, F.; Zoller, J.E. Accuracy of peri-implant bone evaluation using cone beam ct, digital intra-oral radiographs and histology. *Dentomaxillofac. Radiol.* **2014**, *43*, 20130088. [CrossRef]

97. Fleiner, J.; Hannig, C.; Schulze, D.; Stricker, A.; Jacobs, R. Digital method for quantification of circumferential periodontal bone level using cone beam ct. *Clin. Oral Investig.* **2013**, *17*, 389–396. [CrossRef]

98. Kuhl, S.; Zurcher, S.; Zitzmann, N.U.; Filippi, A.; Payer, M.; Dagassan-Berndt, D. Detection of peri-implant bone defects with different radiographic techniques—A human cadaver study. *Clin. Oral Implants Res.* **2016**, *27*, 529–534. [CrossRef] [PubMed]

99. Tyndall, D.A.; Price, J.B.; Tetradis, S.; Ganz, S.D.; Hildebolt, C.; Scarfe, W.C. Position statement of the American Academy of Oral and Maxillofacial Radiology on selection criteria for the use of radiology in dental implantology with emphasis on cone beam computed tomography. *Oral Surg. Oral Med. Oral Pathol. Oral Radiol.* **2012**, *113*, 817–826. [CrossRef] [PubMed]

100. Chan, H.L.; Sinjab, K.; Li, J.; Chen, Z.; Wang, H.L.; Kripfgans, O.D. Ultrasonography for noninvasive and real-time evaluation of peri-implant tissue dimensions. *J. Clin. Periodontol.* **2018**, *45*, 986–995. [CrossRef] [PubMed]

101. Bloch, S.H.; Dayton, P.A.; Ferrara, K.W. Targeted imaging using ultrasound contrast agents. *IEEE Eng. Med. Biol. Mag.* **2004**, *23*, 18–29. [CrossRef] [PubMed]

102. Marotti, J.; Heger, S.; Tinschert, J.; Tortamano, P.; Chuembou, F.; Radermacher, K.; Wolfart, S. Recent advances of ultrasound imaging in dentistry—A review of the literature. *Oral Surg. Oral Med. Oral Pathol. Oral Radiol.* **2013**, *115*, 819–832. [CrossRef] [PubMed]

103. Wang, L.V.; Hu, S. Photoacoustic Tomography: In Vivo Imaging from Organelles to Organs. *Science* **2012**, *335*, 1458–1462. [CrossRef] [PubMed]

104. Xu, M.; Wang, L.V. Photoacoustic imaging in biomedicine. *Rev. Sci. Instrum.* **2006**, *77*, 041101. [CrossRef]

105. Hariri, A.; Lemaster, J.; Wang, J.; Jeevarathinam, A.S.; Chao, D.L.; Jokerst, J.V. The characterization of an economic and portable LED-based photoacoustic imaging system to facilitate molecular imaging. *Photoacoustics* **2018**, *9*, 10–20. [CrossRef]

106. Asao, Y.; Hashizume, Y.; Suita, T.; Nagae, K.-I.; Fukutani, K.; Sudo, Y.; Matsushita, T.; Kobayashi, S.; Tokiwa, M.; Yamaga, I.; et al. Photoacoustic mammography capable of simultaneously acquiring photoacoustic and ultrasound images. *J. Biomed. Opt.* **2016**, *21*, 116009. [CrossRef]

107. Mozaffarzadeh, M.; Hariri, A.; Moore, C.; Jokerst, J.V. The double-stage delay-multiply-and-sum image reconstruction method improves imaging quality in a LED-based photoacoustic array scanner. *Photoacoustics* **2018**, *12*, 22–29. [CrossRef]

108. Hoelen, C.; de Mul, F.; Pongers, R.; Dekker, A. Three-dimensional photoacoustic imaging of blood vessels in tissue. *Opt. Lett.* **1998**, *23*, 648–650. [CrossRef] [PubMed]

109. Köstli, K.P.; Beard, P.C. Two-dimensional photoacoustic imaging by use of Fourier-transform image reconstruction and a detector with an anisotropic response. *Appl. Opt.* **2003**, *42*, 1899–1908. [CrossRef] [PubMed]

110. Xu, M.; Wang, L.V. Universal back-projection algorithm for photoacoustic computed tomography. *Phys. Rev. E* **2005**, *71*, 016706. [CrossRef] [PubMed]

111. Lovell, J.F.; Liu, T.W.; Chen, J.; Zheng, G. Activatable photosensitizers for imaging and therapy. *Chem. Rev.* **2010**, *110*, 2839–2857. [CrossRef] [PubMed]

112. Hariri, A.; Wang, J.; Kim, Y.; Jhunjhunwala, A.; Chao, D.L.; Jokerst, J.V. In vivo photoacoustic imaging of chorioretinal oxygen gradients. *J. Biomed. Opt.* **2018**, *23*, 036005. [CrossRef] [PubMed]

113. Luke, G.P.; Emelianov, S.Y. Label-free Detection of Lymph Node Metastases with US-guided Functional Photoacoustic Imaging. *Radiology* **2015**, *277*, 435–442. [CrossRef] [PubMed]

114. Kircher, M.F.; de la Zerda, A.; Jokerst, J.V.; Zavaleta, C.L.; Kempen, P.J.; Mittra, E.; Pitter, K.; Huang, R.; Campos, C.; Habte, F.; et al. A Brain Tumor Molecular Imaging Strategy Using A New Triple-Modality MRI-Photoacoustic-Raman Nanoparticle. *Nat. Med.* **2012**, *18*, 829–834. [CrossRef]

115. Guan, T.; Shang, W.; Li, H.; Yang, X.; Fang, C.; Tian, J.; Wang, K. From Detection to Resection: Photoacoustic Tomography and Surgery Guidance with Indocyanine Green Loaded Gold Nanorod@liposome Core–Shell Nanoparticles in Liver Cancer. *Bioconjugate Chem.* **2017**, *28*, 1221–1228. [CrossRef]

116. Wang, J.; Chen, F.; Arconada-Alvarez, S.J.; Hartanto, J.; Yap, L.-P.; Park, R.; Wang, F.; Vorobyova, I.; Dagliyan, G.; Conti, P.S. A Nanoscale Tool for Photoacoustic-based Measurements of Clotting Time and Therapeutic Drug Monitoring of Heparin. *Nano Lett.* **2016**, *16*, 6265–6271. [CrossRef]

117. Cash, K.J.; Li, C.; Xia, J.; Wang, L.V.; Clark, H.A. Optical Drug Monitoring: Photoacoustic Imaging of Nanosensors to Monitor Therapeutic Lithium in Vivo. *ACS Nano* **2015**, *9*, 1692–1698. [CrossRef]

118. Zackrisson, S.; van de Ven, S.; Gambhir, S. Light in and sound out: Emerging translational strategies for photoacoustic imaging. *Cancer Res.* **2014**, *74*, 979–1004. [CrossRef] [PubMed]

119. Luke, G.P.; Yeager, D.; Emelianov, S.Y. Biomedical applications of photoacoustic imaging with exogenous contrast agents. *Ann. Biomed. Eng.* **2012**, *40*, 422–437. [CrossRef] [PubMed]

120. Mariotti, A.; Hefti, A.F. Defining periodontal health. *BMC Oral Health* **2015**, *15*, S6. [CrossRef] [PubMed]

121. Perry, D.A.; Beemsterboer, P.; Essex, G. *Periodontology for the Dental Hygienist*, 4th ed.; Elsevier/Saunders: St. Louis, MO, USA, 2014.

122. Araujo, M.W.; Benedek, K.M.; Benedek, J.R.; Grossi, S.G.; Dorn, J.; Wactawski-Wende, J.; Genco, R.J.; Trevisan, M. Reproducibility of probing depth measurements using a constant-force electronic probe: Analysis of inter-and intraexaminer variability. *J. Periodontol.* **2003**, *74*, 1736–1740. [CrossRef]

123. Larsen, C.; Barendregt, D.S.; Slot, D.E.; van der Velden, U.; van der Weijden, F. Probing pressure, a highly undervalued unit of measure in periodontal probing: A systematic review on its effect on probing pocket depth. *J. Clin. Periodontol.* **2009**, *36*, 315–322. [CrossRef]

124. Biddle, A.J.; Palmer, R.M.; Wilson, R.F.; Watts, T.L. Comparison of the validity of periodontal probing measurements in smokers and non-smokers. *J. Clin. Periodontol.* **2001**, *28*, 806–812. [CrossRef] [PubMed]

125. Listgarten, M.A. Periodontal probing: What does it mean? *J. Clin. Periodontol.* **1980**, *7*, 165–176. [CrossRef]

126. Holtfreter, B.; Albandar, J.M.; Dietrich, T.; Dye, B.A.; Eaton, K.A.; Eke, P.I.; Papapanou, P.N.; Kocher, T. Standards for reporting chronic periodontitis prevalence and severity in epidemiologic studies: Proposed standards from the Joint EU/USA Periodontal Epidemiology Working Group. *J. Clin. Periodontol.* **2015**, *42*, 407–412. [CrossRef]

127. Karadottir, H.; Lenoir, L.; Barbierato, B.; Bogle, M.; Riggs, M.; Sigurdsson, T.; Crigger, M.; Egelberg, J. Pain experienced by patients during periodontal maintenance treatment. *J. Periodontol.* **2002**, *73*, 536–542. [CrossRef]

128. Van Wijk, A.; Hoogstraten, J. Experience with dental pain and fear of dental pain. *J. Dent. Res.* **2005**, *84*, 947–950. [CrossRef]

129. Cole, A.; McMichael, A. Audit of dental practice record-keeping: A PCT-coordinated clinical audit by Worcestershire dentists. *Prim. Dent. Care* **2009**, *16*, 85–93. [CrossRef] [PubMed]

130. McFall, W.T., Jr.; Bader, J.D.; Rozier, R.G.; Ramsey, D. Presence of periodontal data in patient records of general practitioners. *J. Periodontol.* **1988**, *59*, 445–449. [CrossRef] [PubMed]

131. Morgan, R.G. Quality evaluation of clinical records of a group of general dental practitioners entering a quality assurance programme. *Br. Dent. J.* **2001**, *191*, 436–441. [CrossRef] [PubMed]

132. Schou, S.; Holmstrup, P.; Stoltze, K.; Hjørting-Hansen, E.; Fiehn, N.E.; Skovgaard, L.T. Probing around implants and teeth with healthy or inflamed peri-implant mucosa/gingiva: A histologic comparison in cynomolgus monkeys (Macaca fascicularis). *Clin. Oral Implants Res.* **2002**, *13*, 113–126. [CrossRef] [PubMed]

133. Koka, S. The implant-mucosal interface and its role in the long-term success of endosseous oral implants: A review of the literature. *Int. J. Prosthodont.* **1998**, *11*, 421–432. [PubMed]

134. Rakic, M.; Galindo-Moreno, P.; Monje, A.; Radovanovic, S.; Wang, H.-L.; Cochran, D.; Sculean, A.; Canullo, L. How frequent does peri-implantitis occur? A systematic review and meta-analysis. *Clin. Oral Investig.* **2018**, *22*, 1805–1816. [CrossRef] [PubMed]

135. Giraldo, V.M.; Duque, A.; Aristizabal, A.G.; Hernández, R.D.M. Prevalence of Peri-implant Disease According to Periodontal Probing Depth and Bleeding on Probing: A Systematic Review and Meta-Analysis. *Int. J. Oral Maxillofac. Implants* **2018**, *33*, e89–e105. [CrossRef]

136. Lin, C.; Chen, F.; Hariri, A.; Chen, C.; Wilder-Smith, P.; Takesh, T.; Jokerst, J. Photoacoustic Imaging for Noninvasive Periodontal Probing Depth Measurements. *J. Dent. Res.* **2018**, *97*, 23–30. [CrossRef]

137. Moore, C.; Bai, Y.; Hariri, A.; Sanchez, J.B.; Lin, C.-Y.; Koka, S.; Sedghizadeh, P.; Chen, C.; Jokerst, J.V. Photoacoustic imaging for monitoring periodontal health: A first human study. *Photoacoustics* **2018**, *12*, 67–74. [CrossRef]

11

Factors Influencing Early Marginal Bone Loss around Dental Implants Positioned Subcrestally: A Multicenter Prospective Clinical Study

Teresa Lombardi [1], Federico Berton [2], Stefano Salgarello [3], Erika Barbalonga [4], Antonio Rapani [2], Francesca Piovesana [2], Caterina Gregorio [5], Giulia Barbati [2], Roberto Di Lenarda [2] and Claudio Stacchi [2,*]

[1] Private Practice, 87011 Cassano allo Ionio, Italy
[2] Department of Medical, Surgical and Health Sciences, University of Trieste, 34129 Trieste, Italy
[3] Department of Medical and Surgical Specialties, Radiological Sciences and Public Health, University of Brescia, 25123 Brescia, Italy
[4] Private Practice, 6600 Locarno, Switzerland
[5] Department of Statistics, University of Padova, 35121 Padova, Italy
* Correspondence: claudio@stacchi.it

Abstract: Early marginal bone loss (MBL) is a non-infective remodeling process of variable entity occurring within the first year after implant placement. It has a multifactorial etiology, being influenced by both surgical and prosthetic factors. Their impact remains a matter of debate, and controversial information is available, particularly regarding implants placed subcrestally. The present multicenter prospective clinical study aimed to correlate marginal bone loss around platform-switched implants with conical connection inserted subcrestally to general and local factors. Fifty-five patients were enrolled according to strict inclusion/exclusion criteria by four clinical centers. Single or multiple implants (AnyRidge, MegaGen, South Korea) were inserted in the posterior mandible with a one-stage protocol. Impressions were taken after two months of healing (T1), screwed metal-ceramic restorations were delivered three months after implant insertion (T2), and patients were recalled after six months (T3) and twelve months (T4) of prosthetic loading. Periapical radiographs were acquired at each time point. Bone levels were measured at each time point on both mesial and distal aspects of implants. Linear mixed models were fitted to the data to identify predictors associated with MBL. Fifty patients (25 male, 25 female; mean age 58.0 ± 12.8) with a total of 83 implants were included in the final analysis. The mean subcrestal position of the implant shoulder at baseline was 1.24 ± 0.57 mm, while at T4, it was 0.46 ± 0.59 mm under the bone level. Early marginal bone remodeling was significantly influenced by implant insertion depth and factors related to biological width establishment (vertical mucosal thickness, healing, and prosthetic abutment height). Deep implant insertion, thin peri-implant mucosa, and short abutments were associated with greater marginal bone loss up to six months after prosthetic loading. Peri-implant bone levels tended to stabilize after this time, and no further marginal bone resorption was recorded at twelve months after implant loading.

Keywords: abutment height; subcrestal implants; marginal bone loss; implant insertion depth; vertical mucosal thickness; biological width

1. Introduction

A complex cascade of biological events occurs after implant insertion. In this type of surgery, wound healing response after surgical trauma is conditioned by the presence of foreign material in the host bone. According to studies by Donath [1,2], a foreign material inside the human body may elicit four types of host response: rejection, dissolution, resorption, or demarcation. Demarcation, which represents a protective reaction aiming to separate a foreign body impossible to dissolute or resorb from healthy tissue, usually results in fibrous encapsulation. However, when biocompatible material is surrounded by bone in a protected environment (with neither infection nor micromovements), bone encapsulation usually occurs, forming a robust bone-to-implant interface, which can be used for clinical purposes: the osseointegration phenomenon [3]. The majority of osseointegrated implants show successful long-term clinical outcomes due to the establishment of steady-state bone remodeling activity. However, the condition of foreign-body equilibrium may be compromised by various factors at different times. The main clinical sign of imbalance between bone apposition and resorption is a marginal bone loss (MBL) [4]. Marginal bone stability around dental implants has always been considered one of the main criteria for defining implant success [5].

Early MBL is a non-infective remodeling process of variable entity occurring within the first year after implant placement. It has a multifactorial etiology, being influenced by both surgical factors (insufficient crestal width and/or implant malpositioning, bone overheating during implant site preparation, implant crest module characteristics, excessive cortical compression) and prosthetic variables (type of implant/abutment connection, entity and location of implant/abutment microgap, number of abutment disconnections, abutment height, residual cement, early loading) [6–9]. Early MBL represents an adaptive response of peri-implant marginal bone to the combined effect of these factors and has been considered to have an important prognostic value for predicting long-term implant success. A recent study on implants positioned at the crestal level suggested that early MBL >0.44 mm in the first six months after prosthetic loading is a risk indicator for peri-implant bone loss progression [10].

Modifications of horizontal and vertical relationships between implant-abutment junction (IAJ) and bone crest have been suggested to influence the entity of early MBL. The horizontal displacement of the microgap location far from the bone crest using an abutment narrower than the implant neck (platform switching) has been demonstrated to be effective in reducing early MBL [11,12]. Conversely, controversial information is available regarding implants placed subcrestally. Some authors recommended placement of the implant platform 1 or 2 mm below the alveolar crest to better maintain marginal bone levels [13,14]. However, other studies reported an increased extension of inflammatory infiltrate due to deep positioning of the IAJ, resulting in greater MBL compared to implants placed equicrestally [15,16].

Therefore, the primary aim of the present multicenter prospective clinical study was to analyze factors potentially influencing early MBL around platform-switched implants with conical connection inserted subcrestally, up to 15 months after implant placement.

2. Material and Methods

2.1. Study Protocol

This multicenter prospective clinical study was reported in strict adherence to the criteria of the STROBE (Strengthening the Reporting of Observational Studies in Epidemiology) checklist. All procedures were performed per the recommendations of the Declaration of Helsinki, as revised in Fortaleza (2013), for investigations with human subjects. The study protocol was approved by the relevant Ethical Committee (Regione Calabria, Sezione Area Nord, No. 46/2016), and was recorded in a public register of clinical trials (www.clinicaltrials.gov-NCT03077880). All eligible patients were thoroughly informed of the study protocol (including surgical and prosthetic procedures, follow-up visits, potential risks involved, and possible therapeutic alternatives), and signed an informed consent form. Patients authorized the use of their data for research purposes.

2.2. Selection Criteria

Any partially edentulous patient requiring implant therapy for fixed prosthetic rehabilitation in the posterior mandible was eligible for this study, subject to the following inclusion and exclusion criteria.

General inclusion criteria were: (I) age >18 years; (II) good general health; (III) patient willing and fully capable to comply with the study protocol; (IV) written informed consent given.

Local inclusion criteria were: (I) presence of keratinized mucosa with a minimum buccolingual width of 4 mm; (II) bone crest with at least 6 mm width and 8 mm height above the mandibular canal in the site when the implant was planned; (III) healed bone crest (at least 6 months elapsed from tooth extraction); (IV) no grafted bone; (V) full mouth plaque score (FMPS) <25% and full mouth bleeding score (FMBS) <20%; (VI) implant insertion torque (IT) >20 Ncm; (VII) presence of the opposing dentition; (VIII) subcrestal positioning. Exclusion criteria were: (I) history of head or neck radiation therapy; (II) uncontrolled diabetes (hemoglobinA1c >7.5%); (III) immunocompromised patients (HIV infection or chemotherapy within the past 5 years); (IV) present or past treatment with intravenous bisphosphonates; (V) patient pregnancy or lactating at any time during the study; (VI) psychological or psychiatric problems; (VII) alcohol or drugs abuse; (VIII) participating in other studies, if the present protocol could not be properly followed.

All patients, selected consecutively between April 2016 and October 2017, were treated independently by four operators (T.L., S.S., E.B., and C.S.) in four private offices. Data collection was performed by a single independent examiner (F.B.).

All patients received oral hygiene instructions and underwent deplaquing 1 week before surgery. Cone beam computed tomography (CBCT) was performed to analyze available bone volume and to plan implant insertion.

2.3. Surgical and Restorative Procedures

All patients were administered with antibiotic prophylaxis (amoxicillin 2 g) one hour before surgery. A mid-crestal incision was performed under local anesthesia, preserving an adequate quantity of keratinized tissue on both buccal and lingual sides. A full-thickness buccal flap was elevated, and vertical mucosal thickness of the undetached lingual flap was measured with a periodontal probe at the center of the programmed implant site, as described elsewhere [17]. The lingual flap was subsequently elevated, and implant site preparation was performed under abundant irrigation of cold saline solution following the manufacturer's recommendations for subcrestal placement. Platform-switched implants with conical connection (AnyRidge, MegaGen, Gyeongbuk, South Korea) were inserted under bone level, and peak IT values were recorded by the surgical motor (Implantmed, W&H, Burmoos, Austria). Implants were immediately connected to healing or transepithelial abutments (Octa, MegaGen, Gyeongbuk, South Korea), adapting their length to the site-specific soft tissue vertical thickness. Flaps were sutured with single stitches and Sentineri technique using synthetic monofilament [18]. Patients were prescribed post-surgical antibiotic therapy (amoxicillin 1 g twice a day) for six days, and nonsteroidal anti-inflammatory drugs (ibuprofen 600 mg), when necessary. Sutures were removed 10–14 days after surgery. Patients were instructed not to use removable prostheses during the entire healing period.

After two months of healing, implants were clinically and radiographically evaluated, and final impressions were taken. Prosthetic abutments height was chosen, adapting their length to the site-specific soft tissue vertical thickness. After functional and aesthetic try-in, screw-retained metal-ceramic rehabilitations were delivered.

Periodontal status was assessed using the modified plaque index (mPI) and modified sulcus bleeding index (mSBI) at prosthesis delivery and after 6 and 12 months of functional loading [19]. The mean of the four values recorded for each implant (mesial, distal, buccal, and lingual) was subsequently analyzed.

2.4. Radiographic Measurements

Digital radiographs were taken using a long-cone paralleling technique with a Rinn-type film holder at the time of implant placement (baseline—T0), at impression taking (2 months after implant placement—T1), at prosthetic restoration delivery (3 months after implant placement—T2), and after 6 and 12 months of prosthetic loading (T3 and T4, respectively) (Figure 1).

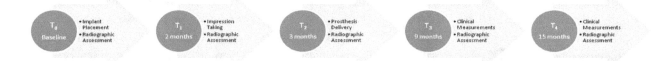

Figure 1. Summary of the visits.

The distance between IAJ and bone crest was measured at each time interval, on both mesial and distal aspects of the implant. A positive value was assigned when the bone crest was coronal to the IAJ, whereas a negative value was assigned when the bone crest was apical to the IAJ.

Any radiograph showing signs of deformation or poor image quality was immediately repeated. All measurements were taken by a single calibrated examiner (F.P.), on a 30-inch led-backlit color diagnostic display, using measuring software (Image J 1.52a, National Institutes of Health, USA) (Figure 2). Each measurement was repeated three times at three different time points, as proposed by Gomez-Roman and Launer [20]. Examiner calibration was performed by assessing ten radiographs, with a different author (F.B.) serving as a reference examiner. Intra-examiner and inter-examiner concordances were 91.9% and 85.2%, respectively, for linear measurements within ±0.1 mm.

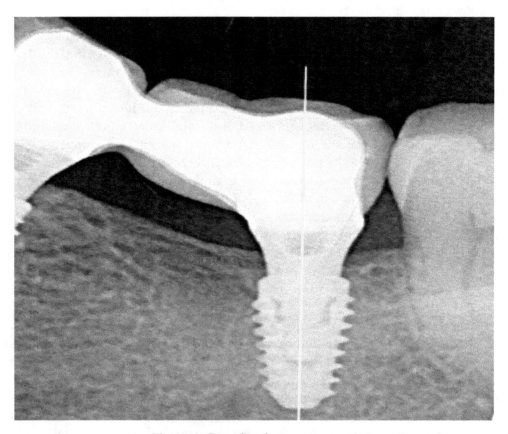

Figure 2. Bone level measurement.

2.5. Predictor and Outcome Variables

Primary predictor variables and their respective period of activity were evaluated as follows: (i) vertical mucosal thickness (thick >2 mm vs. thin ≤2 mm; from T0 to T4); (ii) implant insertion torque (>50 Ncm vs. ≤50 Ncm; from T0 to T1); (iii) depth of implant insertion (mm; from T0 to T4); (iv) healing abutment height (long ≥3 mm vs. short <3 mm; from T0 to T2); (v) number of abutment disconnections (zero vs. multiple; from T0 to T4); (vi) prosthetic abutment height (long ≥3 mm vs. short <3 mm; from T2 to T4); (vii) type of prosthetic restoration (single crown vs. short-span bridge; from T2 to T4). The influence of the following patient-related variables, possibly correlated with the predictor and outcome variables, were also evaluated from T0 to T4: (i) age; (ii) gender; (iii) smoking status (smoker vs. no smoker); (iv) periodontal status (periodontal health vs. chronic periodontitis).

Primary outcome (dependent variable):

- early MBL (up to 12 months from prosthetic loading).

Secondary outcomes:

- implant failure: implant mobility or implant removal due to progressive marginal bone loss. Implant stability was tested by tightening abutment screws (35 N/cm) at prosthesis delivery.
- any complication or adverse event.

2.6. Statistical Analysis

Statistical analysis was performed using R software version 3.5.3 (nlme package; version 3.1.140). Early MBL at each time point was defined as the difference between the depth of implant insertion at the time and depth of implant insertion at baseline.

The means of mesial and distal early MBL at each follow-up were compared using a t-test for paired data. No significant differences were found (T1: Toss = 0.413, d.f. (degrees of freedom) = 82, $p = 0.68$; T2: Toss = 0.002, d.f. = 82, $p = 1$; T3: Toss = −0.143, d.f. = 82, $p = 0.89$; T4: Toss = −0.027, d.f. = 82, $p = 0.98$), hence the mean between mesial and distal MBL was used as a primary outcome in subsequent analysis.

Linear mixed models were fitted to the data to identify predictors associated with MBL. Since not all variables were active at all time-points, four different models were estimated. First, a global model (Model A) was built, considering all four follow-up time points. Preliminary models with only one covariate at a time, plus time and peri-implant bone level at T0, were estimated to select the covariates to be included in the final multivariable model. Only covariates with $p < 0.05$ entered the final model. Covariates taken into account were those that might have affected the primary outcome over the whole follow-up period: age, gender, smoking status, periodontal status, vertical mucosal thickness, and multiple abutment disconnections. Time was considered a continuous variable measured in months, and was modeled using a linear spline function with one knot at T3, as indicated by graphical preliminary exploratory analyses. Subsequently, models considering different follow-up times were estimated:

- Model B: T1
- Model C: T1, T2
- Model D: T2, T3, T4

In these models, in addition to the covariates used in Model A, other independent variables active only at specific time points were added (implant insertion torque in Model B; healing abutment height in Model C; prosthetic abutment height and type of prosthetic restoration in Model D).

In models C and D, time was used as a categorical variable. Time was not included in Model B as only one MBL measurement was involved. Covariate selection was performed using preliminary models, as explained above.

The random-effects structure of each model was evaluated using the Likelihood Ratio Test. For all models, the most suitable structure was random intercept on the subject and random intercept on the operator, except for Model B, in which only random intercept on the operator was included.

3. Results

3.1. Demographics and Clinical Outcomes

Of a total of 228 patients evaluated for eligibility, 55 consecutive patients (T.L. 20; S.S. 9; E.B. 6; C.S. 20) fulfilled all inclusion/exclusion requirements and were enrolled in the present study. Included patients (27 male, 28 female; mean age 57.3 ± 12.6, age-range 32–85) were treated between June 2016 and March 2017 with the insertion of a total of 91 implants in the posterior mandible. Two implants in two patients were not placed subcrestally (negative value of the mean between mesial and distal measurements). Three implants in three patients failed to osseointegrate and were removed before taking impressions (primary failure rate of 3.3%). Two patients (three implants) were lost at 6-month follow-up (one patient of T.L. was jailed, and one patient of C.S. moved abroad). Finally, fifty patients (25 male, 25 female; mean age 58.0 ± 12.8, age-range 32–85), with a total of 83 implants that received single or short-span screwed metal-ceramic restorations, completed all phases of the study and were included in the final analysis. The final sample was balanced in terms of age and gender distribution. Complete demographics and characteristics of the included patients are summarized in Table 1.

Table 1. Characteristics of the included patients.

	Total	%
Age		
Male	56.2 ± 13.8	-
Female	59.2 ± 12.3	-
Gender		
Male	25	50
Female	25	50
Smoking Status		
Smoker	7	14
Non Smoker	43	86
Periodontal Status		
Periodontal Health	37	74
Chronic Periodontitis	13	26

No complications or adverse effects were recorded, and no additional implants were lost. All 83 implants were functioning satisfactorily 6 months and 12 months after prosthetic loading. Although slight increases in mPI and mSBI values were recorded at 15-month follow up, no significant differences were recorded between T3 and T4.

3.2. Marginal Bone Level Changes

The mean subcrestal position of the implant shoulder at T0 was 1.24 ± 0.57 mm under bone level, while at T4, it was 0.46 ± 0.59 mm. At the end of the follow-up period, out of a total of 83 implants, the platform of 63 implants remained subcrestal (75.9%), four resulted in equicrestal (4.8%), and 16 resulted in supracrestal (19.3%).

The pattern of marginal bone resorption over time was the following: mean MBL at T1 was 0.5 ± 0.34 mm. An additional mean MBL of 0.18 ± 0.22 mm was registered at T2. A further increase in mean MBL of 0.11 ± 0.20 mm occurred at T3, while complete marginal bone stabilization was observed at T4 (mean MBL compared to T3 = 0.00 ± 0.19 mm). Marginal bone levels at the different time-points are represented in Figure 3.

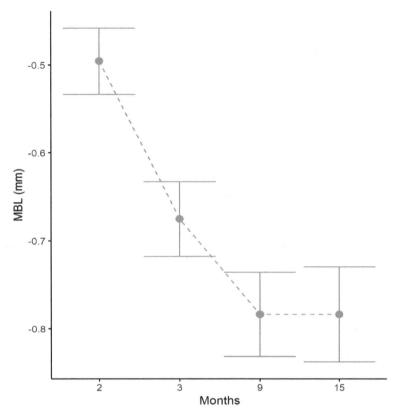

Figure 3. Marginal bone variations at different time points. MBL: marginal bone loss.

Results of preliminary linear mixed models analyzing factors possibly influencing MBL from T0 and T4 are reported in Table 2. From T0 to T4, no significant relationships between early MBL and patient age, gender, smoking status, periodontal status, and multiple abutment disconnections were demonstrated. By contrast, implant insertion depth and presence of thin peri-implant mucosa demonstrated significant negative influence upon early MBL from T0 to T4 ($p < 0.01$ and $p = 0.01$, respectively). Complete results of the multivariable analysis are reported in Table 3.

Table 2. Preliminary univariable linear mixed models, analyzing factors possibly influencing marginal bone loss from implant insertion to 12-months after prosthetic loading.

	MBL (mm)	Std. Error	d.f.	t-Value	p-Value
Age	0.00	0.00	49	−0.49	0.63
Gender	−0.02	0.08	49	−0.21	0.83
Smoking Status	0.12	0.10	49	1.15	0.26
Periodontal Status	−0.02	0.09	49	−0.25	0.80
Multiple Abutment Disconnections	0.03	0.08	30	0.43	0.67

MBL: marginal bone loss; Std: standard; DF: degrees of freedom. Adjusted for time effect and depth of implant insertion.

Table 3. Multivariable linear mixed models, analyzing factors influencing marginal bone loss from implant insertion to 12-months after prosthetic loading.

	MBL (mm)	Std. Error	d.f.	t-Value	p-Value	95% CI
Vertical Mucosal Thickness	0.24	0.08	30	2.91	0.01	0.07; 0.41
Depth of Implant Insertion	−0.23	0.07	30	−3.37	<0.01	−0.37; −0.09

MBL: marginal bone loss; Std: standard; DF: degrees of freedom; CI: confidence interval. Adjusted for time effect.

MBL variability within patients and operators was evaluated by a random-effects model and, from T0 to T1, was observed to be 0.25 mm (0.19; 0.34) and 0.21 mm (0.13; 0.35), respectively.

Preliminary linear mixed models analyzing factors possibly influencing MBL within specific time frames showed no significant associations between implant insertion torque and MBL (from T0 to T1; $p = 0.62$) or between type of prosthetic restoration (single crown vs. short-span bridge) and marginal bone levels (from T2 to T4; $p = 0.92$). Conversely, healing abutment height (from T0 to T2) and prosthetic abutment height (from T2 to T4) had a significant influence on early MBL. In particular, short healing and prosthetic abutments (<3 mm height) were correlated with greater MBL ($p < 0.01$ for both variables). Results of multivariable analysis analyzing factors influencing MBL within specific time frames are reported in Table 4.

Table 4. Multivariable linear mixed models, analyzing factors influencing marginal bone loss within specific time frames.

	Time Interval	MBL (mm)	Std. Error	d.f.	t-Value	p-Value	95% CI
Healing Abutment Height Short (vs. Long)	T0–T2	−0.27	0.07	29	−3.83	<0.01	−0.41; −0.13
Prosthetic Abutment Height Short (vs. Long)	T2–T4	−0.44	0.07	29	−6.42	<0.01	−0.58; −0.3

MBL: marginal bone loss; Std: standard; DF: degrees of freedom; CI: confidence interval; T0: baseline; T1: 2-month visit; T2: 3-month visit; T4: 15-month visit. Adjusted for time effect, depth of implant insertion, and vertical mucosal thickness.

4. Discussion

The present multicenter prospective clinical study showed that platform-switched implants with internal conical connection placed subcrestally presented a reduction in marginal bone levels during the first year of function. Thoroughly analyzing this result, early MBL occurred in the first six months after prosthetic loading. At 15-month follow-up, peri-implant marginal bone levels remained unaltered (difference T4–T3: 0.00 ± 0.19 mm). This finding is in accordance with previous studies on subcrestal implants, showing that MBL mainly occurs in the first period of function [14,21], followed by stabilization of marginal bone levels or even slight marginal bone gain [22].

In the present investigation, a statistically significant positive correlation was demonstrated between the depth of implant insertion and early MBL ($p < 0.01$), confirming a tendency shown in previous studies [22,23]. To be exact, our statistical model suggested that a 1-mm depth increase below the mean implant position at T0 (1.24 mm subcrestal) led to a greater MBL of 0.23 mm at T4. However, from a clinical point of view, it should be underlined that implants with deeper apico-coronal positioning at T0 (>1.5 mm under bone level) resulted in a more subcrestal position at T4, when compared with implants placed more superficially at baseline (<1.5 mm under bone level) (Table 5). Further studies are needed to establish the ideal insertion depth for subcrestal implants, balancing the amount of MBL with the biological shield offered by the presence of bone coronal to the implant shoulder.

Table 5. Bone loss variations in groups with different implant insertion depth.

Insertion Depth	N° Of Implants	Mean Depth At T0	Mean Depth At T4
>1.5 mm	20	2.01 ± 0.48 mm	0.94 ± 0.76 mm
<1.5 mm	63	1.00 ± 0.34 mm	0.31 ± 0.42 mm

T0: baseline; T4: 15-month visit.

General variables, such as age, gender, periodontal status, and smoking habits, appeared not to play a significant role in influencing MBL during the first months of healing. Even if smoking and history of periodontitis are well-known risk factors for the long-term success of implant therapy, their action is time-dependent and often is not predictive for early bone loss after 1-year follow-up [24,25]. Additionally, the one abutment-one time protocol did not have a significant protective action on MBL in comparison to multiple abutment disconnections (three times, in the present study), in agreement with a recent prospective study [26]. This outcome is also consistent with a recent meta-analysis concluding that favorable changes in peri-implant marginal bone level associated with the one abutment-one time protocol should be viewed with caution as its clinical significance remains uncertain [27].

In the present study, the greatest MBL occurred within two months after implant insertion (mean 0.5 ± 0.34 mm), likely due to bone remodeling following surgical trauma and biological width establishment around one-stage implants.

In our sample, variations in implant insertion torque ($>$50 Ncm vs. $\leq$50 Ncm) did not influence MBL during the early healing period. This finding is in accordance with some previous clinical trials [28,29] and is in contrast with other studies, showing a negative impact of high torques on marginal bone stability [30–32]. However, the relationship between insertion torque and cortical compression, possibly leading to marginal bone resorption, is strictly dependent upon some crucial factors, which were not always adequately controlled in the aforementioned studies: implant crest module design, implant diameter, and cortical bone thickness around implants [6,33,34]. In the present investigation, detrimental distribution of compressive forces to cortical bone following implant insertion was reduced by the subcrestal positioning of implants (not compressing the most coronal part of the cortical bone) and by the crest module design of the fixture used in this study, the platform of which was significantly narrower than the wider part of the implant body (3.3 mm vs. 4.3 mm).

Conversely, all investigated variables involved in biological width establishment (vertical mucosal thickness, healing abutment height, and prosthetic abutment height) had a significant influence on marginal bone remodeling. Biological width is the three-dimensional space necessary for the establishment of a soft tissue barrier around dental implants once they become exposed to the oral cavity [35]. Peri-implant soft tissue can be divided into two main zones: a coronal epithelial portion and a more apical fiber-rich connective tissue [35,36]. Recently, the biological width around two-piece dental implants placed at the crestal level has been measured in human histologic studies. Vertical dimensions varied from 3.26 to 3.6 mm, representing the minimum space required to create an optimal seal and protect the underlying tissue from external agents [37,38]. When vertical space is insufficient for biological width establishment, the healing process includes marginal bone resorption.

In the present study, thin vertical mucosal thickness ($\leq$2 mm), short healing abutments ($<$3 mm), and short prosthetic abutments ($<$3 mm) were significantly associated with greater marginal bone resorption (Figure 4). These data are in accordance with numerous clinical trials and a meta-analysis conducted with implants placed at crestal level [17,39–43], even if this matter has been widely debated. In clinical practice and also in the present study, abutment height is adapted to site-specific soft tissue thickness, with the consequence that short abutments have usually been selected in the presence of thin peri-implant mucosa. This condition could represent a confounding factor when analyzing the real influence of both factors on MBL. Recent studies conducted on separate groups (thick mucosa with long and short abutments; thin mucosa with long and short abutments) indicate that MBL during biological width establishment around dental implants placed at crestal level is influenced by abutment height irrespective of vertical mucosal thickness [9,44].

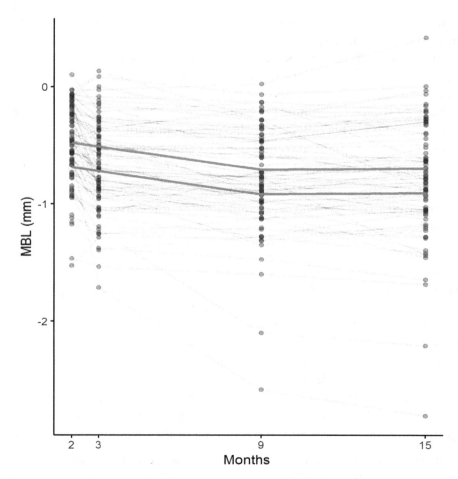

Figure 4. Marginal bone remodeling at different time points estimated by the statistical model: pattern of thick (green) and thin (pink) peri-implant mucosa in the entire sample. MBL: marginal bone loss.

Very few data on these topics are present in literature for subcrestal implants. Some authors suggested adapting the vertical position of implants in relation to soft tissue thickness in order to prevent early MBL [45,46]. The rationale behind this proposal is that subcrestal implant placement could provide additional space for biologic width formation, from the bone crest to the implant platform, resulting in reduced marginal bone remodeling in the presence of thin peri-implant mucosa. However, further clinical and histological studies are necessary to confirm this hypothesis.

Some limitations must be considered when interpreting the outcomes of the present study. These results are not to be generalized for all types of implants: fixtures with a flat-to-flat connection placed subcrestally showed persistent acute inflammation at the microgap between implant and abutment, resulting in increased MBL [15]. The platform-switched conical connection is currently to be considered the pattern of choice to minimize marginal bone remodeling when planning subcrestal implant placement [47].

Another limitation is the use of periapical radiographs to assess marginal bone levels: this method, allowing evaluation of only mesial and distal aspects of peri-implant bone, reduces sensitivity in detecting marginal bone changes.

Moreover, thresholds adopted in the present study to define an abutment as short or long (long: ≥3 mm height; short: <3 mm height) were arbitrary. Future studies should confirm the suitability of these values to define abutment length for implants placed subcrestally.

Finally, the present study collected data from a limited pool of patients in a specific site (posterior mandible): therefore, further trials are needed to generalize these results to a broader population and different areas of the mouth.

5. Conclusions

Early marginal bone remodeling around platform-switched implants with conical connection inserted subcrestally was significantly influenced by implant insertion depth and factors related to biological width establishment (vertical mucosal thickness, healing, and prosthetic abutment height). Deep implant insertion, thin peri-implant mucosa, and short abutments were associated with greater marginal bone loss up to six months after prosthetic loading. Peri-implant bone levels tended to stabilize after this time, and no further marginal bone resorption was recorded at twelve months after implant loading.

The outcomes of this study should be confirmed and generalized by further clinical trials with greater numerosity and conducted in different areas of the mouth.

Finally, further investigations are needed to establish the ideal insertion depth for subcrestal implants, balancing the amount of MBL with the biological shield offered by the presence of bone coronal to the implant shoulder.

Author Contributions: Conceptualization, T.L. and C.S.; Data curation, F.B., A.R., and F.P.; Formal analysis, C.G., G.B., and C.S. Investigation, T.L., S.S., E.B., and C.S.; Methodology, C.G., G.B., and R.D.L.; Project administration, R.D.L.; Resources, T.L. and R.D.L.; Software, F.P.; Supervision, G.B. and C.S.; Validation, F.B. and E.B.; Visualization, S.S.; Writing—original draft, T.L. and C.S.; Writing—review and editing, F.B., S.S., E.B., and A.R.

Acknowledgments: The authors wish to thank Sergio Spinato and Richard de Roeck for their help in reviewing and editing the final manuscript.

References

1. Donath, K. Pathogenesis of bony pocket formation around dental implants. *J. Dent. Assoc. S. Afr.* **1992**, *47*, 204–208. [PubMed]

2. Donath, K.; Laass, M.; Günzl, H.J. The histopathology of different foreign body reactions in oral soft tissue and bone tissue. *Virchows Arch. A Pathol. Anat. Histopathol.* **1992**, *420*, 131–137. [CrossRef] [PubMed]

3. Albrektsson, T.; Chrcanovic, B.; Jacobsson, M.; Wennerberg, A. Osseointegration of implants—A biological and clinical overview. *JSM Dent. Surg.* **2017**, *2*, 1022–1027.

4. Trindade, R.; Albrektsson, T.; Tengvall, P.; Wennerberg, A. Foreign body reaction to biomaterials: On mechanisms for buildup and breakdown of osseointegration. *Clin. Implant Dent. Relat. Res.* **2016**, *18*, 192–203. [CrossRef] [PubMed]

5. Albrektsson, T.; Zarb, G.; Worthington, P.; Eriksson, A.R. The long-term efficacy of currently used dental implants: A review and proposed criteria of success. *Int. J. Oral Maxillofac. Implant.* **1986**, *1*, 11–25.

6. Oh, T.J.; Yoon, J.; Misch, C.E.; Wang, H.-L. The causes of early implant bone loss: Myth or science? *J. Periodontol.* **2002**, *73*, 322–333. [CrossRef] [PubMed]

7. Tatarakis, N.; Bashutski, J.; Wang, H.-L.; Oh, T.J. Early implant bone loss: Preventable or inevitable? *Implant Dent.* **2012**, *21*, 379–386. [CrossRef]

8. Qian, J.; Wennerberg, A.; Albrektsson, T. Reasons for marginal bone loss around oral implants. *Clin. Implant Dent. Relat. Res.* **2012**, *14*, 792–807. [CrossRef]

9. Spinato, S.; Stacchi, C.; Lombardi, T.; Bernardello, F.; Messina, M.; Zaffe, D. Biological width establishment around dental implants is influenced by abutment height irrespective of vertical mucosal thickness: A cluster randomized controlled trial. *Clin. Oral Implant. Res.* **2019**, *30*, 649–659. [CrossRef]

10. Galindo-Moreno, P.; León-Cano, A.; Ortega-Oller, I.; Monje, A.; O'Valle, F.; Catena, A. Marginal bone loss as success criterion in implant dentistry: Beyond 2 mm. *Clin. Oral Implant. Res.* **2015**, *26*, e28–e34. [CrossRef]

11. Santiago, J.F., Jr.; Batista, V.E.; Verri, F.R.; Honório, H.M.; de Mello, C.C.; Almeida, D.A.; Pellizzer, E.P. Platform-switching implants and bone preservation: A systematic review and meta-analysis. *Int. J. Oral Maxillofac. Surg.* **2016**, *45*, 332–345. [CrossRef] [PubMed]

12. Hsu, Y.T.; Lin, G.H.; Wang, H.L. Effects of platform-switching on peri-implant soft and hard tissue outcomes: A systematic review and meta-analysis. *Int. J. Oral Maxillofac. Implant.* **2017**, *32*, e9–e24. [CrossRef] [PubMed]

13. Donovan, R.; Fetner, A.; Koutouzis, T.; Lundgren, T. Crestal bone changes around implants with reduced abutment diameter placed non-submerged and at subcrestal positions: A 1-year radiographic evaluation. *J. Periodontol.* **2010**, *81*, 428–434. [CrossRef] [PubMed]

14. Aimetti, M.; Ferrarotti, F.; Mariani, G.M.; Ghelardoni, C.; Romano, F. Soft tissue and crestal bone changes around implants with platform-switched abutments placed nonsubmerged at subcrestal position: A 2-year clinical and radiographic evaluation. *Int. J. Oral Maxillofac. Implant.* **2015**, *30*, 1369–1377. [CrossRef] [PubMed]

15. Broggini, N.; McManus, L.M.; Hermann, J.S. Periimplant inflammation defined by the implant-abutment interface. *J. Dent. Res.* **2006**, *85*, 473–478. [CrossRef] [PubMed]

16. Gatti, C.; Gatti, F.; Silvestri, M.; Mintrone, F.; Rossi, R.; Tridondani, G.; Piacentini, G.; Borrelli, P. A prospective multicenter study on radiographic crestal bone changes around dental implants placed at crestal or subcrestal level: One-year findings. *Int. J. Oral Maxillofac. Implant.* **2018**, *33*, 913–918. [CrossRef] [PubMed]

17. Linkevicius, T.; Apse, P.; Grybauskas, S.; Puisys, A. The influence of soft tissue thickness on crestal bone changes around implants: A 1-year prospective controlled clinical trial. *Int. J. Oral Maxillofac. Implant.* **2009**, *24*, 712–719.

18. Sentineri, R.; Lombardi, T.; Berton, F.; Stacchi, C. Laurell-Gottlow suture modified by Sentineri for tight closure of a wound with a single line of sutures. *Br. J. Oral Maxillofac. Surg.* **2016**, *54*, e18–e19. [CrossRef]

19. Mombelli, A.; van Oosten, M.A.; Schurch, E.; Lang, N. The microbiota associated with successful or failing implants. *Oral Microbiol. Immunol.* **1987**, *2*, 145–151. [CrossRef]

20. Gomez-Roman, G.; Launer, S. Peri-implant bone changes in immediate and non-immediate root-analog stepped implants-a matched comparative prospective study up to 10 years. *Int. J. Implant Dent.* **2016**, *2*, 15. [CrossRef]

21. Fickl, S.; Zuhr, O.; Stein, J.M.; Hurzeler, M.B. Peri-implant bone level around implants with platform-switched abutments. *Int. J. Oral Maxillofac. Implant.* **2010**, *25*, 577–581.

22. Froum, S.J.; Cho, S.C.; Suzuki, T.; Yu, P.; Corby, P.; Khouly, I. Epicrestal and subcrestal placement of platform-switched implants: 18 month-result of a randomized, controlled, split-mouth, prospective clinical trial. *Clin. Oral Implant. Res.* **2018**, *29*, 353–366. [CrossRef] [PubMed]

23. Koutouzis, T.; Neiva, R.; Nonhoff, J.; Lundgren, T. Placement of implants with platform-switched Morse taper connections with the implant-abutment interface at different levels in relation to the alveolar crest: A short-term (1-year) randomized prospective controlled clinical trial. *Int. J. Oral Maxillofac. Implant.* **2013**, *28*, 1553–1563. [CrossRef] [PubMed]

24. Collaert, B.; De Bruyn, H. Immediate functional loading of TiOblast dental implants in full-arch edentulous maxillae: A 3-year prospective study. *Clin. Oral Implant. Res.* **2008**, *19*, 1254–1260. [CrossRef] [PubMed]

25. Vervaeke, S.; Collaert, B.; Cosyn, J.; De Bruyn, H. A 9-year prospective case series using multivariate analyses to identify predictors of early and late peri-implant bone loss. *Clin. Implant Dent. Relat. Res.* **2016**, *18*, 30–39. [CrossRef] [PubMed]

26. Borges, T.; Leitão, B.; Pereira, M.; Carvalho, Á.; Galindo-Moreno, P. Influence of the abutment height and connection timing in early peri-implant marginal bone changes: A prospective randomized clinical trial. *Clin. Oral Implant. Res.* **2018**, *29*, 907–914. [CrossRef]

27. Atieh, M.A.; Tawse-Smith, A.; Alsabeeha, N.H.M.; Ma, S.; Duncan, W.J. The one abutment-one time protocol: A systematic review and meta-analysis. *J. Periodontol.* **2017**, *88*, 1173–1185. [CrossRef]

28. Khayat, P.G.; Arnal, H.M.; Tourbah, B.I.; Sennerby, L. Clinical outcome of dental implants placed with high insertion torques (up to 176 Ncm). *Clin. Implant Dent. Relat. Res.* **2013**, *15*, 227–233. [CrossRef]

29. Grandi, T.; Guazzi, P.; Samarani, R.; Grandi, G. Clinical outcome and bone healing of implants placed with high insertion torque: 12-month results from a multicenter controlled cohort study. *Int. J. Oral Maxillofac. Surg.* **2013**, *42*, 516–520. [CrossRef]

30. Duyck, J.; Roesems, R.; Cardoso, M.V.; Ogawa, T.; De Villa Camargos, G.; Vandamme, K. Effect of insertion torque on titanium implant osseointegration: An animal experimental study. *Clin. Oral Implant. Res.* **2015**, *26*, 191–196. [CrossRef]

31. Barone, A.; Alfonsi, F.; Derchi, G.; Tonelli, P.; Toti, P.; Marchionni, S.; Covani, U. The effect of insertion torque on the clinical outcome of single implants: A randomized clinical trial. *Clin. Implant Dent. Relat. Res.* **2016**, *18*, 588–600. [CrossRef] [PubMed]

32. Marconcini, S.; Giammarinaro, E.; Toti, P.; Alfonsi, F.; Covani, U.; Barone, A. Longitudinal analysis on the effect of insertion torque on delayed single implants: A 3-year randomized clinical study. *Clin. Implant Dent. Relat. Res.* **2018**, *20*, 322–332. [CrossRef] [PubMed]

33. Norton, M. Primary stability versus viable constraint—A need to redefine. *Int. J. Oral Maxillofac. Implant.* **2013**, *28*, 19–21.

34. Spray, J.R.; Black, C.G.; Morris, H.F.; Ochi, S. The influence of bone thickness on facial marginal bone response: Stage 1 placement through stage 2 uncovering. *Ann. Periodontol.* **2000**, *5*, 119–128. [CrossRef] [PubMed]

35. Berglundh, T.; Lindhe, J.; Ericsson, I.; Marinello, C.P.; Liljenberg, B.; Thomsen, P. The soft tissue barrier at implants and teeth. *Clin. Oral Implant. Res.* **1991**, *2*, 81–90. [CrossRef]

36. Abrahamsson, I.; Berglundh, T.; Wennström, J.; Lindhe, J. The peri-implant hard and soft tissues at different implant systems. A comparative study in the dog. *Clin. Oral Implant. Res.* **1996**, *7*, 212–219. [CrossRef]

37. Judgar, R.; Giro, G.; Zenobio, E.; Coelho, P.G.; Feres, M.; Rodrigues, J.A.; Mangano, C.; Iezzi, G.; Piattelli, A.; Shibli, J.A. Biological width around one-and two-piece implants retrieved from human jaws. *BioMed Res. Int.* **2014**, *2014*, 850120. [CrossRef]

38. Tomasi, C.; Tessarolo, F.; Caola, I.; Wennström, J.; Nollo, G.; Berglundh, T. Morphogenesis of peri-implant mucosa revisited: An experimental study in humans. *Clin. Oral Implant. Res.* **2014**, *25*, 997–1003. [CrossRef]

39. Galindo-Moreno, P.; León-Cano, A.; Ortega-Oller, I.; Monje, A.; Suárez, F.; O'Valle, F.; Spinato, S.; Catena, A. Prosthetic abutment height is a key factor in peri-implant marginal bone loss. *J. Dent. Res.* **2014**, *93*, 80S–85S. [CrossRef]

40. Vervaeke, S.; Dierens, M.; Besseler, J.; De Bruyn, H. The influence of initial soft tissue thickness on peri-implant bone remodeling. *Clin. Implant Dent. Relat. Res.* **2014**, *16*, 238–247. [CrossRef]

41. Galindo-Moreno, P.; León-Cano, A.; Monje, A.; Ortega-Oller, I.; O'Valle, F.; Catena, A. Abutment height influences the effect of platform switching on peri-implant marginal bone loss. *Clin. Oral Implant. Res.* **2016**, *27*, 167–173. [CrossRef] [PubMed]

42. Spinato, S.; Galindo-Moreno, P.; Bernardello, F.; Zaffe, D. Minimum abutment height to eliminate bone loss: Influence of implant neck design and platform switching. *Int. J. Oral Maxillofac. Implant.* **2018**, *33*, 405–411. [CrossRef] [PubMed]

43. Chen, Z.; Lin, C.Y.; Li, J.; Wang, H.L.; Yu, H. Influence of abutment height on peri-implant marginal bone loss: A systematic review and meta-analysis. *J. Prosthet. Dent.* **2019**, *122*, 14–21.e2. [CrossRef] [PubMed]

44. Blanco, J.; Pico, A.; Caneiro, L.; Nóvoa, L.; Batalla, P.; Martín-Lancharro, P. Effect of abutment height on interproximal implant bone level in the early healing: A randomized clinical trial. *Clin. Oral Implant. Res.* **2018**, *29*, 108–117. [CrossRef] [PubMed]

45. Vervaeke, S.; Matthys, C.; Nassar, R.; Christiaens, V.; Cosyn, J.; De Bruyn, H. Adapting the vertical position of implants with a conical connection in relation to soft tissue thickness prevents early implant surface exposure: A 2-year prospective intra-subject comparison. *J. Clin. Periodontol.* **2018**, *45*, 605–612. [CrossRef] [PubMed]

46. Pico, A.; Martín-Lancharro, P.; Caneiro, L.; Nóvoa, L.; Batalla, P.; Blanco, J. Influence of abutment height and implant depth position on interproximal peri-implant bone in sites with thin mucosa: A 1-year randomized clinical trial. *Clin. Oral Implant. Res.* **2019**, *30*, 595–602. [CrossRef] [PubMed]

47. Palaska, I.; Tsaousoglou, P.; Vouros, I.; Konstantinidis, A.; Menexes, G. Influence of placement depth and abutment connection pattern on bone remodeling around 1-stage implants: A prospective randomized controlled clinical trial. *Clin. Oral Implant. Res.* **2016**, *27*, e47–e56. [CrossRef] [PubMed]

12

Is Peri-Implant Probing Causing Over-Diagnosis and Over-Treatment of Dental Implants?

Pierluigi Coli [1] and Lars Sennerby [1,2,*]

[1]   Edinburgh Dental Specialists, Edinburgh EH2 4BA, UK
[2]   Department of Maxillofacial Surgery, University of Gothenburg, 413 90 Gothenburg, Sweden
*   Correspondence: lars.sennerby@gu.se

Abstract: Pocket probing depth (PPD) and bleeding on probing (BOP) measurements are useful indices for the assessment of periodontal conditions. The same periodontal indices are commonly recommended to evaluate the dental implant/tissue interface to identify sites with mucositis and peri-implantitis, which, if not treated, are anticipated to lead to implant failure. The aim of the present narrative review is to discuss the available literature on the effectiveness of probing at dental implants for identification of peri-implant pathology. There is substantial clinical evidence that PPD and BOP measurements are very poor indices of peri-implant tissue conditions and are questionable surrogate endpoints for implant failure. On the contrary, the literature suggests that frequent disturbance of the soft tissue barrier at implants may instead induce inflammation and bone resorption. Moreover, over-diagnosis and subsequent unnecessary treatment may lead to iatrogenic damage to the implant-tissue interface. Despite this, the recommendations from recent consensus meetings are still promoting the use of probing at dental implants. For evaluation of implants, for instance at annual check-ups, the present authors recommend a clinical examination that includes (i) a visual inspection of the peri-implant tissues for the assessment of oral hygiene and the detection of potential redness, swelling, (ii) palpation of the peri-implant tissues for assessment of the potential presence of swelling, bleeding, suppuration. In addition, (iii) radiography is recommended for the assessment of crestal bone level for comparison with previous radiographs to evaluate potential progressive bone loss even if there is a need for more scientific evidence of the true value of the first two clinical testing modes.

Keywords: dental implants; mucositis; peri-implantitis; diagnosis; over-treatment; iatrogenic damage

1. Introduction

The ultimate goals of the maintenance phase of implant treatment are to preserve the function and the aesthetics of the rehabilitation as well as the stability /health of the peri-implant tissues for as long as possible. From a research point of view, the goal is to monitor the treatment outcomes: implant survival and success/failure. One evident problem is that the definitions of survival, success/failure used in more recent publications do not necessarily reflect the patient/clinician perceived successful maintenance of the function and aesthetics of the treatment. In other words, the definitions of disease, which would motivate a clinical intervention to cure the disease, do not seem to reflect the clinical reality. Thus, the first questions to be answered are "what should be considered pathology at a dental implant?" and "what diagnostic tools are available?" With regards to the natural dentition, there has been a wide agreement within the scientific community in relation to disease definitions and available diagnostic tools [1]. Despite the recent World Consensus meeting in Chicago [1], a similar consensus with regards to definition of pathologies and available diagnostic tools does not seem to exist for peri-implant tissue conditions [2–5]. The controversy regarding the application of periodontal indices to dental implants is not a recent one [6]. The basis for the disagreement can be found in the difference in the viewing of the peri-implant tissues. Can similar disease definitions and diagnostic tools be used in natural dentition and in situations where the natural dentition has been replaced with implant-retained restorations? The question is logical since there are no doubts that the periodontium and the peri-implant tissues ought to be regarded as two very different entities [5,7,8].

Is it correct to assume that similar reactions to infection, occlusal trauma, trauma from probing can be expected for the periodontium and the peri-implant tissues? Is there a similar pattern of disease progression? And if these aspects differ between the two entities, is it correct to use similar diagnostic tools? There is evidence in the literature that the peri-implant tissues are more susceptible to inflammatory reactions, a phenomenon also confirmed immunohistochemically with increase of inflammatory infiltrate in comparison to teeth [9] that lesions around implants and teeth have critical histopathologic differences [10], and that there are differences in the onset and progression of the periodontal and peri-implant diseases [11]. Becker and co-workers examined the differences and similarities between peri-implantitis and periodontitis underlying disease mechanisms [12]. On the basis of quantitative transcriptome analysis, peri-implantitis and periodontitis exhibited significantly different mRNA signatures, supporting the hypothesis of peri-implantitis being a complex inflammatory disorder with a unique pathophysiology. While in peri-implantitis tissue, the regulation of transcripts related to innate immune responses and defense responses were dominating, in periodontitis tissues, bacterial response systems prevailed [12]. Several authors questioned the role of infection as a principal cause of peri-implant diseases. For instance, Koka and Zarb questioned whether peri-implantitis is a disease entity at all. The Authors refuted the bacterial implications and suggested terms such as osseoinsufficiency or osseoseparation to describe problematic implants [13]. Moreover, in a review article, Qian and co-workers failed to find evidence that primary infection causes marginal bone resorption around implants [14]. Osseointegration has been suggested to represent a foreign body reaction to biomaterials and its long-term clinical function depending on a foreign body equilibrium that, if disturbed, may lead to impaired clinical function of the implant [15]. Recently, dental implants have been suggested having more in common to orthopaedic implants in terms of foreign body reaction and failure pattern than to teeth [16]. Given these fundamental differences between the periodontal and peri-implant tissues, can periodontal indices be used as reliable diagnostic tools for peri-implant tissues?

2. The Risk of Using Surrogate Endpoints for Prediction of Fatal Events

In the most recent definition and diagnosis requirements for peri-mucositis and peri-implantitis, the use of probing around dental implants has been recommended for the detection of presence of bleeding on probing (BOP), of increases in pocket probing depth (PPD) or of presence of PPD equal or more than 6 mm [17]. Thus, periodontal indices are recommended as biologic measures to distinguish between health and disease conditions and as surrogate endpoints as substitutes for fatal events (implant failures) in clinical trial designs. The underlying assumption is that an improvement in the surrogates would benefit the patient and that it is equivalent to reducing the rate of implant losses [18]. Whenever surrogate endpoints (or biological markers) are used, the link between the surrogate and the true clinical event is critical since the use of non-validated endpoints may be more harmful than beneficial. A classic example in the field of medicine is the clinical investigation carried out on the assumption that arrhythmia is a risk factor for acute myocardial infarction and that, as a consequence, the suppression of arrhythmia would reduce the risk of death by infarction. The investigation had to be stopped when it became clear that the antiarrhythmic agents successfully reduced the number of arrhythmia episodes but increased the risk of dying by infarction. Clearly, the reduction of arrhythmia was not a good surrogate of treatment benefit to the patient [19]. One can question whether the high prevalence of periodontal diseases claimed in more recent years and the alarming possibility of peri-implantitis becoming a major future health problem [20] is correct or whether it is based on the wrong choice of surrogate endpoints (biologic markers), and therefore cause unnecessary alarmism and overtreatments which are of no benefit to the patients.

3. The Use of Periodontal Indices to Diagnose Peri-Implant Disease

A systematic review of peri-implantitis therapy published in 2010 showed that PPD, BOP and clinical attachment level (CAL) were the most frequently reported surrogate markers for important clinical events such as implant failure, despite the fact that these surrogate markers/endpoints had not yet been validated [18]. Has anything changed in the last nine years? Has the use of periodontal indices around dental implants been validated since then? Periodontal probing has been a common basic diagnostic tool around teeth since investigations in the 1970s demonstrated that PPD measurements around teeth provide information regarding the ability of the periodontium to withstand probe penetration as a measure of the inflammatory conditions of the tissues. In case of an inflamed periodontium, the tip of the probe penetrates the epithelium into the connective tissue, overestimating the depth of the histological pocket. In case of a healthy gingiva, the tip of the probe fails to reach the most apical cell of the epithelium due to the increased resistance of the periodontal tissues, thus underestimating the depth of the histological pocket [21–23]. Ericsson and Lindhe confirmed this finding in animals but also showed that in healthy soft tissues conditions, probe penetration was more advanced at implants than at teeth and concluded that the differences between the attachment structure of teeth versus peri-implant mucosa makes the conditions for PPD measurements at teeth and implants different [24]. In contrast, Lang and co-workers reported that in healthy and mucositis sites, the probe tip was located at the most apical cell of the junctional epithelium, whereas in the case of ligature-induced peri-implantitis sites, the probe tip penetrated into the connective tissue. They concluded that probing around implants represents a good technique for assessing the status of peri-implant mucosal health or disease. The difference in results between the two studies was attributed to the lower probing forces in the last study, which was 0.2 N versus 0.5 N [25].

More relevantly, on an evidence-based scale, investigations in humans failed to detect a positive correlation between the presence of periodontal signs of inflammation (PPD, BOP) and peri-implant bone loss. In a cross-sectional study by Lekholm and co-workers with a mean follow-up time of 7.6 years of 125 implants placed in 20 partially edentulous patients reported that 60% of the pockets measured more than 4 mm and that 80% of the sites were positive for BOP despite a limited mean bone loss of 0.07 mm annually. The microflora was periodontally non-pathogenic in nature in 94% of the samples and soft tissue biopsies showed a healthy mucosa in 95% of the cases. Thus, bleeding of the peri-implant tissues and deep pockets had no correlation to crestal bone loss or to the presence of a pathogenic microflora or to histological changes indicative for signs of periodontitis [26]. These findings were confirmed several years later by Dierens and co-workers, who reported of lack of correlations between PPD or BOP and crestal bone loss around single implants functional for 16–22 years. PPD and BOP were found to be of poor diagnostic value [27]. Recently also Winitsky and co-workers confirmed these observations, reporting of a lack of correlation between radiographically-detected crestal bone loss and periodontal indices such as PPD >6 mm and BOP in a 14–20 follow-up of 48 single anterior maxillary implants with a survival rate of 96%. The authors concluded by raising the question of whether PPD and BOP should be used as diagnostic measurements of implant health [28].

4. Evidences That Pocket Probing Depth Is a Poor Indicator of Ongoing Peri-Implant Pathology

The thickness of the healthy soft tissues surrounding implants has been reported to range between 1.85 and 5.75 mm in beagle dogs [29]. A clinical study showed values ranging from of 0.85 to 6.85 mm, but even papillae of 7–9 mm were observed [30]. Often, deeper PPDs are found at implant sites inserted in partially edentulous ridges compared to edentulous ridges [31]. Kan and co-workers reported the interproximal thickness of healthy peri-implant mucosa to be roughly 6 mm (SD 1.2) in maxillary anterior single implant with a mean functional time of 3 years [32]. Long-term clinical investigations have clearly shown that the probing depth of healthy peri-implant mucosa is often more than 4 mm (60% to 63%) [26,28,33] and up and over 6 mm (15% to 23%) [27,28] and that successful implants with over 18 years of function might have a history of PPD up to 9 mm [28,33]. From animal and human studies, it is evident that PPD depends on the thickness of the soft tissue at the time of implant placement and on the anatomical circumstances. For these reasons, there is no specific pocket depth that can indicate disease conditions. This fact is acknowledged in the new classification scheme for periodontal and peri-implant diseases and conditions, where in the peri-implant health definition it is stated that "it is not possible to define a range of probing depths compatible with peri-implant health" [1], and it is reflected in the fact that for the diagnosis of peri-implant health, it is mentioned that probing depths depend on the height of the soft tissue at the location of the implant [17]. Unfortunately, in the same paper, it is stated that in the absence of previous examination data, diagnosis of peri-implantitis requires the presence of bleeding and/or suppuration on gentle probing, probing depths ≥6 mm, and bone levels ≥3 mm apical of the most coronal portion of the intraosseous part of the implant.

Obviously, in light of what was discussed so far, the recommendation of using a 6-mm deep pocket (which appears to be an arbitrary choice) as one of the indicators of peri-implantitis appears to be highly questionable.

In the same paper, it is stated that for the diagnosis of peri-implantitis among other parameters, "an increased probing depth compared to previous examinations" is required.

The use of changes in PPD to establish a diagnosis of peri-implantitis has been questioned [5]. Schou and co-workers have shown in animal studies that PPD assessments could not distinguish between peri-implant sites with or without crestal bone loss and that the only correct indication of bone level stability was obtained by radiographs [34]. Furthermore, even mild inflammation was associated with deeper probe penetration around implants in comparison to teeth with no correlation to presence of bone loss [35]. In a more relevant 5-year clinical prospective investigation, Weber and co-workers assessed the ability of several clinical parameters (Suppuration, PI. BOP, PPD, PAL, mobility) to predict crestal bone loss as detected on radiographs in 112 ITI implants [36]. The authors reported no bone changes between years one and five in comparison to increasing PPD values during the five years. The cumulative predictive power of the six clinical parameters with regards to bone loss was reported to range from 2.8% to 14.3%. It was concluded that "the low levels of correlation between the individual and cumulative clinical parameters with radiographically measured bone loss, suggests that these measures are of limited clinical value in assessing and predicting future peri-implant bone loss". Healthy peri-implant soft tissues have been reported in sites with increased PPD values by Giannopoulou and co-workers in a 9-year follow-up of 61 maxillary anterior implants using clinical, microbiologic and biochemical parameters, thus showing a very poor correlation between PPD changes and the presence of pathology at the peri-implant tissues [37]. From the above discussed data, it appears that an increase in probing depth around implants does not necessarily mean that loss of bone or clinical attachment has occurred. Since the key parameter for establishing a diagnosis of peri-implantitis is bone loss and since the latter cannot be properly identified by a specific, pre-established PPD value or by changes in PPD, the use of probing for PPD assessments around implants does not appear to be a validated diagnostic tool.

5. Evidences That Bleeding on Probing Is a Poor Indicator of Ongoing Peri-Implant Pathology

For the detection of pathology and consequent treatment needs, BOP is a key parameter, according to the most recent recommendations, since BOP is used as a diagnostic parameter for the detection of both peri-mucositis and peri-implantitis [17]. This recommendation assumes that healthy peri-implant soft tissues do not test positive to BOP, whereas only diseased sites do (or, at least, that there is a statistically significant clinical difference between healthy and diseased sites when it comes to BOP positivity test). While Lang and co-workers' Beagle dog investigation detected constant increases in BOP from healthy peri-implant sites to ligature-induced peri-mucositis sites to ligature-induced peri-implantitis [25], Ericsson and Lindhe's Beagle dog investigation reported of the presence of

BOP for the majority of the healthy peri-implant sites [24]. One investigation comparing teeth and implants with respect to soft tissue healing revealed that peri-implant healing as determined by crevicular molecular composition differs from periodontal healing and suggested that peri-implant tissues represent a higher pro-inflammatory state [38]. Thus, the peri-implant soft tissues could be considered to be in a state of subclinical chronic inflammation. In fact, cross-sectional studies have shown that BOP can be detected at the majority of sites, showing stable peri-implant tissues.

With a definition of peri-implantitis as an association of BOP and any bone-level alterations at implant sites occurring between the 1-year and the 5-year (up to 23 years) follow-up examinations, Fransson and co-workers reported the presence of BOP in 93.9% of the 197 implants with "progressive" bone loss and in 90.9% of the 285 implants with stable bone level [39].

Roos-Jansåker et al reported that peri-implant mucositis, diagnosed by BOP, was detected in approximately 70% of functioning implants after 9 to 14 years. The prevalence of peri-implantitis, defined as bone loss of at least 1.8 mm following the first year of function, combined with BOP and/or pus, was 16% at patient level and 6.6% at implant level. Interestingly, 42.2% of the implants had stable bone levels and still showed BOP or suppuration, and 8.4% of the implants showed bone level gain even in the presence of BOP or suppuration [40]. A very poor correlation between presence of BOP and presence of peri-implant diseases has been reported in several long-term clinical studies. Lekholm at al reported the BOP of 80% around implants, showing an annual bone loss of 0.07 mm and a 95% healthy mucosa at biopsies [26]. Dierens and coworkers reported 81% BOP around implants, showing stable conditions for 16 to 22 years of function [27]. Winitsky and co-workers reported 71% BOP around implants, showing stable conditions for 14 to 20 years of function [28]. French and co-workers, in a large cohort study including 4591 Straumann implants from 2060 subjects evaluated up to ten-year follow-up, reported that BOP was a common finding, detected in more than 40% of the implants during the study. Despite the high prevalence of bleeding, less than 3% of implants exhibited more than 1 mm crestal bone. The presented data indicated that minimal bleeding did not correlate with bone loss, whereas profuse bleeding or suppuration did [41].

The type of implant, two-piece vs. one-piece, may affect the soft tissue bleeding response to probing. The presence of a chronic infiltrate at the implant-abutment interface of two-piece implants has been reported and has been attributed to the microgap between the implant and the abutment [42,43]. In contrast, the connective tissue surrounding one-piece implants has been reported to be inflammation-free, possibly due to the absence of a microgap [44]. This could partially explain the high BOP prevalence detected at stable peri-implant sites in investigations on two-piece implants [26–28,39,40] and the lower percentage of BOP (40%) detected at stable peri-implant sites around one-piece implants. In case of one-piece implants, the presence of profuse BOP had a higher correlation to crestal bone loss compared to the poor correlation of minimal BOP [41].

The type of abutment material has been demonstrated to have an effect on BOP values in a recent systematic review, where increased BOP values over time were demonstrated for Ti when compared to Zi abutments [45]. Implant position (anterior v posterior), gender and PPD have been shown to be factors affecting the probability of a peri-implant site to be positive to BOP. In 112 patients, data related to 1725 peri-implant sites showed that the probability to bleed on probing increases for implants placed in anterior compared to posterior areas of the dentition, for implants placed in female patients compared to male patients, and that for each mm increase in PPD, there is a corresponding 10% increase in the probability of detecting BOP at the site [46].

Thus, BOP seems to depend on the implant type (two-piece/one-piece), the type of abutment material, the implant position (anterior/posterior), the patient's gender and the PPD of the probed site without correlation to disease presence.

It has been shown that BOP can be detected in the majority of healthy peri-implant sites and cannot therefore be reasonably used to distinguish between peri-implant health and disease.

The investigations that attempted to establish the validity of the use of BOP as a predictor of future crestal bone loss around implants have failed to produce convincing result to justify the use of BOP as an appropriate diagnostic test. Jepsen and co-workers reported no difference in BOP between sites with progressive peri-implant PAL loss (rather than progressive bone loss) or stable sites. The authors pointed out that probing might provoke a nonspecific bleeding that is unrelated to the amount of inflammation. Thus, BOP as a diagnostic test for progressive PAL loss had a sensitivity of 70% and a specificity of 32%. In other words, BOP was of limited value in the implant-specific diagnosis when examined as positive predictors for peri-implant attachment loss. However, BOP demonstrated a higher negative predictive value and it was concluded that negative scores can serve as indicators of stable peri-implant conditions [47]. Monje and co-workers found that the diagnostic accuracy of BOP was not enough to distinguish healthy from peri-implantitis sites (defined as presence of inflammation and 2 mm crestal bone loss). A visual sign, such as mucosa redness, was reported having a much better diagnostic accuracy in monitoring the presence of pathology. For the clinical parameters investigated (PPD, BPO, mucosa redness, PI), it was found that, as diagnostic tests, their specificity surpasses their sensitivity in the detection of peri-implant diseases. The authors therefore concluded that the diagnosis of peri-implant diseases cannot rely on a single clinical parameter but rather requires a combination. More interestingly, it was pointed out that progressive radiographic bone loss must be cautiously examined to reach definitive diagnosis and avoid overtreatment [48]. Weber and co-workers reported that the cumulative predictive power of six clinical parameters (Suppuration, PI. BOP, PPD, PAL) with regards to bone loss ranges from 2.8% to 14.3% and concluded that "these measures are of limited clinical value in assessing and predicting future peri-implant bone loss" [36]. A recent systematic review and meta-analysis demonstrated that for BOP-positive implants, there was a 24.1% chance of being diagnosed with peri-implantitis, while for BOP-positive patients, there was a 33.8% probability of being diagnosed with peri-implantitis. It was concluded that clinicians should be aware of the considerable false-positive rate of BOP to diagnose peri-implantitis [49].

6. Mismatch between Known Clinical Facts and Recommendations from Consensus Meetings

It is interesting to note that review articles [5,49,50] and prospective studies [36,48] conclude that periodontal indices are unreliable tools for examining implants. Yet, the consensus meetings that often commission the reports keep recommending the use of periodontal indices around implants.

As discussed by Coli and co-workers, the efficacy of a diagnostic test is affected by the prevalence of the disease in the investigated population [5]. With increases in the disease prevalence, the probability that a person with a positive test result does in fact have the disease increases. Thus, two factors are of importance in order to properly establish an accurate disease diagnosis and avoid high figures of false positives. The first factor is the availability of a diagnostic test with high sensitivity and specificity. This has not yet been proven to be the case for any of the periodontal indices usually applied around dental implants. The second factor is the application of the diagnostic test to a population that has a high prevalence of the disease. Studies using the presence of BOP and a pre-established amount of crestal bone loss can result in high prevalence of peri-mucositis and peri-implantitis, however, if more stringent values of crestal bone loss are applied, much lower prevalence values are presented [50].

Long-term clinical investigations on machined implants are showing that despite the presence of several clinical parameters that would be considered indicative of pathology in the case of natural dentition (BOP, increases in PPD, suppuration), peri-implant tissue conditions were generally stable for over 18 years with only 2.5%–5% of implants showing progressive bone loss [27,28,33,51,52]. A review including ten different publications on three brands of moderately rough surfaces with ten- year or longer follow-up times reported a 2.7% peri-implantitis prevalence [7]. Jemt and co-workers reported that the incidence of surgery related to peri-implantitis problems carried out at the Branemark clinic was on an average 1.2% of followed-up patients per year (on an average, 1294 patients per year) during an 8-years period [53]. Thus, long-term clinical studies on machined as well as on modern micro-rough implant surfaces are indicative of a low 1.2%–5% prevalence of peri-implantitis and implant losses due to peri-implantitis. With such low peri-implantitis prevalence figures and with clinical parameters with poor accuracy as diagnostic tests, the probability of a dental implant being correctly diagnosed as suffering from peri-implant diseases appears to be very low and the risk of overtreatment very high.

Two investigations highlight the poor accuracy of periodontal indices causing overdiagnosis in several cases and failing to correctly identify implants that will suffer crestal bone loss in the future. In a follow-up study based on the population described by Fransson and co-workers [39,54], Jemt and co-workers showed that 9 years after the initial diagnosis of peri-implantitis, 31% of the patients presented with implants with bone loss >2mm/year or with implant failures, whereas 69% of them showed no problems with their implants [55]. A total of 91.4% of the implants in the peri-implantitis diagnosed patients showed no or smaller annual bone loss than <0.2mm during the 9 years from the diagnosis. The authors reported a low prevalence of obvious bone loss at implants (>0.2 mm/year) with a comparable distribution between "affected" and "not affected" implants. Hence, the definition of peri-implantitis used in the Fransson and co-workers study [39], bone loss associated with BOP, was shown to be a poor predictor of future bone loss and implant failure and, consequently, a poor indicator of treatment needs. In a follow-up study based on the population described by Roos-Jansåker and co-workers in 2006 [40], Renvert and co-workers reported that 12 years after the initial diagnosis of peri-implantitis and surgical treatment, 23% of the patients presented with implants with further bone loss ≥3 threads. In the remaining 77% of the subjects, bone gains (15%) or no further bone loss or bone loss <3 threads were detected [56]. Out of the subjects that at the first examination did not have peri-implantitis, 15% were diagnosed as having at least one implant with bone loss of ≥3 threads in the 21–26-year examination. For the 9–14 years examination, 58% of the individuals had been diagnosed with mucositis. Of those, 14% were found to have developed peri-implantitis at the 21–26-year examination. On the other hand, 22% of the patients without any sign of mucositis after 9–14 years had developed peri-implantitis at a later stage. Thus, a diagnosis of mucositis established after 9–14 years was not predictive for development of peri-implantitis after 21–26 years, nor was the diagnosis of peri-implantitis after 9–14 years predictive of further bone loss at 21–26 years. It seems evident that the use of a dichotomous diagnostic criterion (bleeding yes or no) for the definition of peri-mucositis and the arbitrary choice of a defined bone loss in association with BOP (surrogate endpoints) for the definition of peri-implantitis, does not capture the long-term true outcome (endpoint) in the form of implant failure and could result in massive overtreatment of implant patients. In fact, patients treated by oral hygienists and/or had experienced peri-implantitis surgery did not seem to show any more favourable progression of bone loss as compared with non-treated patients [55,56].

7. The Risk of Iatrogenic Damage by Probing of Dental Implants

One important aspect that has not been debated in the literature and that has not yet been properly tested is the fact that probing around implants could potentially result in trauma to the peri-implant soft tissues with consequent inflammation, apical proliferation of the epithelium and consequent bone loss. There is strong evidence in the literature that the mechanical disruption of the mucosal barrier around an implant should be considered as a connective tissue wound resulting in epithelial proliferation to cover the wound and in bone resorption to allow a connective tissue barrier of proper dimensions to reform in order to re-establish a "biological width". Repeated abutment dis/reconnections with a consequent disruption of the peri-implant soft tissue barrier have been shown to cause crestal bone resorption around dental implants in animal studies [57,58] and in short-term and long-term clinical investigations, as confirmed in several meta-analysis reports [59–61]. Although this limited crestal bone resorption does not seem to be clinically relevant, this established fact should at least raise the doubt that regular peri-implant tissue probing assessments might repeatedly disrupt the soft tissue barrier with consequent serious iatrogenic effects on the stability of the peri-implant tissues in the long term.

Another serious aspect to be considered is the overdiagnosis and overtreatment caused by the use of periodontal indices. In periodontology, it is well established that the presence of BOP is not an indicator of future periodontal tissue loss, but rather that the absence of BOP is a good predictor of periodontal stability [62]. For this reason, during the active and maintenance phases of periodontal treatment, 4-mm-deep or deeper sites showing BOP are treated by scaling and root planing. This zero-tolerance approach certainly results in overtreatment in several cases but does not result in damages to the periodontal tissues and is therefore accepted and recommended. The same approach in the case of dental implants seems to be unjustified and potentially dangerous. As discussed above, there is no evidence in the literature that the presence of BOP at an implant site is a sign of pathology (peri-mucositis or peri-implantitis) with a consequent treatment needed. The zero-tolerance approach to bleeding in the case of dental implants could not only result in overtreatment, but, in fact, in the triggering and the establishment of a difficult-to-manage inflammation in the soft tissues and excruciate into a foreign-body reaction.

Different techniques are used to achieve decontamination of the abutment/implant surfaces. Calculus is removed by manual debridement, such as conventional or ultrasonic scaling, resulting in the release of Ti particles in the surrounding tissues and in surface changes affecting the corrosion resistance of the material [63–67]. Orthopaedic studies have shown that the presence of titanium particles from wear of limb prosthesis could over-express pro-inflammatory cytokines, that are related to the osteolysis process, culminating in bone loss around the implant and prosthesis failure [68]. A recent review concluded that Ti particles and corrosion products from dental implants can have adverse effects on biological tissue [69]. Titanium particles released by ultrasonic scaling on dental implants have been shown to activate inflammatory responses in in vitro studies: activating the DNA damage response pathway in oral epithelial cells [70] or resulting in an increased secretion of IL-1β, IL-6, and TNF-α in cultured human macrophages [71–73], inducing bone resorption [71]. In vivo, titanium particles have been found in soft and hard tissue biopsies retrieved from sites with peri-implantitis [74,75]. Peri-implantitis tissues have been shown to contain high concentrations of Ti compared to controls from periodontitis tissues, leading to the conclusion that the high Ti content in peri-implant mucosa has the potential to aggravate inflammation [76]. Furthermore, greater levels of dissolved titanium have been detected in submucosal plaque around implants with peri-implantitis compared with healthy implants, indicating an association between titanium dissolution and peri-implantitis [77].

Since Ti particles can be released from surfaces of dental implants because of mechanical wear and because of contact to chemical agents and/or with substances produced by adherent biofilm and inflammatory cells, Mombelli and co-workers suggested that rather than being the trigger of disease, the observed higher concentration of Ti particles in inflamed peri-implant tissues could be the consequence of the presence of biofilms and inflammation [78]. However, in a recent animal model, it was shown that Ti particles induce an inflammatory response with consequent bone loss and that both inflammation and bone loss can be inhibited by the use of blockers targeting specific inflammatory cytokines. The specific role of inflammatory cytokines in the development of Ti particle-induced peri-implantitis was therefore clearly demonstrated [79]. Another investigation using a different animal model further confirms that Ti particles can induce inflammatory bone loss even in the absence of a bacteria infection and that the inflammatory response can be inhibited by blocking macrophage activity [80]. Thus, there is increasing evidence that dental implant degradation products released by corrosion and/or abrasion during mechanical debridement can act as foreign bodies, initiating the release of inflammatory mediators associated with bone resorption, as already described in the case of orthopaedic implants [81]. Hence, non-surgical implant debridement, incorrectly triggered by the detection of BOP at one otherwise healthy and stable implant site, could result in alterations of the implant surface, with the release of Ti particles (at the time of debridement and/or as a later consequence of the surface corrosion) and initiation of a foreign-body reaction.

8. Conclusions and Recommendations Regarding Evaluation of the Implant-Tissue Interface

Periodontal indices do not seem to be reliable indicators for appropriate diagnosis and treatment needs around dental implants. Apparently, they do not provide better information than visual inspection and detection of mucosa redness. Probing around dental implant is more uncomfortable for the patient compared to probing around teeth. Probing around implants could potentially create a trauma in the peri-implant scar tissue that could become difficult to manage. All the information gathered from probing (BOP, PPD, CAL) needs to be associated to the radiographic assessment of crestal bone levels to establish a definitive diagnosis and avoid overtreatment. Therefore, it appears to be more logical to avoid any risks of disturbing the peri-implant tissues with probing and instead proceeding with a clinical examination that includes (1) a visual inspection of the peri-implant tissues for the assessment of oral hygiene and the detection of potential redness, swelling, (2) palpation of the peri-implant tissues for assessment of the potential presence of swelling, bleeding, and suppuration, and (3) radiography for the assessment of crestal bone level for comparison with previous radiographs to evaluate potential progressive bone loss even if there is a need for more scientific evidence of the true value of the first two clinical testing modes.

References

1. Caton, J.G.; Armitage, G.; Berglundh, T.; Chapple, I.L.C.; Jepsen, S.; Kornman, K.S.; Mealey, B.L.; Papapanou, P.N.; Sanz, M.; Tonetti, M.S. A new classification scheme for periodontal and peri-implant diseases and conditions—Introduction and key changes from the 1999 classification. *J. Clin. Periodontol.* **2018**, *45* (Suppl. 20), S1–S8. [CrossRef] [PubMed]

2. Tomasi, C.; Derks, J. Clinical research of peri-implant diseases—Quality of reporting, case definitions and methods to study incidence, prevalence and risk factors of peri-implant diseases. *J. Clin. Periodontol.* **2012**, *39* (Suppl. 12), 207–223. [CrossRef]

3. Derks, J.; Tomasi, C. Peri-implant health and disease. A systematic review of current epidemiology. *J. Clin. Periodontol.* **2015** *42* (Suppl. 16), S158–S171. [CrossRef] [PubMed]

4. Albrektsson, T.; Chrcanovic, B.; Ostman, P.O.; Sennerby, L. Initial and long-term crestal bone responses to modern dental implants. *Periodontology 2000* **2017**, *73*, 41–50. [CrossRef] [PubMed]

5. Coli, P.; Christiaens, V.; Sennerby, L.; Bruyn, H. Reliability of periodontal diagnostic tools for monitoring peri-implant health and disease. *Periodontology 2000* **2017**, *73*, 203–217. [CrossRef] [PubMed]

6. Brånemark, P.I.; Hansson, B.O.; Adell, R.; Breine, U.; Lindström, J.; Hallén, O.; Ohman, A. Osseointegrated implants in the treatment of the edentulous jaw. Experience from a 10-year period. *Scand. J. Plast. Reconstr. Surg. Suppl.* **1977**, *16*, 1–132. [PubMed]

7. Albrektsson, T.; Buser, D.; Sennerby, L. Crestal bone loss and oral implants. *Clin. Implant Dent. Relat. Res.* **2012**, *14*, 783–791. [CrossRef]

8. Albrektsson, T.; Dahlin, C.; Jemt, T.; Sennerby, L.; Turri, A.; Wennerberg, A. Is marginal bone loss around oral implants the result of a provoked foreign body reaction? *Clin. Implant Dent. Relat. Res.* **2014**, *16*, 155–165. [CrossRef]

9. Degidi, M.; Artese, L.; Piattelli, A.; Scarano, A.; Shibli, J.A.; Piccirilli, M.; Perrotti, V.; Iezzi, G. Histological and immunohistochemical evaluation of the peri-implant soft tissues around machined and acid-etched titanium healing abutments: A prospective randomised study. *Clin. Oral Investig.* **2012**, *16*, 857–866. [CrossRef]

10. Carcuac, O.; Berglundh, T. Composition of Human Peri-implantitis and Periodontitis Lesions. *J. Dent. Res.* **2014**, *93*, 1083–1088. [CrossRef]

11. Lang, N.P.; Berglundh, T. Periimplant diseases: Where are we now? Consensus of the Seventh European Workshop on periodontology. *J. Clin. Periodontol.* **2011**, *38*, 178–181. [CrossRef] [PubMed]

12. Becker, S.T.; Beck-Broichsitter, B.E.; Graetz, C.; Dörfer, C.E.; Wiltfang, J.; Häsler, R. Peri-implantitis versus periodontitis: Functional differences indicated by transcriptome profiling. *Clin. Implant Dent. Relat. Res.* **2014**, *16*, 401–411. [CrossRef] [PubMed]

13. Koka, S.; Zarb, G. On osseointegration: The healing adaptation principle in the context of osseosufficiency, osseoseparation, and dental implant failure. *Int. J. Prosthodont.* **2012**, *25*, 48–52. [PubMed]

14. Qian, J.; Wennerberg, A.; Albrektsson, T. Reasons for marginal bone loss around oral implants. *Clin. Implant Dent. Relat. Res.* **2012**, *14*, 792–807. [CrossRef] [PubMed]

15. Trindade, R.; Albrektsson, T.; Tengvall, P.; Wennerberg, A. Foreign Body Reaction to Biomaterials: On Mechanisms for Buildup and Breakdown of Osseointegration. *Clin. Implant Dent. Relat. Res.* **2016**, *18*, 192–203. [CrossRef] [PubMed]

16. Albrektsson, T.; Becker, W.; Coli, P.; Jemt, T.; Mölne, J.; Sennerby, L. Bone loss around oral and orthopedic implants: An immunologically based condition. *Clin. Implant Dent. Relat. Res.* **2019**. [CrossRef]

17. Berglundh, T.; Armitage, G.; Araujo, M.G.; Avila-Ortiz, G.; Blanco, J.; Camargo, P.M.; Chen, S.; Cochran, D.; Derks, J.; Figuero, E.; et al. Peri-implant diseases and conditions: Consensus report of workgroup 4 of the 2017 World Workshop on the Classification of Periodontal and Peri-Implant Diseases and Conditions. *J. Clin. Periodontol.* **2018**, *45* (Suppl. 20), S286–S291. [CrossRef]

18. Faggion, C.M., Jr.; Listl, S.; Tu, Y.K. Assessment of endpoints in studies on peri-implantitis treatment—A systematic review. *J. Dent.* **2010**, *38*, 443–450. [CrossRef]

19. Echt, D.S.; Liebson, P.R.; Mitchell, L.B.; Peters, R.W.; Obias-Manno, D.; Barker, A.H.; Arensberg, D.; Baker, A.; Friedman, L.; Greene, H.L.; et al. Mortality and Morbidity in Patients Receiving Encainide, Flecainide, or Placebo—The Cardiac Arrhythmia Suppression Trial. *N. Engl. J. Med.* **1991**, *324*, 781–788. [CrossRef]

20. Giannobile, W.V.; Lang, N.P. Are Dental Implants a Panacea or Should We Better Strive to Save Teeth? *J. Dent. Res.* **2016**, *95*, 5–6. [CrossRef]

21. Listgarten, M.A.; Mao, R.; Robinson, P.J. Periodontal probing and the relationship of the probe tip to periodontal tissues. *J. Periodontol.* **1976**, *47*, 511–513. [CrossRef]

22. Armitage, G.C.; Svanberg, G.K.; Loë, H. Microscopic evaluation of clinical measurements of connective tissue attachment levels. *J. Clin. Periodontol.* **1977**, *4*, 173–190. [CrossRef]

23. Spray, J.R.; Garnick, J.J.; Doles, L.R.; Klawitter, J.J. Microscopic demonstration of the position of periodontal probes. *J. Periodontol.* **1978**, *49*, 148–152. [CrossRef]

24. Ericsson, I.; Lindhe, J. Probing depth at implants and teeth. An experimental study in the dog. *J. Clin. Periodontol.* **1993**, *20*, 623–627. [CrossRef]

25. Lang, N.P.; Wetzel, A.C.; Stich, H.; Caffesse, R.G. Histologic probe penetration in healthy and inflamed peri-implant tissues. *Clin. Oral Implants Res.* **1994**, *5*, 191–201. [CrossRef]

26. Lekholm, U.; Adell, R.; Lindhe, J.; Brånemark, P.I.; Eriksson, B.; Rockler, B.; Lindvall, A.M.; Yoneyama, T. Marginal tissue reactions at osseointegrated titanium fixtures. (II) A cross-sectional retrospective study. *Int. J. Oral Maxillofac. Surg.* **1986**, *15*, 53–61. [CrossRef]

27. Dierens, M.; Vandeweghe, S.; Kisch, J.; Nilner, K.; De Bruyn, H. Long-term follow-up of turned single implants placed in periodontally healthy patients after 16–22 years: Radiographic and peri-implant outcome. *Clin. Oral Implants Res.* **2012**, *23*, 197–204. [CrossRef]

28. Winitsky, N.; Olgart, K.; Jemt, T.; Smedberg, J.I. A retro-prospective long-term follow-up of Brånemark single implants in the anterior maxilla in young adults. Part 1: Clinical and radiographic parameters. *Clin. Implant Dent. Relat. Res.* **2018**, *20*, 937–944. [CrossRef]

29. Berglundh, T.; Lindhe, J.; Ericsson, I.; Marinello, C.P.; Liljenberg, B.; Thomsen, P. The soft tissue barrier at implants and teeth. *Clin. Oral Implants Res.* **1991**, *2*, 81–90. [CrossRef]

30. Choquet, V.; Hermans, M.; Adriaenssens, P.; Daelemans, P.; Tarnow, D.P.; Malevez, C. Clinical and radiographic evaluation of the papilla level adjacent to single-tooth dental implants. A retrospective study in the maxillary anterior region. *J. Periodontol.* **2001**, *72*, 1364–1371. [CrossRef]

31. Serino, G.; Turri, A.; Lang, N.P. Probing at implants with peri-implantitis and its relation to clinical peri-implant bone loss. *Clin. Oral Implants Res.* **2013**, *24*, 91–95. [CrossRef]

32. Kan, J.Y.; Rungcharassaeng, K.; Umezu, K.; Kois, J.C. Dimensions of peri-implant mucosa: An evaluation of maxillary anterior single implants in humans. *J. Periodontol.* **2003**, *74*, 557–562. [CrossRef]

33. Bergenblock, S.; Andersson, B.; Fürst, B.; Jemt, T. Long-term follow-up of CeraOne single-implant restorations: An 18-year follow-up study based on a prospective patient cohort. *Clin. Implant Dent. Relat. Res.* **2012**, *14*, 471–479. [CrossRef]

34. Schou, S.; Holmstrup, P.; Stoltze, K.; Hjørting-Hansen, E.; Kornman, K.S. Ligature-induced marginal inflammation around osseointegrated implants and ankylosed teeth. *Clin. Oral Implants Res.* **1993**, *4*, 12–22. [CrossRef]

35. Schou, S.; Holmstrup, P.; Stoltze, K.; Hjørting-Hansen, E.; Fiehn NESkovgaard, L.T. Probing around implants and teeth with healthy or inflamed peri-implant mucosa/gingiva. A histologic comparison in cynomolgus monkeys (Macaca fascicularis). *Clin. Oral Implants Res.* **2002**, *13*, 113–126. [CrossRef]

36. Weber, H.P.; Crohin, C.C.; Fiorellini, J.P. A 5-year prospective clinical and radiographic study of non-submerged dental implants. *Clin. Oral Implants Res.* **2000**, *11*, 144–153. [CrossRef]

37. Giannopoulou, C.; Bernard, J.P.; Buser, D.; Carrel, A.; Belser, U.C. Effect of intracrevicular restoration margins on peri-implant health: Clinical, biochemical, and microbiologic findings around esthetic implants up to 9 years. *Int. J. Oral Maxillofac. Implants* **2003**, *18*, 173–181.

38. Emecen-Huja, P.; Eubank, T.D.; Shapiro, V.; Yildiz, V.; Tatakis, D.N.; Leblebicioglu, B. Peri-implant versus periodontal wound healing. *J. Clin. Periodontol.* **2013**, *40*, 816–824. [CrossRef]

39. Fransson, C.; Wennström, J.; Berglundh, T. Clinical characteristics and implant with a history of progressive bone loss. *Clin. Oral Implants Res.* **2008**, *19*, 142–147. [CrossRef]

40. Roos-Jansåker, A.M.; Lindahl, C.; Renvert, H.; Renvert, S. Nine to fourteen-year follow-up of implant treatment. Part II: Presence of peri-implant lesions. *J. Clin. Periodontol.* **2006**, *33*, 290–295. [CrossRef]

41. French, D.; Cochran, D.L.; Ofec, R. Retrospective cohort study of 4591 Straumann implants placed in 2060 patients in private practice with up to 10-year follow-up: The relationship between crestal bone level and soft tissue condition. *Int. J. Oral Maxillofac. Implants* **2016**, *31*, e168–e178. [CrossRef]

42. Broggini, N.; McManus, L.M.; Hermann, J.S.; Medina, R.U.; Oates, T.W.; Schenk, R.K.; Buser, D.; Mellonig, J.T.; Cochran, D.L. Persistent acute inflammation at the implant-abutment interface. *J. Dent. Res.* **2003**, *82*, 232–237. [CrossRef]

43. Broggini, N.; McManus, L.M.; Hermann, J.S.; Medina, R.; Schenk, R.K.; Buser, D.; Cochran, D.L. Peri-implant inflammation defined by the implant-abutment interface. *J. Dent. Res.* **2006**, *85*, 473–478. [CrossRef]

44. Buser, D.; Weber, H.P.; Donath, K.; Fiorellini, J.P.; Paquette, D.W.; Williams, R.C. Soft tissue reactions to non-submerged unloaded titanium implant in beagle dogs. *J. Periodontol.* **1992**, *63*, 225–235. [CrossRef]

45. Sanz-Martín, I.; Sanz-Sánchez, I.; Carrillo de Albornoz, A.; Figuero, E.; Sanz, M. Effects of modified abutment characteristics on peri-implant soft tissue health: A systematic review and meta-analysis. *Clin. Oral Implants Res.* **2018**, *29*, 118–129. [CrossRef]

46. Farina, R.; Filippi, M.; Brazzioli, J.; Tomasi, C.; Trombelli, L. Bleeding on probing around dental implants: A retrospective study of associated factors. *J. Clin. Periodontol.* **2017**, *44*, 115–122. [CrossRef]

47. Jepsen, S.; Rühling, A.; Jepsen, K.; Ohlenbusch, B.; Albers, H.K. Progressive peri-implantitis. Incidence and prediction of peri-implant attachment loss. *Clin. Oral Implants Res.* **1996**, *7*, 133–142. [CrossRef]

48. Monje, A.; Caballé-Serrano, J.; Nart, J.; Peñarrocha, D.; Wang, H.L.; Rakic, M. Diagnostic accuracy of clinical parameters to monitor peri-implant conditions: A matched case-control study. *J. Periodontol.* **2018**, *89*, 407–417. [CrossRef]

49. Hashim, D.; Cionca, N.; Combescure, C.; Mombelli, A. The diagnosis of peri-implantitis: A systematic review on the predictive value of bleeding on probing. *Clin. Oral Implants Res.* **2018**, *29* (Suppl. 16), 276–293. [CrossRef]

50. Doornewaard, R.; Jacquet, W.; Cosyn, J.; De Bruyn, H. How do peri-implant biologic parameters correspond with implant survival and peri-implantitis? A critical review. *Clin. Oral Implants Res.* **2018**, *29* (Suppl. 18), 100–123. [CrossRef]

51. Attard, N.J.; Zarb, G.A. Long-term treatment outcomes in edentulous patients with implant-fixed prostheses: The Toronto study. *Int. J. Prosthodont.* **2004**, *17*, 417–424. [CrossRef]

52. Astrand, P.; Ahlqvist, J.; Gunne, J.; Nilson, H. Implant treatment of patients with edentulous jaws: A 20-year follow-up. *Clin. Implant Dent. Relat. Res.* **2008**, *10*, 207–217. [CrossRef]

53. Jemt, T.; Gyzander, V.; Britse, A.Ö. Incidence of surgery related to problems with peri-implantitis: A retrospective study on patients followed up between 2003 and 2010 at one specialist clinic. *Clin. Implant Dent. Relat. Res.* **2015**, *17*, 209–220. [CrossRef]

54. Fransson, C.; Lekholm, U.; Jemt, T.; Berglundh, T. Prevalence of subjects with progressive bone loss at implants. *Clin. Oral Implants Res.* **2005**, *16*, 440–446. [CrossRef]

55. Jemt, T.; Sundén Pikner, S.; Gröndahl, K. Changes of marginal bone level in patients with progressive bone loss at Brånemark System®implants: A radiographic follow-up study over an average of 9 years. *Clin. Implant Dent. Relat. Res.* **2015**, *17*, 619–628. [CrossRef]

56. Renvert, S.; Lindahl, C.; Persson, G.R. Occurrence of cases with peri-implant mucositis or peri-implantitis in a 21-26 year follow up study. *J. Clin. Periodontol.* **2018**, *45*, 233–240. [CrossRef]

57. Abrahamsson, I.; Berglundh, T.; Lindhe, J. The mucosal barrier following abutment dis/reconnection. An experimental study in dogs. *J. Clin. Periodontol.* **1997**, *24*, 568–572. [CrossRef]

58. Rodríguez, X.; Vela, X.; Méndez, V.; Segalà, M.; Calvo-Guirado, J.L.; Tarnow, D.P. The effect of abutment dis/reconnections on peri-implant bone resorption: A radiologic study of platform-switched and non-platform-switched implants placed in animals. *Clin. Oral Implants Res.* **2013**, *24*, 305–311. [CrossRef]

59. Koutouzis, T.; Gholami, F.; Reynolds, J.; Lundgren, T.; Kotsakis, G.A. Abutment Disconnection/Reconnection Affects Peri-implant Marginal Bone Levels: A Meta-Analysis. *Int. J. Oral Maxillofac. Implants* **2017**, *32*, 575–581. [CrossRef]

60. Wang, Q.Q.; Dai, R.; Cao, C.Y.; Fang, H.; Han, M.; Li, Q.L. One-time versus repeated abutment connection for platform-switched implant: A systematic review and meta-analysis. *PLoS ONE* **2017**, *12*, e0186385. [CrossRef]

61. Tallarico, M.; Caneva, M.; Meloni, S.M.; Xhanari, E.; Covani, U.; Canullo, L. Definitive Abutments Placed at Implant Insertion and Never Removed: Is It an Effective Approach? A Systematic Review and Meta-Analysis of Randomized Controlled Trials. *J. Oral Maxillofac. Surg.* **2018**, *76*, 316–324. [CrossRef]

62. Lang, N.P.; Adler, R.; Joss, A.; Nyman, S. Absence of bleeding on probing. An indicator of periodontal stability. *J. Clin. Periodontol.* **1990**, *17*, 714–721. [CrossRef]

63. Louropoulou, A.; Slot, D.E.; van der Weijden, F.A. Titanium surface alterations following the use of different mechanical instruments: A systematic review. *Clin. Oral Implants Res.* **2012**, *23*, 643–658. [CrossRef]

64. Ruhling, A.; Kocher, T.; Kreusch, J.; Plagmann, H.C. Treatment of subgingival implant surfaces with TeflonR-coated sonic and ultrasonic scaler tips and various implant curettes. An in vitro study. *Clin. Oral Implant Res.* **1994**, *5*, 19–29. [CrossRef]

65. Hallmon, W.W.; Waldrop, T.C.; Meffert, R.M.; Wade, B.W. A comparative study of the effects of metallic, nonmetallic, and sonic instrumentation on titanium abutment surfaces. *Int. J. Oral Maxillofac. Implants* **1996**, *11*, 96–100. [CrossRef]

66. Homiak, A.W.; Cook, P.A.; DeBoer, J. Effect of hygiene instrumentation on titanium abutments: A scanning electron microscopy study. *J. Prosthet. Dent.* **1992**, *67*, 364–369. [CrossRef]

67. Cross-Poline, G.N.; Shaklee, R.L.; Stach, D.J. Effect of implant curettes on titanium implant surfaces. *Am. J. Dent.* **1997**, *10*, 41–45.

68. Souza, P.P.; Lerner, U.H. The role of cytokines in inflammatory bone loss. *Immunol. Investig.* **2013**, *42*, 555–622. [CrossRef]

69. Noronha Oliveira, M.; Schunemann, W.V.H.; Mathew, M.T.; Henriques, B.; Magini, R.S.; Teughels, W.; Souza, J.C.M. Can degradation products released from dental implants affect peri-implant tissues? *J. Periodontal Res.* **2018**, *53*, 1–11. [CrossRef]

70. Suarez-Lopez del Amo, F.; Rudek, I.E.; Wagner, V.P.; Martins, M.D.; O'Valle, F.; Galindo-Moreno, P.; Giannobile, W.V.; Wang, H.L.; Castilho, R.M. Titanium activates the DNA damage response pathway in oral epithelial cells: A pilot study. *Int. J. Oral Maxillofac. Implants* **2017**, *32*, 1413–1420. [CrossRef]

71. Eger, M.; Sterer, N.; Liron, T.; Kohavi, D.; Gabet, Y. Scaling of titanium implants entrains inflammation-induced osteolysis. *Sci. Rep.* **2017**, *7*, 39612. [CrossRef] [PubMed]

72. Pettersson, M.; Kelk, P.; Belibasakis, G.N.; Bylund, D.; Molin Thoren, M.; Johansson, A. Titanium ions form particles that activate and execute interleukin-1beta release from lipopolysaccharide-primed macrophages. *J. Periodontal Res.* **2017**, *52*, 21–32. [CrossRef] [PubMed]

73. Dodo, C.G.; Meirelles, L.; Aviles-Reyes, A.; Ruiz, K.G.S.; Abranches, J.; Cury, A.A.D.B. Pro-inflammatory Analysis of Macrophages in Contact with Titanium Particles and Porphyromonas gingivalis. *Braz. Dent. J.* **2017**, *28*, 428–434. [CrossRef] [PubMed]

74. Wilson, T.G., Jr.; Valderrama, P.; Burbano, M.; Blansett, J.; Levine, R.; Kessler, H.; Rodrigues, D.C. Foreign bodies associated with peri-implantitis human biopsies. *J. Periodontol.* **2015**, *86*, 9–15. [CrossRef] [PubMed]

75. Fretwurst, T.; Buzanich, G.; Nahles, S.; Woelber, J.P.; Riesemeier, H.; Nelson, K. Metal elements in tissue with dental peri-implantitis: A pilot study. *Clin. Oral Implants Res.* **2016**, *27*, 1178–1186. [CrossRef] [PubMed]

76. Pettersson, M.; Pettersson, J.; Johansson, A.; Molin Thorén, M. Titanium release in peri-implantitis. *J. Oral Rehabil.* **2019**, *46*, 179–188. [CrossRef] [PubMed]

77. Safioti, L.M.; Kotsakis, G.A.; Pozhitkov, A.E.; Chung, W.O.; Daubert, D.M. Increased Levels of Dissolved Titanium Are Associated with Peri-Implantitis. A Cross-Sectional Study. *J. Periodontol.* **2017**, *88*, 436–442. [CrossRef]

78. Mombelli, A.; Hashim, D.; Cionca, N. What is the impact of titanium particles and biocorrosion on implant survival and complications? A critical review. *Clin. Oral Implants Res.* **2018**, *29* (Suppl. 18), 37–53. [CrossRef]

79. Eger, M.; Hiram-Bab, S.; Liron, T.; Sterer, N.; Carmi, Y.; Kohavi, D.; Gabet, Y. Mechanism and Prevention of Titanium Particle-Induced Inflammation and Osteolysis. *Front. Immunol.* **2018**, *18*, 2963. [CrossRef]

80. Wang, X.; Li, Y.; Feng, Y.; Cheng, H.; Li, D. Macrophage polarization in aseptic bone resorption around dental implants induced by Ti particles in a murine model. *J. Periodontal Res.* **2019**, *54*, 329–338. [CrossRef]

81. Purdue, P.E.; Koulouvaris, P.; Potter, H.G.; Nestor, B.J.; Sculco, T.P. The cellular and molecular biology of periprosthetic osteolysis. *Clin. Orthop. Relat. Res.* **2007**, *454*, 251–261. [CrossRef] [PubMed]

13

Carbon Fiber Reinforced PEEK Composites Based on 3D-Printing Technology for Orthopedic and Dental Applications

Xingting Han [1], Dong Yang [2], Chuncheng Yang [2], Sebastian Spintzyk [1], Lutz Scheideler [1], Ping Li [1], Dichen Li [2,*], Jürgen Geis-Gerstorfer [1] and Frank Rupp [1]

[1] Section Medical Materials Science and Technology, University Hospital Tübingen, Osianderstr. 2–8, D-72076 Tübingen, Germany; xingting.han@student.uni-tuebingen.de (X.H.); Sebastian.Spintzyk@med.uni-tuebingen.de (S.S.); lutz.scheideler@med.uni-tuebingen.de (L.S.); ping.li@uni-tuebingen.de (P.L.); juergen.geis-gerstorfer@med.uni-tuebingen.de (J.G.-G.); Frank.Rupp@med.uni-tuebingen.de (F.R.)

[2] State Key Laboratory for Manufacturing System Engineering, School of Mechanical Engineering, Xi'an Jiaotong University, Xi'an 710054, China; yangdong2015@stu.xjtu.edu.cn (D.Y.); yang.chun.cheng@stu.xjtu.edu.cn (C.Y.)

* Correspondence: dcli@mail.xjtu.edu.cn

Abstract: Fused deposition modeling (FDM) is a rapidly growing three-dimensional (3D) printing technology and has great potential in medicine. Polyether-ether-ketone (PEEK) is a biocompatible high-performance polymer, which is suitable to be used as an orthopedic/dental implant material. However, the mechanical properties and biocompatibility of FDM-printed PEEK and its composites are still not clear. In this study, FDM-printed pure PEEK and carbon fiber reinforced PEEK (CFR-PEEK) composite were successfully fabricated by FDM and characterized by mechanical tests. Moreover, the sample surfaces were modified with polishing and sandblasting methods to analyze the influence of surface roughness and topography on general biocompatibility (cytotoxicity) and cell adhesion. The results indicated that the printed CFR-PEEK samples had significantly higher general mechanical strengths than the printed pure PEEK (even though there was no statistical difference in compressive strength). Both PEEK and CFR-PEEK materials showed good biocompatibility with and without surface modification. Cell densities on the "as-printed" PEEK and the CFR-PEEK sample surfaces were significantly higher than on the corresponding polished and sandblasted samples. Therefore, the FDM-printed CFR-PEEK composite with proper mechanical strengths has potential as a biomaterial for bone grafting and tissue engineering applications.

Keywords: fused deposition modeling; polyether ether ketone; biocomposite; orthopedic implant; oral implant; mechanical properties; wettability; topography; biocompatibility; cell adhesion

1. Introduction

Cranio-maxillofacial defects related to tumors, traumas, infections, or congenital deformities are highly challenging tasks for oral and maxillofacial surgeons to reconstruct [1,2]. When bone losses are too severe for human body routine mechanisms to regenerate, autologous grafts are the first considerations due to the simultaneous osteogenic, osteoinductive, and osteoconductive properties [3]. However, the shape of the donor sites, bone graft resorption, and infection restrict the application of autografts [4]. Currently, the most popular orthopedic/dental artificial materials are metals like titanium (Ti) and its alloys. These materials have many advantages, such as excellent biocompatibility, corrosion resistance, and mechanical strength [5]. However, there are some critical drawbacks of Ti, one of which is stress-shielding, which may occur at the interface between Ti and bone during load transfer and result in surrounding bone loss [6]. In addition, the radiopacity of Ti alloys in the CT and MR scan images and the release of harmful metal ions hinder the application of metals [7]. Due to the limitations observed in metallic biomaterials, polymers have been explored in recent years as potential alternative materials for bone replacement.

In the last few years, polyether ether ketone (PEEK) has been investigated widely in oral and cranio-maxillofacial surgery. Possible applications are dental implants, skull implants, osteosynthesis plates, and bone replacement material for nasal, maxillary, or mandibular reconstructions (Figure 1) [8–11]. PEEK is considered an alternative material for Ti due to its excellent biocompatibility, radiolucency, chemical resistance, low density (1.32 g/cm^3), and mechanical properties resembling human bone. PEEK is a polyaromatic semi-crystalline thermoplastic polymer with an elastic modulus of 3–4 GPa (Table 1), which is much lower than that of Ti (102–110 GPa) and very close to the human trabecular bone (1 GPa) [8,12]. Moreover, the mechanical strengths of PEEK can be enhanced by the incorporation of other materials (e.g., carbon fibers) [8]. Normally, carbon fiber reinforced polyether ether ketone (CFR-PEEK) has an elastic modulus close to the human cortical bone (14 GPa), depending on the amount of reinforced carbon fiber and manufacturing methods. CFR-PEEK is considered as a promising candidate to replace metallic materials because of the inherited advantages of PEEK and improved mechanical properties [13,14].

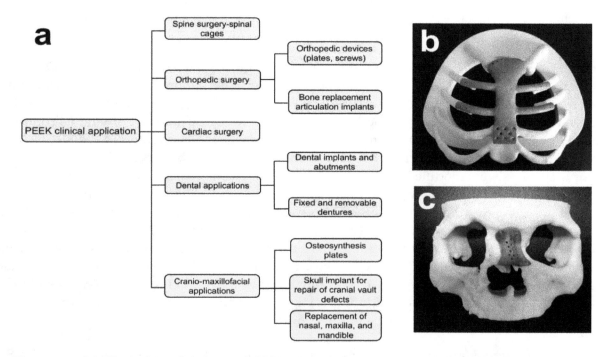

Figure 1. (a) Clinical applications of PEEK; Fused deposition modeling (FDM)-printed PEEK (b) breastbone and (c) nasal reconstructions.

Table 1. The elastic modulus of different materials and human tissues.

Materials	Elastic Modulus (GPa)	References
PEEK	3–4	[8]
Ti	102–110	[8]
Zirconia	210	[15]
Cortical bone	14	[8]
Trabecular bone	1	[15]

Additive manufacturing (AM) is a layer-by-layer manufacturing method, fabricating specimens by fusing or depositing materials, such as metals, ceramics, plastics, or even living cells [16]. This technique is becoming popular in orthopedic surgery for fabricating patient-specific implants due to the low cost, the feasibility of complex architectures, and the short production time [17]. Selective laser sintering (SLS) has been the most popular AM technology for fabricating PEEK in the past decades [18,19]. Compared with SLS, fused deposition modeling (FDM) is one of the fastest growing three-dimensional (3D) printing methods due to the lower costs, easier use (filament vs. powder), and reduced risk of material contamination or degradation. Furthermore, it has increasingly been applied to the manufacturing of PEEK and its composites in recent years [20]. However, due to the semicrystalline structure and high melting temperature of PEEK (compared with other FDM filament materials like polylactic acid (PLA) and acrylonitrile butadiene styrene (ABS)), it is difficult to process PEEK objects by FDM printing and the process is liable to cause excessive thermal stress and thermal cracks [8,18]. Yang et al. and Wu et al. have already measured the mechanical properties of FDM-printed pure PEEK and found that compared with some traditional manufacturing methods (i.e., injection molding), FDM-printed PEEK had lower mechanical strengths, which were influenced by layer thickness, printing speed, ambient temperature, nozzle temperature, and heat treatment [21,22] FDM-printed PEEK composites, to the best of our knowledge, have not yet been studied.

Compared with Ti, the unmodified PEEK is bioinert and has limited osteoconductive properties, which may influence the osseointegration after implantation [23,24]. Surface topographical modification is one of the mechanical surface modification methods to increase the biological performance of cranio-maxillofacial implants [25]. Surface roughness may influence cell adhesion, and a roughened surface usually has a more extensive surface area which offers more binding sites for cell attachment [26]. Some studies have already analyzed the influence of surface roughness on the bioactivity of PEEK and its composites [26–28]. However, in these reports, PEEK and its composites were all manufactured by traditional techniques like milling, injection modeling, and compression molding. For the FDM-manufactured PEEK, most studies only analyzed the manufacturing process and mechanical properties of pure PEEK, without PEEK composites [17,18,22]. According to our knowledge, tests of the mechanical properties of FDM-printed CFR-PEEK are still lacking. Therefore, the aim of this study was to evaluate the mechanical properties and microstructures of PEEK and CFR-PEEK samples manufactured by FDM. Specific attention was paid to the question of whether the FDM printing process has introduced or produced toxic substances and to the influence of surface treatments on the cell adhesion on sample surfaces.

2. Materials and Methods

2.1. Sample Preparation and Surface Modification

2.1.1. Sample Preparation

A 3D printing system for PEEK material and its composite from Jugao-AM Tech. Corp. (Xi'an, China) was used to prepare all test specimens. In the printing process, the PEEK material was heated and transformed into a semi-liquid state inside the nozzle. Then, the feedstock filament was forced to pass through the nozzle where it was melted and deposited in the form of a thin layer onto the platform. After one layer was finished, the platform went down along the z-axis equal to the pre-setting layer thickness. The desired geometry of the final complex objects was built layer-by-layer under the control of a computer. The extrusion temperature was set at 420 °C, and the printing speed was 40 mm/s. The bead width of each printing line was 0.4 mm, and the layer thickness was 0.2 mm (Table 2). Moreover, the PEEK filaments, as the material for 3D printing in this paper, were reprocessed from pellets (450G, VICTREX Corp., Thornton Cleveleys, UK), and 5% milled carbon fibers with a length of 80–150 μm and a diameter of 7 μm (Nanjing WeiDa Composite Material Co. Ltd., Nanjing, China) were chosen as the reinforcements. Before printing, a special fixative paper (Mingtai 3D Technology Co., Ltd., Shenzhen, China) was applied to the print bed for the objects' adhesion and warping improvement. After printing the samples and cooling them down to room temperature, the samples were placed into a furnace (101-0 s, Shaoxing SuPo Instrument Corp., Shaoxing, China) for the heat treatment (tempering) process. After heating for 2 h at 300 °C, the samples were cooled down to room temperature to decrease shrinkage distortion and residual stress to obtain good mechanical performance of the parts.

Table 2. Technical specifications of the FDM printer.

Parameters	Technical Specifications
Nozzle diameter	0.4 mm
Bead width	0.4 mm
Layer thickness	0.2 mm
Printing speed	40 mm/s
Raster angle	Consistent with the longest edge
Ambient temperature	20 °C
Nozzle temperature	420 °C

The dimension of the PEEK and CFR-PEEK samples for testing the mechanical properties (tensile, bending, and compressive tests) was according to ISO standards. The dog-bone shape tensile testing specimens (90 mm × 5 mm × 4 mm) were printed according to ISO 527-1 standard [29], and the cuboid bending specimens (80 mm × 10 mm × 4 mm) were printed according to ISO 178 standard (Figure 2) [30]. According to ISO 604 standard, two sample groups were manufactured for testing compressive strength and compressive modulus, respectively [31]. The round-shaped PEEK and CFR-PEEK disc samples for the wettability, roughness, microstructure, and biological tests were produced with a diameter of 14 mm and a thickness of 1 mm.

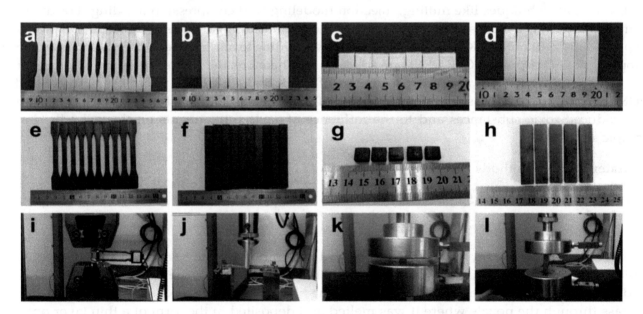

Figure 2. Pure PEEK and CFR-PEEK samples for testing mechanical properties: (**a,e**) tensile samples of PEEK and CFR-PEEK; (**b,f**) bending samples of PEEK and CFR-PEEK; (**c,g**) compressive samples (compressive strength) of PEEK and CFR-PEEK; (**d,h**) compressive samples (compressive modulus) of PEEK and CFR-PEEK; (**i**) tensile test; (**j**) bending test; (**k,l**) compressive tests of strength and modulus.

Ti disc samples (Grade: 4, Straumann AG, Basel, Switzerland) with 15 mm diameter and 1 mm thickness were prepared from Ti sheet metal (Straumann AG, Basel, Switzerland) with a punching tool. The Ti samples were used as an additional control group for the wettability, roughness, and biological tests. All titanium discs underwent a surface treatment, which was consistent with the polished PEEK and CFR-PEEK.

2.1.2. Sample Surface Modification

After printing, the PEEK and CFR-PEEK disc samples for wettability, roughness, microstructure, and biological tests were divided into three groups: as-printed (untreated) group, polished group, and sandblasted group (n = 12 per group). The untreated group included the directly printed samples, without any surface treatment. For the polished and sandblasted groups, all the discs were manually polished with a series of SiC abrasive papers up to P4000 (Buehler, Lake Bluff, IL, USA) by a polisher (Buehler, Coventry, UK). Then, the samples of the sandblasted group were further modified using a sandblasting machine (P-G 400, Harnisch + Rieth, Winterbach, Germany) with 120 μm alumina (Al_2O_3) particles (Cobra, Renfert, Hilzingen, Germany) under the pressure of 0.1 MPa at a distance of 50 mm for 15 s.

All Ti disc surfaces were modified using the same processes as for PEEK and CFR-PEEK samples by a series of SiC abrasive papers (1200, 2500, 4000 grit, Buehler, Lake Bluff, IL, USA) by a polisher (Buehler, Coventry, UK). After polishing, all the samples were cleaned with deionized (DI) water by an ultrasonic cleaner (Sonorex Super RK102H, Bandelin, Berlin, Germany) to remove residual Al_2O_3 particles on the sample surfaces.

2.2. Mechanical Properties Test

Mechanical tests were carried out using an electro-hydraulic servo mechanical testing machine (CMT4304, MTS Corp., Eden Prairie, MN, USA) according to ISO standards. ISO 527-1: 2012 (Plastics—Determination of tensile properties), ISO 178: 2010 (Plastics—Determination of flexural properties), and ISO 604: 2002 (Plastics—Determination of compressive properties) were applied for the tensile, bending, and compressive tests, respectively [29–31]. Six samples were tested for each batch with a 1 mm/min testing speed, and the test was performed at an ambient temperature of 20 °C.

2.3. Surface Characterization

To determine the surface morphology, samples of PEEK and CFR-PEEK from the untreated, polished, and sandblasted groups (n = 2 per group) were sputtered with a 20 nm thick Au–Pd coating (SCD 050, Baltec, Lübeck, Germany) and characterized by a scanning electron microscope (SEM) (LEO 1430, Zeiss, Oberkochen, Germany) at 200× and 2000× magnification.

The surface topography of the discs (n = 6 per group) was analyzed by a profilometer (Perthometer Concept S6P, Mahr, Göttingen, Germany). For each sample, 121 profiles were measured over a 3 mm × 3 mm area. The arithmetic mean height (Sa) and root mean square height (Sq) were calculated based on these topographies by software (MountainsMap Universal 7.3, Digital Surf, Besançon, France).

The water contact angle (WCA) was measured at room temperature on six samples per group using a drop shape analyzer (DSA 10-MK 2, Kruess, Hamburg, Germany). Drops of 2 μL of distilled water were deposited on the respective disc surfaces using an automatic pipette. After 20 s wetting time, the contact angle at the air–water–substrate interface was quantified from the drop geometry using DSA software (version 1.90.0.11, Kruess, Hamburg, Germany).

2.4. Biological Tests

Biological tests consisted of an extract test and a direct contact test to analyze the cytotoxicity and of the investigation of cell attachment to the different samples (n = 9 per group). Two materials (PEEK and CFR-PEEK) with three different surfaces each (untreated, polished, and sandblasted) were tested. In each test, n = 3 samples were used for each surface modification. All tests were performed three times in independent experiments. Directly before the biological tests, samples were ultrasonically cleaned with DI water for 15 min and sterilized with 70% ethanol and 100% ethanol (15 min each). Subsequently, the samples were dried on filter paper in a sterile workbench (Lamin Air HB2472, Burgdorf, Switzerland).

2.4.1. Cell Culture

L929 fibroblasts (DSMZ GmbH, Braunschweig, Germany) were cultured in DMEM medium (21063-029, Gibco, Paisley, UK) containing 10% fetal bovine serum (FBS, Life Technologies, Carlsbad, CA, USA), 1% penicillin/streptomycin (15140-122, Life Technologies Co., Carlsbad, CA, USA), and 1% GlutaMAX (Life Technologies Co., Paisley, UK) in 75 cm^2 sterile cell culture flasks (Costar, Corning, Tewksbury, MA, USA). The cells were maintained in an incubator under a humidified atmosphere with 5% CO_2 at 37 °C. The DMEM culture medium was renewed twice a week. When cells reached confluence, Trypsin (GIBCO, Paisley, UK) was used to detach cells from the bottom of flasks, and 1/10 of the total cells were transferred into a new flask.

2.4.2. Test for In Vitro Cytotoxicity

The in vitro cytotoxicity test of PEEK and CFR-PEEK was performed by an extract method based on ISO 10993-5 [32]. Extracts were derived from soaking the samples with DMEM cell culture medium for 24 h at 37 °C. The ratio between the sample surface area and extraction vehicle volume was 3 cm^2/mL. In the meantime, the cells were precultured for 24 h. The seeding concentration of L929 cells was 30,000 cells/cm^2 in 200 μL DMEM medium per well in a 96-well plate (Cellstar 655180, Greiner Bio-One, Frickenhausen, Germany). After 24 h, the culture medium was removed from the cells and replaced by 150 μL extracts obtained from the respective sample groups. Three concentrations of each extract were tested: (a) undiluted (150 μL extracts), (b) 1:3 diluted with medium (50 μL extracts + 100 μL medium), and (c) 1:10 diluted (15 μL extracts + 135 μL medium). Ti samples were used as the negative control, and copper (Cu) samples were used as the positive control. After culturing for an additional 24 h, the extracts in all groups were replaced by 100 μL fresh DMEM medium to avoid artifacts in the following assay caused by blue color in the Cu extracts. The cytotoxicity was quantitatively analyzed by CCK-8 assay (Dojindo Molecular Technologies, Inc., Rockville, MD, USA). The volume of CCK-8 solution added to each test well was 10 μL. After incubating for 2 h, the optical density (OD) value was measured by a microplate ELISA reader (Tecan F50, Tecan Austria, Groedig, Austria) at 450 nm wavelength. The metabolic activity of L929 cells in the different test groups in comparison to the negative control was calculated according to the following formula:

$$\text{Cell metabolic activity (\%)} = (OD_t - OD_b)/(OD_{nc} - OD_b)\ 100\%, \qquad (1)$$

where the OD value is the absorbance value of the respective test group (OD_t), blank control group (OD_b), and negative control group (OD_{nc}).

2.4.3. Cell Adhesion and Spreading

L929 cells were seeded on PEEK, CFR-PEEK, and Ti samples in 12-well plates (REF 3512, Costar, Kennebunk, ME, USA) with a density of 30,000 cells/cm^2 and incubated in 2.4 mL DMEM medium at 37 °C and 5% CO_2. After incubation for 24 h, cell adhesion was terminated by rinsing with Hank's balanced salt solution (HBSS, Biochrom AG, Berlin, Germany). Adhering cells were vital stained for 10 min in a solution of 25 μg/mL fluorescein diacetate (FDA) and 1.25 μg/mL ethidium bromide (EB) (Sigma-Aldrich Chemie GmbH, Taufkirchen, Germany) in HBSS. For each sample, a minimum of six typical surface areas of every magnification (25×, 100×, 200×, and 400×) was documented by an Optishot-2 fluorescence microscope (Nikon, Tokyo, Japan) equipped with a digital camera (550D, Canon, Tokyo, Japan). Cell adhesion and spreading were assessed by measuring the density of the vital-stained cells (cells/cm^2) and the mean area of sample surface covered by cells (% of Ti) using a photo editing software (ImageJ, v1.8.0, National Institutes of Health, Bethesda, MD, USA).

2.5. Statistical Analysis

SPSS Version 21 (SPSS INC, Chicago, IL, USA) was used for analyzing the data. Shapiro–Wilk and Levene tests were applied to assess the assumptions of data normal distribution and homogeneity of variances. The results of the mechanical properties of each parameter were tested using the Student's *t*-test of unpaired data with equal variance. One-way analysis of variance (ANOVA) was used for the cell density, and cell adhesion and spreading followed by Tukey post-hoc test ($\alpha = 0.05$). The contact angle and roughness data were analyzed by Kruskal–Wallis analysis ($\alpha = 0.05$) for the disobedience of the data normality or homogeneity of variances.

3. Results

3.1. Mechanical Properties

Table 3 shows the results of mechanical tests for the FDM-printed PEEK and CFR-PEEK samples. From Table 3, it is observed that the PEEK samples with reinforced carbon fiber had significantly better strengths than the bare PEEK in the tensile and bending tests ($p < 0.05$). As for the compressive test, there was no statistical difference between the two materials in compressive strength.

Table 3. Mechanical properties (means ± standard deviation) of PEEK and CFR-PEEK.

Groups	Tensile Strength (MPa)	Tensile Modulus (GPa)	Bending Strength (MPa)	Bending Modulus (GPa)	Compressive Strength (MPa)	Compressive Modulus (GPa)
PEEK	95.21 ± 1.86 [a]	3.79 ± 0.27 [a]	140.83 ± 1.97 [a]	3.56 ± 0.13 [a]	138.63 ± 2.69 [a]	2.79 ± 0.11 [a]
CFR-PEEK	101.41 ± 4.23 [b]	7.37 ± 1.22 [b]	159.25 ± 13.54 [b]	5.41 ± 0.51 [b]	137.11 ± 3.43 [a]	3.51 ± 2.12 [b]

Different lowercase letters in the same column indicate significantly different groups ($p < 0.05$).

3.2. Surface Characterization

To understand how topological factors affect cell adhesion and spreading, the surface morphology of PEEK and CFR-PEEK composite was determined using SEM. Figure 3 presents the SEM images of untreated, polished, and sandblasted PEEK and CFR-PEEK samples. Printing borders, as shown in Figure 3a,d were formed on the surface due to the deposition between two printing lines. The clear peaks and valleys, which completely disappeared after polishing and sandblasting, could be identified on both untreated PEEK and CFR-PEEK sample surfaces. The polished surfaces displayed the smoothest morphology, although a few defects remained on the polished CFR-PEEK surfaces (Figure 3b,e). The surfaces of specimens, however, after sandblasting treatment possessed surface topography features in the micrometer scale with a homogeneous distribution of protuberances and cavities (Figure 3c,f).

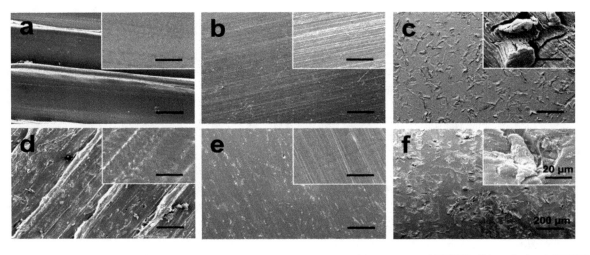

Figure 3. SEM images of PEEK and CFR-PEEK composite: (**a**) untreated PEEK; (**b**) polished PEEK; (**c**) sandblasted PEEK; (**d**) untreated CFR-PEEK; (**e**) polished CFR-PEEK; (**f**) sandblasted CFR-PEEK. Bars represent 200 μm and 20 μm (inserts), respectively.

Figure 4 illustrates the roughness of specimens of different groups. It is obvious that the untreated specimens displayed the roughest surfaces, both for PEEK and CFR-PEEK materials with the Sa value of 17.67 ± 5.7 μm and 32.36 ± 17.02 μm, which were significantly higher than the values of the polished and sandblasted groups ($p < 0.05$). The Sa values of sandblasted PEEK (0.85 ± 0.14 μm) and CFR-PEEK (0.97 ± 0.26 μm) samples were slightly higher than those of the polished surfaces (0.42 ± 0.26 μm and 0.67 ± 0.42 μm). In contrast, the polished Ti samples showed a very smooth surface (0.2 ± 0.04 μm), which was more homogenous compared with that of the polished PEEK and CFR-PEEK samples. The same trend could also be seen in the Sq data.

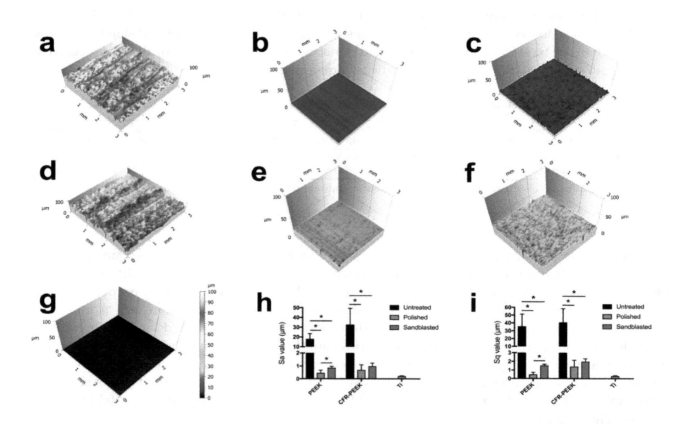

Figure 4. Reconstructed three-dimensional (3D) surface topographies of analyzed samples, and Sa and Sq values: (**a**) untreated PEEK; (**b**) polished PEEK; (**c**) sandblasted PEEK; (**d**) untreated CFR-PEEK; (**e**) polished CFR-PEEK; (**f**) sandblasted CFR-PEEK; (**g**) polished Ti; (**h,i**) Sa and Sq values of as-printed, polished, and sandblasted PEEK and CFR-PEEK samples, the polished Ti was used as an additional reference. The data are presented as means ± standard deviation, * $p < 0.05$.

The result of contact angle analysis is shown in Figure 5. Data revealed that the untreated surfaces of pure PEEK reflected an obvious hydrophobic response to water with a mean contact angle of 105 ± 26°. The polished PEEK specimens exhibited a hydrophilic behavior (78 ± 3°). After sandblasting, the contact angle rose slightly (88 ± 7°), but the difference was not significant ($p > 0.05$). As for the CFR-PEEK samples, the untreated group also indicated the most hydrophobic sample surface (92 ± 12°) compared with polished (82 ± 5°) and sandblasted (75 ± 3°) specimens. Both PEEK and CFR-PEEK samples, whether with or without surface modifications, revealed a more hydrophobic response to water compared to Ti (51 ± 5°).

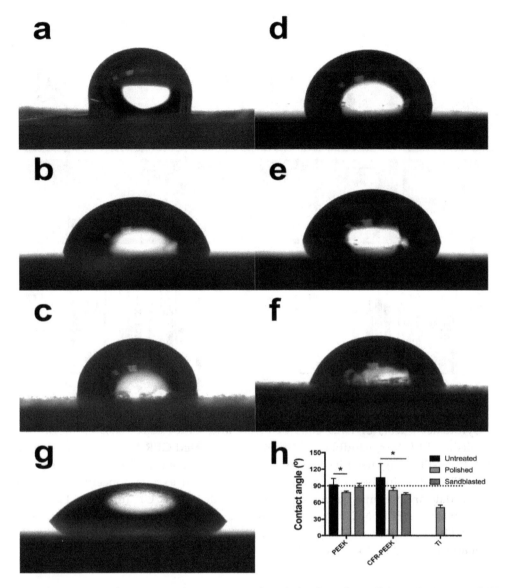

Figure 5. Water contact angle measured on untreated, polished, and sandblasted PEEK and CFR-PEEK samples: (**a**) untreated PEEK; (**b**) polished PEEK; (**c**) sandblasted PEEK; (**d**) untreated CFR-PEEK; (**e**) polished CFR-PEEK; (**f**) sandblasted CFR-PEEK. (**g**) Ti (additional reference); (**h**) quantitative contact angle values (means ± standard deviation). The dotted line indicates the contact angle of 90°, which is the division of hydrophilicity and hydrophobicity, * $p < 0.05$.

3.3. Cytotoxicity

Cell metabolic activity is expressed as a percentage of the mean OD value of cells cultured with extracts of the negative control (Ti), as displayed in Figure 6i,j. The data showed high cell viability in the cultures treated with 1:1, 1:3, and 1:10 extract concentrations of both tested materials, PEEK and CFR-PEEK, independent of the respective surface treatment (PEEK: untreated: 98 ± 23%, 106 ± 17%, 97 ± 22%; polished: 105 ± 25%, 106 ± 16%, 102 ± 15%; sandblasted: 106 ± 33%, 114 ± 27%, 98 ± 37%; CFR-PEEK: untreated: 98 ± 20%, 100 ± 28%, 97 ± 23%; polished: 102 ± 27%, 97 ± 31%, 105 ± 25%; sandblasted: 99 ± 38%, 100 ± 33%, 96 ± 23%). All extracts of PEEK and CFR-PEEK samples showed no toxicity after 24 h incubation. Cell viability in all cultures was significantly above the 70% level regarded as toxicity threshold according to ISO 10993-5 [32]. The results were confirmed by morphology analysis as seen in Figure 6a–h. Cells in the 100% extracts of the PEEK and CFR-PEEK groups exhibited a similar appearance as the negative control (Ti) group with distinct fibroblastic profiles. On the contrary, a large number of dead cells appeared in the positive group with a cell survival rate of $1 \pm 2\%$.

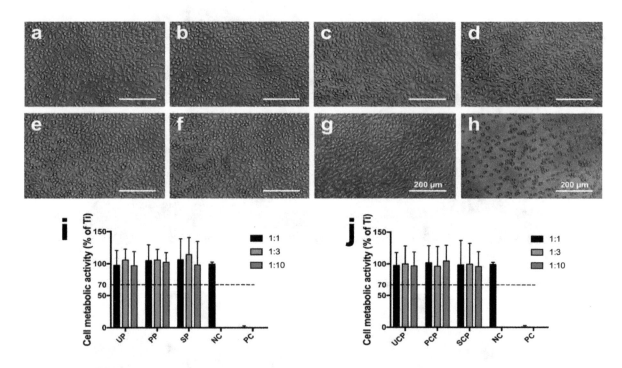

Figure 6. Cytotoxicity tests of L929 cells of PEEK and CFR-PEEK 100% extracts: (**a**) untreated PEEK; (**b**) polished PEEK; (**c**) sandblasted PEEK; (**d**) untreated CFR-PEEK; (**e**) polished CFR-PEEK; (**f**) sandblasted CFR-PEEK; (**g**) negative control (Ti); (**h**) positive control (Cu). (**i,j**) shows the quantitative result of the CCK-8 test in the culture media with different extract concentrations of PEEK and CFR-PEEK. The data are presented as means ± standard deviation. UP: untreated PEEK; PP: polished PEEK; SP: sandblasted PEEK; NC: negative control; PC: positive control; UCP: untreated CFR-PEEK; PCP: polished CFR-PEEK; SCP: sandblasted CFR-PEEK. The dotted line indicates the toxicity threshold of 70% cell viability according to ISO 10993-5.

3.4. Cell Adhesion and Spreading

Cell viability, attachment, and spreading were examined through a LIVE/DEAD staining assay, as shown in Figure 7. Compared with polished and sandblasted samples, untreated samples indicated more attached cells on the surfaces, both for PEEK and CFR-PEEK materials (Figure 7a–f). In addition, many cells attached in lines in the valleys resulting from the FDM manufacturing process (Figure 7a,d). Figure 7h,i reveals the quantitative cell density and quantification of the mean surface area covered by cells. Cell density on the sample surfaces of untreated PEEK and CFR-PEEK was significantly higher than on the corresponding polished and sandblasted groups ($p < 0.05$), where density was close to the Ti group. Moreover, the untreated groups showed higher cell coverage compared to the modified surfaces. The polished groups showed the lowest cell attachment for PEEK as well as CFR-PEEK samples.

Figure 8 shows the attached L929 cells around PEEK (Figure 8a–c), CFR-PEEK (Figure 8d–f), and Ti (Figure 8g) samples of the direct contact test after culturing for 24 h. The cells on PEEK and CFR-PEEK samples showed fibroblastic features and distinct profiles unaffected by the different materials and surface modifications. Moreover, the cell number was also similar to the negative control (Ti), which confirmed that the PEEK and CFR-PEEK materials were not toxic.

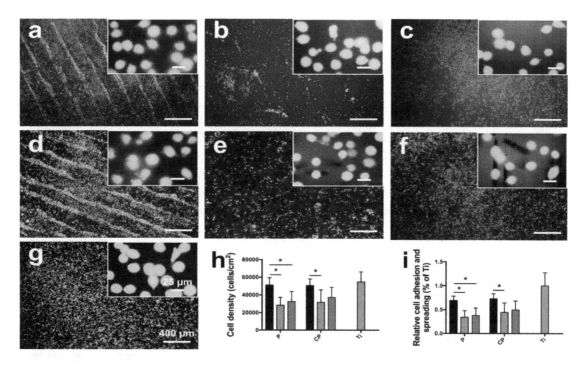

Figure 7. LIVE/DEAD staining of L929 cells on PEEK and CFR-PEEK samples after culturing for 24 h, with Ti as an additional control. (**a**) untreated PEEK; (**b**) polished PEEK; (**c**) sandblasted PEEK; (**d**) untreated CFR-PEEK; (**e**) polished CFR-PEEK; (**f**) sandblasted CFR-PEEK; (**g**) Ti. (**h**,**i**) shows the quantitative cell density and quantification of the mean surface area covered by cells. The data are presented as means ± standard deviation, * $p < 0.05$. P: PEEK; CP: CFR-PEEK; black bar: untreated group; orange bar: polished group; blue bar: sandblasted group. Cytotoxic effects, indicated by dead (red stained) cells, are not detectable.

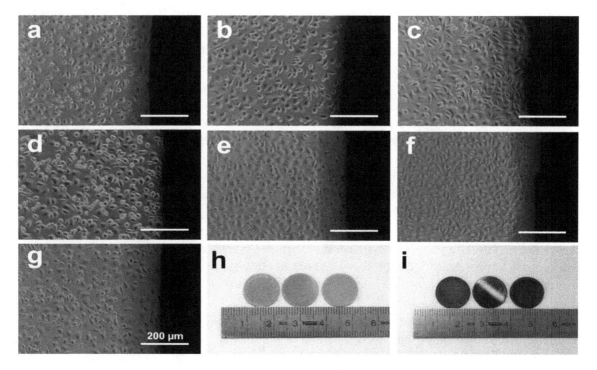

Figure 8. Microscopic images of L929 cells observed around samples of direct contact test after culturing for 24 h. (**a**) untreated PEEK; (**b**) polished PEEK; (**c**) sandblasted PEEK; (**d**) untreated CFR-PEEK; (**e**) polished CFR-PEEK; (**f**) sandblasted CFR-PEEK; (**g**) Ti; (**h**) PEEK samples (untreated, polished, and sandblasted); (**i**) CFR-PEEK samples (untreated, polished, and sandblasted).

4. Discussion

This study aimed to investigate the mechanical properties of FDM-printed PEEK composite, the influence of manufacturing on the materials' cytotoxicity, and the impact of surface topography and wettability on cell adhesion. To the best of our knowledge, there is currently no literature on these topics, whereas the manufacturing parameters and mechanical properties of FDM-processed bare PEEK and the SLS-printed PEEK composite have already been published elsewhere [18,21,33–35]. According to the manufacturing principles of FDM, only thermoplastic filaments can be used, like PLA, ABS, and PEEK [33]. However, it is a great challenge to fabricate ideal-performance PEEK objects through FDM equipment due to its high melting temperature (above 300 °C), high melting expansion, and especially the semicrystalline property, in particular for PEEK composites [22,34]. In this study, FDM-printed CFR-PEEK composite was successfully fabricated, and the mechanical properties were first measured. Moreover, the influence of the surface topography and roughness on biocompatibility and cell adhesion of FDM-printed PEEK and CFR-PEEK was also estimated for the first time.

The mechanical results indicated that the pure PEEK showed low strength in tensile, bending, and compressive tests. However, the addition of 5% carbon fiber into the PEEK matrix improved the mechanical strengths (Table 3), showing values similar to those of human cortical bone (elastic modulus: 14 GPa) [8] Normally, the mechanical properties of additively manufactured PEEK were obviously lower than the traditionally produced parts (i.e., injection molding) [21]. Although some studies have been done on PEEK composites by adding reinforcement fillers using SLS technology, the mechanical properties of FDM-printed PEEK composites were still insufficient, compared with their cast counterparts as a bone replacement material for severe cranio-maxillofacial defects [34,35]. The manufacturing conditions of the FDM process, such as layer thickness, printing speed, ambient temperature, nozzle temperature, and heat treatment, can produce a significant impact on the mechanical properties of PEEK samples [21,22]. In this study, the tensile strength of bare PEEK was 95.21 ± 1.86 MPa with an elastic modulus of 3.79 ± 0.27 GPa, which was comparable to the injection-molded pure PEEK (100 MPa and 4 GPa) [21]. While the tensile strength and elastic modulus of CFR-PEEK composites reached 101.41 ± 4.23 MPa and 7.37 ± 1.22 GPa, which were much higher than the injection-molded pure PEEK, the similar trend could also be seen in the bending and compressive tests. This result indicates that the printing conditions used in this study were suitable for PEEK and CFR-PEEK manufacturing. Deng et al. and Wu et al. have measured the mechanical properties of FDM-printed pure PEEK and found that the mechanical strength of printed PEEK samples was significantly lower than the traditionally produced objects, whereas in this study the values were quite similar [18,21]. One proper explanation for the excellent mechanical properties in this research is the application of post heat treatment (tempering). Theoretically, heat treatment methods can increase the degree of crystallinity and relieve the residual stress and shrinkage distortion, which will increase the mechanical performance of PEEK parts [22]. Therefore, the mechanical strengths of PEEK composite could be tailored by carbon fibers to mimic human cortical bone, thus avoiding stress shielding [8].

Polishing and sandblasting are common surface processing methods in dentistry to get a smooth or rough surface. However, the FDM-printed sample surfaces were much rougher compared with sandblasted ones, as shown in Figures 3 and 4. This finding can be related to the working principle of FDM. Thermoplastic materials are extruded by the printing nozzle, which can move across the building platform in x- and y-axes, to generate a 2D layer line by line. Then, a 3D object is built up by melting the successive 2D layers together. The crosswise oriented, threadlike inner structure of the specimen results in some unfilled areas between lines and layers, and also in the original printing structures on sample surfaces [36]. In this study, the sandblasted samples showed slightly rougher surfaces than the polished ones. Compared with some previous studies, the sandblasting parameters (i.e., distance and pressure) in this research had to be set lower in order not to perforate the layer-by-layer manufacturing pattern [26,27,37]. In other studies, using traditional methods to fabricate PEEK and its composite samples like injection molding or milling, the interior of the blocks was homogenous without layers or unfilled areas. The samples in this study were produced using FDM technology, laying down objects in layers with a thickness of 0.2 mm. If a higher sandblasting pressure or closer distance were applied to modify the sample, the upper surface layer would be exfoliated (Figure 9). Therefore, based on the parameters used for sandblasting in this study, the sandblasted sample surfaces were slightly rougher than the polished ones, but not obviously different.

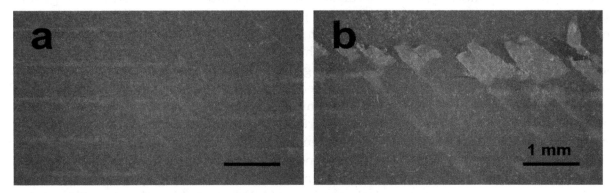

Figure 9. Optical micrographs of sandblasted PEEK samples (**a**) under 0.1 MPa pressure; (**b**) under 0.5 MPa pressure.

It is recognized that the surface wettability of biomaterials is important for their bioactivities, such as cell adhesion and spreading [38]. Therefore, the hydrophilicity of the samples was evaluated by the static sessile drop method, and the results are shown in Figure 5. Both PEEK and CFR-PEEK materials, before surface modification, represented a hydrophobic response to water (contact angle between 90–110°), which is typical for PEEK materials [8,39]. After polishing and sandblasting, both samples exhibited slightly hydrophilic behavior with contact angles below 90°. Commonly, wettability is closely related to the surface topography and chemical composition of a material [39]. The higher water contact angle in the untreated group in this study could be explained by the printing structures produced by FDM (Figures 3 and 4). On highly roughened surfaces, the peaks and valleys prevent the water droplet from spreading on the surface, which can result in increased contact angles since the peaks and valleys on the sample surfaces constitute "geometrical barriers" for the droplet spreading [37,40]. According to the study undertaken by Ourahmoune et al., the surface morphology strongly influences the hydrophilic behavior of PEEK and its composites [37]. For the polished and sandblasted samples, since the differences of roughness values between these two groups were not obvious, the water contact angles were similar.

Due to its chemical inertness, PEEK provides inherent good biocompatibility, and this is also one of its advantages that favors its clinical use [8]. However, for the FDM-printed PEEK using a relatively new technology to fabricate PEEK using AM, studies focusing on the possible introduction of toxic substances during the printing process are still lacking, especially for its composites. According to ISO 10993-5, a reduction of cell viability by more than 30% indicates a cytotoxic effect [32]. In this study (Figure 6), the cell metabolic test of PEEK and CFR-PEEK samples showed that more than 96% of cells survived in all sample groups tested, independent of the respective surface modification. This result was comparable to the negative control group (Ti). The cytotoxicity results indicated that there were no toxic effects generated by the printing process. Moreover, after surface treatment, some carbon fibers were exposed on the surface of CFR-PEEK samples. However, this exposure has not led to increased cytotoxicity. Zhao et al. investigated FDM-printed pure PEEK and obtained a similar result that no toxic substances were introduced during the printing process [17].

Cell adhesion and spreading are closely related to surface properties, that is, composition, roughness, morphology, and wettability [41]. In addition to chemical composition, surface roughness and morphology play a critical role in the biological responses of biomaterial surfaces. In this study, the untreated PEEK and CFR-PEEK sample surfaces exhibited significantly more cell attachment than the polished and sandblasted samples, where the attachment level was close to the Ti surfaces. The as-printed PEEK and CFR-PEEK showed a higher cell density which might be due to the special 3D-printed structures. As shown in Figure 3a,d and Figure 4a,d, the clear ridges and valleys on the surfaces could be identified on both PEEK and CFR-PEEK sample surfaces. These special printing structures could enlarge the surface area significantly compared with polished and sandblasted surfaces. Significantly more spaces are available for cells to attach and spread on this geometrical morphology. For many engineering applications, a post-printing process is always needed to eliminate the manufactured structures [39]. However, to improve the cell attachment and spreading, a rough surface as generated by FDM seems beneficial, which could not be achieved by sandblasting. It was obvious that the cells accumulated in the surface grooves resulting from the manufacturing process (Figure 7a,d). Figure 4a,d showed the reconstructed 3D surface topographies of the as-printed PEEK and CFR-PEEK samples. The cells could slide into the valleys on the sample surfaces and attach there. As for both the polished and sandblasted surfaces, the originally printed surface structures were removed and the surfaces showed a lower cell density, but the cells appeared more homogeneously attached. After polishing and sandblasting, the exposure of carbon fibers on the surface of CFR-PEEK samples did not improve the cell attachment significantly. This finding confirmed that reinforced carbon fibers could improve the mechanical properties of FDM-printed PEEK, but would not influence the cytotoxicity and cell adhesion. In this study, the biological response of FDM-printed PEEK was investigated at a basic level, including cytotoxicity and cell adhesion. In future studies, more biological tests (e.g., in vitro cell metabolic activity, proliferation, and in vivo osseointegration) should be applied to evaluate bioactivities.

To sum up, the results indicate that the FDM-printed CFR-PEEK has excellent mechanical properties compared with the printed bare PEEK. In addition, no toxic substances were introduced during the FDM printing process. FDM technology can yield a highly roughened surface suitable for cells to attach.

5. Conclusions

In this study, the mechanical properties of FDM-printed, carbon fiber reinforced PEEK composite were systematically studied for the first time, including tensile, bending, and compressive tests. The experimental results confirmed that samples printed from pure PEEK material showed mechanical properties comparable to traditionally manufactured PEEK objects, obtained by extrusion techniques for example. On the contrary, the printed CFR-PEEK specimen represented significantly improved mechanical properties compared to printed pure PEEK. FDM technology could be used to provide more satisfactory mechanical strength of PEEK and its composites. Therefore, it is an appropriate method for matching the mechanical properties of PEEK composites with carbon fibers to mimic human cortical bone and avoid stress shielding in clinical applications, like dental implants, skull implants, osteosynthesis plates, and bone replacement material for nasal, maxillary, or mandibular reconstructions.

Additionally, the impact of the surface topography and roughness of FDM-printed PEEK and its composites on biocompatibility and cell adhesion was also estimated for the first time. Laboratory experiments here clearly showed that no toxic substances were introduced during the FDM manufacturing process of pure PEEK and CFR-PEEK. Surface treatments leading to partial exposure of the fiber compound in the bulk material did not lead to increased cytotoxicity. FDM-manufactured surfaces had highly rough topographies, which could not be achieved by typical dental sandblasting processes. This structure was more suitable for cells to attach and spread compared with polished and sandblasted surfaces, resulting in a cell density comparable to that on Ti sample surfaces. Although tests carried out in this study are limited, it is expected that the CFR-PEEK composite with its enhanced mechanical properties has great potential to be used as an orthopedic or dental implant material in bone repair, regeneration, and tissue engineering applications.

Author Contributions: Conceptualization, S.S., L.S., and F.R.; Formal analysis, X.H.; Methodology, X.H., D.Y., C.Y., and P.L.; Project administration, D.L. and J.G.-G.; Writing—original draft, X.H.; Writing—review and editing, X.H., S.S., L.S., J.G.-G., and F.R.

Acknowledgments: The authors would like to thank Ernst Schweizer for his assistance in the SEM analysis.

References

1. Ren, Z.H.; Wu, H.J.; Tan, H.Y.; Wang, K.; Zhang, S. Transfer of anterolateral thigh flaps in elderly oral cancer patients: Complications in oral and maxillofacial reconstruction. *J. Oral Maxillofac. Surg.* **2015**, *73*, 534–540. [CrossRef] [PubMed]

2. Rohner, D.; Guijarro-Martínez, R.; Bucher, P.; Hammer, B. Importance of patient-specific intraoperative guides in complex maxillofacial reconstruction. *J. Cranio-Maxillofac. Surg.* **2013**, *41*, 382–390. [CrossRef] [PubMed]

3. Bauer, T.W.; Muschler, G.F. Bone Graft Materials: An Overview of the Basic Science. *Clin. Orthop. Relat. Res.* **2000**, *371*, 10–27. [CrossRef]

4. Hallman, M.; Thor, A. Bone substitutes and growth factors as an alternative/complement to autogenous bone for grafting in implant dentistry. *Periodontol. 2000* **2008**, *47*, 172–192. [CrossRef] [PubMed]

5. Zhao, Y.; Wong, S.M.; Wong, H.M.; Wu, S.; Hu, T.; Yeung, K.W.K.; Chu, P.K. Effects of Carbon and Nitrogen Plasma Immersion Ion Implantation on In vitro and In vivo Biocompatibility of Titanium Alloy. *ACS Appl. Mater. Interfaces* **2013**, *5*, 1510–1516. [CrossRef] [PubMed]

6. Bougherara, H.; Bureau, M.N.; Yahia, L. Bone remodeling in a new biomimetic polymer-composite hip stem. *J. Biomed. Mater. Res. Part A* **2010**, *92*, 164–174. [CrossRef]

7. Wang, H.; Lu, T.; Meng, F.; Zhu, H.; Liu, X. Enhanced osteoblast responses to poly ether ether ketone surface modified by water plasma immersion ion implantation. *Colloids Surf. B Biointerfaces* **2014**, *117*, 89–97. [CrossRef]

8. Najeeb, S.; Zafar, M.S.; Khurshid, Z.; Siddiqui, F. Applications of polyetheretherketone (PEEK) in oral implantology and prosthodontics. *J. Prosthodont. Res.* **2016**, *60*, 12–19. [CrossRef]

9. Panayotov, I.V.; Orti, V.; Cuisinier, F.; Yachouh, J. Polyetheretherketone (PEEK) for medical applications. *J. Mater. Sci. Mater. Med.* **2016**, *27*, 118. [CrossRef]

10. Schwitalla, A.; Müller, W.-D. PEEK Dental Implants: A Review of the Literature. *J. Oral Implantol.* **2013**, *39*, 743–749. [CrossRef]

11. Trindade, R.; Albrektsson, T.; Galli, S.; Prgomet, Z.; Tengvall, P.; Wennerberg, A. Bone Immune Response to Materials, Part I: Titanium, PEEK and Copper in Comparison to Sham at 10 Days in Rabbit Tibia. *J. Clin. Med.* **2018**, *7*, 526. [CrossRef] [PubMed]

12. Sandler, J.; Werner, P.; Shaffer, M.S.P.; Demchuk, V.; Altstädt, V.; Windle, A.H. Carbon-nanofibre-reinforced poly (ether ether ketone) composites. *Compos. Part A Appl. Sci. Manuf.* **2002**, *33*, 1033–1039. [CrossRef]

13. Devine, D.M.; Hahn, J.; Richards, R.G.; Gruner, H.; Wieling, R.; Pearce, S.G. Coating of carbon fiber-reinforced polyetheretherketone implants with titanium to improve bone apposition. *J. Biomed. Mater. Res. Part B Appl. Biomater.* **2013**, *101*, 591–598. [CrossRef] [PubMed]

14. Lu, T.; Liu, X.; Qian, S.; Cao, H.; Qiao, Y.; Mei, Y.; Chu, P.K.; Ding, C. Multilevel surface engineering of nanostructured TiO_2 on carbon-fiber-reinforced polyetheretherketone. *Biomaterials* **2014**, *35*, 5731–5740. [CrossRef] [PubMed]

15. Lee, W.; Koak, J.; Lim, Y.; Kim, S.; Kwon, H.; Kim, M. Stress shielding and fatigue limits of poly-ether-ether-ketone dental implants. *J. Biomed. Mater. Res. Part B Appl. Biomater.* **2012**, *100*, 1044–1052. [CrossRef] [PubMed]

16. Ventola, C.L. Medical Applications for 3D Printing: Current and Projected Uses. *Pharm. Ther.* **2014**, *39*, 704–711.

17. Zhao, F.; Li, D.; Jin, Z. Preliminary investigation of poly-ether-ether-ketone based on fused deposition modeling for medical applications. *Materials* **2018**, *11*, 288. [CrossRef]

18. Deng, X.; Zeng, Z.; Peng, B.; Yan, S.; Ke, W. Mechanical properties optimization of poly-ether-ether-ketone via fused deposition modeling. *Materials* **2018**, *11*, 216. [CrossRef]

19. Zhao, X.; Xiong, D.; Liu, Y. Improving surface wettability and lubrication of polyetheretherketone (PEEK) by combining with polyvinyl alcohol (PVA) hydrogel. *J. Mech. Behav. Biomed. Mater.* **2018**, *82*, 27–34. [CrossRef]

20. Punchak, M.; Chung, L.K.; Lagman, C.; Bui, T.T.; Lazareff, J.; Rezzadeh, K.; Jarrahy, R.; Yang, I. Outcomes following polyetheretherketone (PEEK) cranioplasty: Systematic review and meta-analysis. *J. Clin. Neurosci.* **2017**, *41*, 30–35. [CrossRef]

21. Wu, W.; Geng, P.; Li, G.; Zhao, D.; Zhang, H.; Zhao, J. Influence of layer thickness and raster angle on the mechanical properties of 3D-printed PEEK and a comparative mechanical study between PEEK and ABS. *Materials* **2015**, *8*, 5834–5846. [CrossRef] [PubMed]

22. Yang, C.; Tian, X.; Li, D.; Cao, Y.; Zhao, F.; Shi, C. Influence of thermal processing conditions in 3D printing on the crystallinity and mechanical properties of PEEK material. *J. Mater. Process. Technol.* **2017**, *248*, 1–7. [CrossRef]

23. Rabiei, A.; Sandukas, S. Processing and evaluation of bioactive coatings on polymeric implants. *J. Biomed. Mater. Res. Part A* **2013**, *101*, 2621–2629. [CrossRef] [PubMed]

24. Ma, R.; Tang, T. Current strategies to improve the bioactivity of PEEK. *Int. J. Mol. Sci.* **2014**, *15*, 5426–5445. [CrossRef] [PubMed]

25. Gittens, R.A.; Olivares-Navarrete, R.; McLachlan, T.; Cai, Y.; Hyzy, S.L.; Schneider, J.M.; Schwartz, Z.; Sandhage, K.H.; Boyan, B.D. Differential responses of osteoblast lineage cells to nanotopographically-modified, microroughened titanium–aluminum–vanadium alloy surfaces. *Biomaterials* **2012**, *33*, 8986–8994. [CrossRef] [PubMed]

26. Deng, Y.; Liu, X.; Xu, A.; Wang, L.; Luo, Z.; Zheng, Y.; Deng, F.; Wei, J.; Tang, Z.; Wei, S. Effect of surface roughness on osteogenesis in vitro and osseointegration in vivo of carbon fiber-reinforced polyetheretherketone– Nanohydroxyapatite composite. *Int. J. Nanomed.* **2015**, *10*, 1425–1447. [PubMed]

27. Elawadly, T.; Radi, I.A.W.; El Khadem, A.; Osman, R.B. Can PEEK Be an Implant Material? Evaluation of Surface Topography and Wettability of Filled Versus Unfilled PEEK With Different Surface Roughness. *J. Oral Implantol.* **2017**, *43*, 456–461. [CrossRef] [PubMed]

28. Wu, X.; Liu, X.; Wei, J.; Ma, J.; Deng, F.; Wei, S. Nano-TiO$_2$/PEEK bioactive composite as a bone substitute material: In vitro and in vivo studies. *Int. J. Nanomed.* **2012**, *7*, 1215.

29. *ISO 527-1: 2012 Plastics—Determination of Tensile Properties—Part 1: General Principles*; International Organization for Standardization: Geneva, Switzerland, 2012.

30. *ISO 178: 2010 Plastics—Determination of Flexural Properties*; International Organization for Standardization: Geneva, Switzerland, 2010.

31. *ISO 604: 2002 Plastics—Determination of Compressive Properties Plastiques*; International Organization for Standardization: Geneva, Switzerland, 2002.

32. *ISO 10993-5: 2009 Biological Evaluation of Medical Devices—Part 5: Tests for In Vitro Cytotoxicity*; International Organization for Standardization: Geneva, Switzerland, 2009.

33. Rinaldi, M.; Ghidini, T.; Cecchini, F.; Brandao, A.; Nanni, F. Additive layer manufacturing of poly (ether ether ketone) via FDM. *Compos. Part B Eng.* **2018**, *145*, 162–172. [CrossRef]

34. Yan, M.; Tian, X.; Peng, G.; Li, D.; Zhang, X. High temperature rheological behavior and sintering kinetics of CF/PEEK composites during selective laser sintering. *Compos. Sci. Technol.* **2018**, *165*, 140–147. [CrossRef]

35. Stepashkin, A.A.; Chukov, D.I.; Senatov, F.S.; Salimon, A.I.; Korsunsky, A.M.; Kaloshkin, S.D. 3D-printed PEEK-carbon fiber (CF) composites: Structure and thermal properties. *Compos. Sci. Technol.* **2018**, *164*, 319–326. [CrossRef]

36. Xu, Y.; Unkovskiy, A.; Klaue, F.; Rupp, F.; Geis-Gerstorfer, J.; Spintzyk, S.; Xu, Y.; Unkovskiy, A.; Klaue, F.; Rupp, F.; et al. Compatibility of a Silicone Impression/Adhesive System to FDM-Printed Tray Materials—A Laboratory Peel-off Study. *Materials* **2018**, *11*, 1905. [CrossRef] [PubMed]

37. Ourahmoune, R.; Salvia, M.; Mathia, T.G.; Mesrati, N. Surface morphology and wettability of sandblasted PEEK and its composites. *Scanning* **2014**, *36*, 64–75. [CrossRef] [PubMed]

38. Gittens, R.A.; Scheideler, L.; Rupp, F.; Hyzy, S.L.; Geis-Gerstorfer, J.; Schwartz, Z.; Boyan, B.D. A review on the wettability of dental implant surfaces II: Biological and clinical aspects. *Acta Biomater.* **2014**, *10*, 2907–2918. [CrossRef] [PubMed]

39. Al Qahtani, M.S.A.; Wu, Y.; Spintzyk, S.; Krieg, P.; Killinger, A.; Schweizer, E.; Stephan, I.; Scheideler, L.; Geis-Gerstorfer, J.; Rupp, F. UV-A and UV-C light induced hydrophilization of dental implants. *Dent. Mater.* **2015**, *31*, e157–e167. [CrossRef] [PubMed]

40. Rupp, F.; Gittens, R.A.; Scheideler, L.; Marmur, A.; Boyan, B.D.; Schwartz, Z.; Geis-Gerstorfer, J. A review on the wettability of dental implant surfaces I: Theoretical and experimental aspects. *Acta Biomater.* **2014**, *10*, 2894–2906. [CrossRef] [PubMed]

41. Zhu, X.; Chen, J.; Scheideler, L.; Reichl, R.; Geis-Gerstorfer, J. Effects of topography and composition of titanium surface oxides on osteoblast responses. *Biomaterials* **2004**, *25*, 4087–4103. [CrossRef]

14

Treatment of Peri-Implantitis—Electrolytic Cleaning Versus Mechanical and Electrolytic Cleaning—A Randomized Controlled Clinical Trial—Six-Month Results

Markus Schlee [1], Florian Rathe [2], Urs Brodbeck [3], Christoph Ratka [4], Paul Weigl [4] and Holger Zipprich [4,*]

[1]   Private Practice and Department of Maxillofacial Surgery, Goethe University, 60590 Frankfurt am Main, Germany; markus.schlee@32schoenezaehne.de

[2]   Private Practice and Department of Prosthodontics, Danube University, 3500 Krems, Austria; florian.rathe@32schoenezaehne.de

[3]   Private Practice, 8051 Zürich, Switzerland; ursbrodbeck@bluewin.ch

[4]   Department of Prosthodontics, Goethe University, 60590 Frankfurt am Main, Germany; ratka@med.uni-frankfurt.de (C.R.); weigl@em.uni-frankfurt.de (P.W.)

*   Correspondence: zipprich@em.uni-frankfurt.de

Abstract: Objectives: The present randomized clinical trial assesses the six-month outcomes following surgical regenerative therapy of periimplantitis lesions using either an electrolytic method (EC) to remove biofilms or a combination of powder spray and electrolytic method (PEC). Materials and Methods: 24 patients with 24 implants suffering from peri-implantitis with any type of bone defect were randomly treated by EC or PEC. Bone defects were augmented with a mixture of natural bone mineral and autogenous bone and left for submerged healing. The distance from implant shoulder to bone was assessed at six defined points at baseline (T0) and after six months at uncovering surgery (T1) by periodontal probe and standardized x-rays. Results: One implant had to be removed at T1 because of reinfection and other obstacles. None of the other implants showed signs of inflammation. Bone gain was 2.71 ± 1.70 mm for EC and 2.81 ± 2.15 mm for PEC. No statistically significant difference between EC and PEC was detected. Significant clinical bone fill was observed for all 24 implants. Complete regeneration of bone was achieved in 12 implants. Defect morphology impacted the amount of regeneration. Conclusion: EC needs no further mechanical cleaning by powder spray. Complete re-osseointegration in peri-implantitis cases is possible.

Keywords: periimplantitis; electrolytic cleaning; augmentation; air flow; re-osseointegration; classification of bone defects

1. Introduction

Increasing numbers of inserted dental implants cause an increasing number of infected implants [1]. Mucositis is a reversible inflammatory process limited to peri-implant soft tissue. Peri-implantitis (PI) is defined as an inflammatory process affecting peri-implant hard as well as soft tissue. Typical cup-shaped progressive bone defects, pus, and bleeding on probing (BoP) are clinical parameters which have to be verified simultaneously to justify the diagnosis of PI [2,3]. Mucositis and PI are correlated with bacterial biofilms colonizing the surfaces of implants or abutments [4]. In view of the difficulty in differentiating pathologic bleeding from bleeding caused by improper probing, as well as the discordance in the dental community about the acceptable threshold of bone loss, there is no consensus about when pathology starts and how PI can be diagnosed precisely. Hence, prevalence data vary from author to author [5,6]. Based on these data, up to 100 million dental implants may be infected worldwide. As implant surfaces, which are exposed to the oral cavity, are immediately colonized by the individual microbiome, the surfaces need to be re-osseointegrated for positive long-term results [7]. Treatment and replacement of implants cause immense costs and discomfort. Therefore, it is necessary to find more effective approaches to decontaminating infected implants.

Several methods, all of which are ablative for removing biofilms have been discussed. For example, mechanical debridement by hand or ultrasound-driven curettes, brushes, lasers, pellets, cold plasma, or air-powder sprays in conjunction with or without disinfection or antibiotic agents. Re-osseointegration of between 39% and 46% of treated implant surfaces was reported in a review [8]. Re-osseointegration in humans has not yet been proven. A review of the literature demonstrated that none of the assessed methods was superior to any other in removing the biofilm and no method was able to achieve a stable result over time [9]. Up to 100% relapse of the disease for some methods was demonstrated after one year, and evidence for the superiority of any treatment modality is lacking [10]. Powder spray systems (PSS) are commonly used to treat PI. Small particles (erythritol or glycine) are accelerated by air pressure and remove the biofilm when impacting the implant surface. Several animal studies investigating re-osseointegration after cleaning by PSS proved incomplete re-osseointegration [8]. Clinical parameters like BoP, pocket depth (PD), and pus improved. Furthermore, PSS failed to prove superiority to any other treatment modality [11–13]. Possible reasons for this limited efficacy might be craterlike bone defects with compromised access, thus improper working angle and distance of the device, macro- and micro-design of the implant surface, and particles too large for much smaller bacteria hidden in the microstructure of textured implants.

In an in vitro test, two bacterially contaminated implants were embedded in an electro-conductive gelatin block and were loaded with a continuous current of 0-10 mA – one acting as a cathode, the other as an anode. A reduction of bacteria was proved. This approach dramatically changed the pH at both implants [14]. Zipprich et al. covered implants with a mature biofilm, loaded them as cathode, and flooded the implants with a buffered potassium iodine solution which had passed an anode. Complete removal of the biofilm was demonstrated by SEM analysis [15]. The mode of action was investigated by a collaborative working group [16]. In an in vitro test, Ratka et al. used EC versus PSS to treat implants with different surfaces and alloys covered with a mature biofilm. In contrast to PSS, no bacteria could be cultivated in the EC groups. The difference was extremely significant [17]. Based on these findings, an electrolytic device was developed by the authors to remove the biofilm in a clinical setting.

The aim and endpoint of this controlled clinical trial was to compare the effectiveness of two processes of decontamination in terms of bone level changes.

2. Materials and Methods

2.1. Legal

The study was registered (BfArM DA/CA99, DIMDI 00010977) and approved by the "Ethik-Kommission der Bayerischen Landesärztekammer" (BASEC_No. DE/EKBY10) with the registration code 17075.

2.2. Sample Size Calculation

The data presented in this study were collected for a proof of principle study assessing the bacterial load before and after the treatment. This article describes the six-month results of the proof of principle study. Based on previous in vitro tests using a paired t-test with a power of 90% and a level of significance of 5%, a sample size of 12 per group was calculated. The sample size calculation was done using G*Power 3.1 (Heinrich Heine University of Düsseldorf).

2.3. Devices and Mode of Action

For the electrolytic approach (EL) the implant has to be loaded negatively with a voltage and a maximum current of 600 mA. This is achieved by a device (GS1000, GalvoSurge Dental AG, Widnau, Switzerland) providing the voltage and pumping a sodium formiate solution through a spray-head, which has to be pressed into the implant by finger pressure to achieve an electrical contact (Figure 1). Driven by a peristaltic pump, a sodium formiate solution passes an anode inside the spray-head and then covers the implant with a "film" of liquid (Figure 2). The current splits the water into hydrogen anions and cations. The cations penetrate the biofilm and take an electron from the implant. Hydrogen bubbles lift the biofilm off the implant surface.

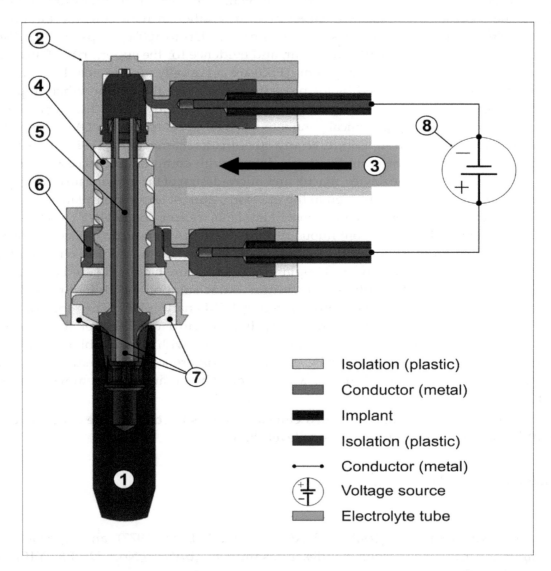

Figure 1. Composition of the spray-head. (1) Implant (loaded as a cathode); (2) spray head; (3) tube for electrolyte; (4) spiral-like threaded isolator; (5) connector (loaded as a cathode); (6) anode; (7) shower head (exit of electrolyte); (8) control unit and voltage source. Application of Figure 1: The spray-head (2) has to be pressed on containment of the implant (1) manually. The electrolyte will be pumped through the tube (3) and passes the spiral of the treaded isolator (4), reaches the anode (6), and will be sprayed by the shower head (7) onto the exposed implant surface. A second pathway branching off from the threaded isolator to the implant connector (5) pumps electrolyte in the implant containment (1). The positive current path derives from the voltage source (8), passes metallic conductors to the anode. The negative current path derives from the voltage source (8), passes metallic conductors to the connector (5), to the implant (1), which acts in the electrolytic process as the cathode.

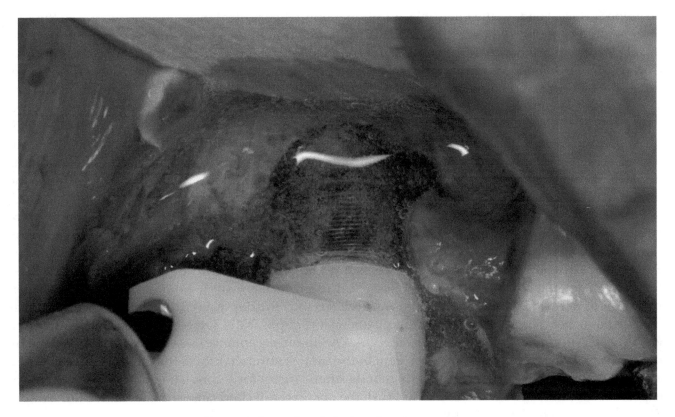

Figure 2. Spray-head during cleaning process.

2.4. Patient and Sample Selection, Randomization

24 patients with at least one titanium implant and diagnosed with periimplantitis (definition according to Berglund et al.) [3] were included in the study. If more than one implant was affected, one implant was chosen randomly. The patients were allocated to test group (EC) or control group (PEC) after randomization by using sealed envelopes immediately before surgery.

2.5. Inclusion Criteria

Patients older than 18 years, capable of understanding and signing an informed consent, smoking fewer than 10 cigarettes per day, without uncontrolled periodontitis, BoP < 20%, Plaque Index < 20%, no allergy to the drugs or materials used, and not pregnant or nursing were suitable to be enrolled in the study.

In contrast to most of the literature, the bone defects were not limited to intraosseous defects. All implants were included independently of their bone defect morphology, three-dimensional implant position, e.g. implant axis, inter-implant distance, etc.

2.6. Procedures and Measurements

Selected patients were instructed and motivated regarding proper oral hygiene and, if necessary, underwent periodontal treatment. Standardized photos were taken (occlusal, buccal, lingual view) and repeated in all appointments listed below. Suprastructures were removed 14 days before surgery. The implants were cleaned by powder spray (Nozzle, EMS, Nyon, Switzerland) and rinsed with chlorhexidine (Chlorhexamed forte, GlaxoSmithKline, Munich, Germany) to reduce soft tissue inflammation in line with standard procedures in periodontal therapy. A cover screw was placed. As a result of this pretreatment, in most cases the soft tissue grew over the implant, leaving a crestal fistula. PD and BoP were assessed at six defined points (m, mb, b, db, d, dl) (Figure 3) using a periodontal probe with a 1 mm scale (PCPUNC 15, HuFridy, Chicago, IL, USA). A crestal incision with releasing incisions was performed to enable a flap to be reflected so that access to the implant could be gained. Buccal and, in the mandible, additional lingual periosteal incisions were made so that the tissues could be mobilized over the implant. The granulation tissues were removed and, if applicable, tartar or cement remnants were removed mechanically by the use of curettes (DSC13/14, HuFridy, Chicago, IL, USA) and/or ultrasonic devices (Dentsply Sirona, Bensheim, Germany). This is necessary because the EC process can only work if the electrolyte is in direct contact with the conductive implant. The distance from implant platform to the most apical position of bone (P-B) was assessed as described in (Figure 3) at the same six points as PD and BoP were measured using the described periodontal probe. In the EC group, the spray-head was pressed into the implant and the GS1000 control unit started. The current was applied 5 s after the peristaltic pump was started and the electrolytic spray was initiated. The cleaning process took 120 s. In the PEC group, the implants were treated according to the manufacturer's manual by a powder spray (Airflow Plus powder, Airflow, EMS, Nyon, Switzerland) for 60 s followed by the treatment described for the EC group. After cleaning, the implants were rinsed with sterile saline and augmented with a mixture of autogenous bone harvested from the ramus area (Micross Safescraper, Zantomed, Duisburg, Germany) and Bio-Oss (Geistlich, Wohlhusen, Switzerland) in a 50:50 ratio. In cases with non-supporting infrabony defects, tenting screws were used for space maintaining (Umbrella-Screw, Ustomed, Tuttlingen, Germany). After placement of a collagen membrane (Bio-Gide, Geistlich, Wohlhusen, Switzerland) the flap was coronally advanced to cover the site passively. The 6-0 propylene monofilaments (Medipac, Kilis, Greece) were removed after two weeks, and wound healing was documented. A VAS (pain, acceptance) assessment was also done by the patients. When no exposure was present at the time of suture removal the patients were checked again four weeks later, then scheduled six months after surgery for second-stage surgery. In the case of exposure, the patients were instructed to brush the area carefully and rinse the site with chlorhexidine. These sites were checked monthly.

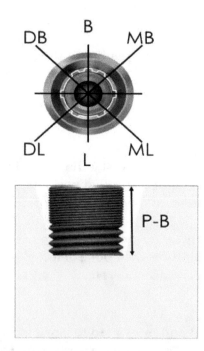

Figure 3. Bone defects were assessed at six defined points from implant shoulder to the most coronal position of the bone.

During the period of healing (six months) the patients were supervised, and exposures or infections were documented. After six months, second-stage surgery was performed. The implants and the surrounding bone were exposed and P-B was assessed under direct vision at the previous points. In cases with exposures, no second-stage surgery was necessary and P-B was assessed by bone sounding under local anesthesia using the described periodontal probe with sufficient pressure. Furthermore infections, BoP, and recessions were documented. For all implants, suprastructures were replaced, photographs were taken, and a standardized x-ray in the right-angle position was performed. Sutures were removed after 14 days, if applicable. Bone levels at baseline and after six months were assessed by two examiners using software (DBS Win, Dürr, Bietigheim-Bissingen, Germany). The examiners, not knowing the aim of the study, were calibrated until their results correlated adequately as measured by Cohen's Kappa (κ ≥ 0.6). In addition, the measurements had to reach 90% agreement for ±0.5 mm as well as exact agreement in 75% of the radiologic measurements before assessment of the x-rays in this study.

Schwarz et al. [18] introduced a classification describing typical peri-implant bone defect anatomy. For clinical purposes, however, a classification providing information about the healing potential of a defect would be more helpful for the practitioner. Therefore, we hereby introduce the RP Classification differentiating the regenerative potential (RP) of a bone defect based on the risk-chance ratio of treatment. We assessed intrabony defects (RP1), intrabony defects with dehiscence defects (RP2) and horizontal bone defects (RP3) (Figure 4) and correlated them to total and median bone fill. Complete regain of bone is dependent on the type of implant. In most of the implants 1 mm remodeling occurs within the first year. It cannot be expected that these implants will re-osseointegrate up to the platform. Implants with a polished neck osseointegrate to the border rough-polished. They are placed at this level very often. More coronal re-osseointegration cannot be expected [19,20].

Therefore, we define bone-to-implant contact with a P-B < 1 mm as complete bone fill. Implants with polished necks are counted as complete bone fill, if the bone fill reaches the border rough-polished being visible at T2 after flap removal.

All the surgical procedures and clinical assessments such as PPD, recessions and BoP were performed by the first-named author.

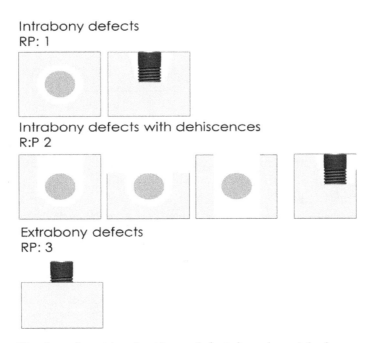

Figure 4. RP Classification of peri-implant bone defects based on risk-chance ratio of treatment.

2.7. Statistics

Quantitative values are presented as mean and standard deviation, and minimum and maximum, as well as quartiles. Gaussian distribution of data was assessed using the Saphiro-Wilk test. Comparisons were performed with the Mann-Whitney U test or *t*-test, as appropriate. The homogeneity of variance was verified by Levene's test before the *t*-tests. The level of significance was set at $\alpha = 0.05$ and all tests were two-sided. The statistical analysis was performed using R 3.6.1 with the package car 3.0-3. R. The package used is available from CRAN at http://CRAN.R-project.org/.

3. Results

The distribution of gender and age was homogeneous (12f/12m; mean age 57.13 y) and there were four smokers (3 EC, 1 PEC) < 10 cigarettes per day. All the sites were infected, BoP was positive, pus drained from pockets, and all sites probed deeper than 5 mm at baseline (Table 1). PD was 6.64 mm in the EC and 7.02 mm in the PEC group. No significant difference was assessable (Fisher's exact test, $p > 0.999$). Thus, the entity was considered to be homogeneous.

Table 1. Qualitative baseline data indicating homogenous data.

General Information	Specific Information	n/Mean Years	Percentage
gender	female	12	50.00%
	male	12	50.00%
age	female	59.2 y	
	male	51.4 y	
jaw	maxilla EL	4	16.67%
	maxilla PEL	8	33.33%
	mandible EL	8	33.33%
	mandible PEL	4	16.67%
	maxilla total	12	50.00%
	mandible total	12	50.00%
smokers	EL	3	12.50%
	PEL	1	4.17%
BoP		24	100.00%
pus		24	100.00%

Nineteen sites were exposed at suture removal, 15 after six months. Nevertheless, no implant was lost during the healing phase. One implant from the PEC group had to be removed after six months because of infection, incomplete bone regeneration, and the presence of infection. Compliance of this female patient was poor, and the implant was placed far too lingually in a compromised axis. The addition of these factors led to the recommendation to remove this implant.

The quality of regained bone was assessed by visual inspection with a microscope (24x magnification), bone sounding with high pressure, and interpretation of x-rays. Complete and solid bone in direct contact with the implant was confirmed.

Bone gain was assessed at six months as a difference between P-B$_{baseline}$ and P-B$_{6\,months}$ (ΔP-B) at the six defined points. There was no statistical significant difference either between the specific points or the median. Bone gain and differences between the EC and PEC groups are visualized in Table 2. Bone gain was 2.71 ± 1.70 mm in the EC group and 2.81 ± 2.15 for PEC. The difference (Δ PEC-EC) was not statistically significant (0.10 mm, p-value 0.87). The related boxplots are displayed in Figures 5 and 6.

The implants in the study population consisted of different implant brands and designs. Their distribution is displayed in Table 3. According to our definition, complete bone fill was achieved if ΔP-B was less than 1 mm. This was observed in nine implants (37.5%). In two cases with a polished implant shoulder (Camlog, Altatec, Wimsheim, Germany), the bone fill reached the border rough-polished (ΔP-B < 2). If those cases are accepted as complete bone fill, a total of 12 implants

(50%) accomplished complete bone fill. The distribution of the different defect morphologies and regenerative potential was four implants RP1, 11 implants RP2, and nine implants RP3. Complete regain of visible and probable bone up to the implant shoulder was achieved in all the RP1 implants. Six implants in RP2 cases and only two implants in RP3 achieved complete bone fill. Median bone gain related to defect morphology was 4.02 ± 0.96 mm in RP1 cases, 2.64 ± 1.58 mm in RP2 and 2.34 ± 1.58 mm in RP3 (Table 4).

Table 2. Bone gain and differences between EC and AFL group.

Location	EC Group [mm]	PEC Group [mm]	AEL-EL	p-Value
			Differences	
db	3.00 ± 1.67	2.50 ± 2.10	−0.50	0.52
b	3.25 ± 1.63	2.83 ± 2.94	−0.42	0.71
mb	3.17 ± 1.61	3.00 ± 2.12	−0.17	0.83
ml	2.58 ± 1.84	3.13 ± 2.25	0.55	0.53
l	2.29 ± 1.79	2.96 ± 1.86	0.67	0.38
dl	1.96 ± 1.57	2.46 ± 1.83	0.50	0.48
Median	2.71 ± 1.70	2.81 ± 2.15	0.10	0.87

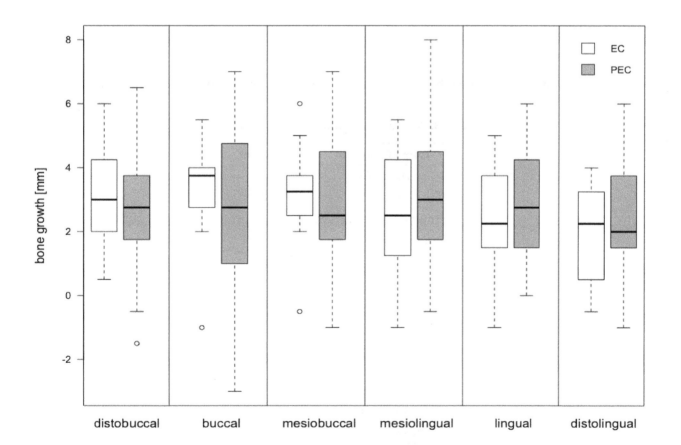

Figure 5. Boxplot indicating the distribution of the assessment points in EC and PEC.

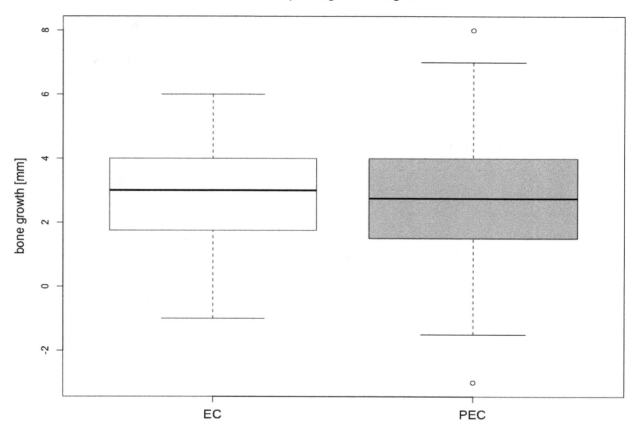

Figure 6. Boxplot indicating the merged distribution of the assessment points in EC and PEC.

Table 3. Allocation of different implant types.

Type of Implant	Number
Astra TX	5
Astra EV	2
Straumann tissue level	2
Straumann bone level	1
Conelog	2
Camlog	2
Ankylos	2
Sky	1
Branemark	2
Xive	1
Steri Oss	1
Zimmer	2
Nobel Active	1

Table 4. Bone gain in relation to RP class.

RP Class	Bone Gain
RP1	4.02 ± 0.96
RP2	2.64 ± 1.58
RP3	2.34 ± 1.58

In one case 1.5 mm bone grew over the top of the implant and 1.5 mm clinically hard and mature bone had to be removed to get access to the implant (Figures 7 and 8) [21]. In two cases, (both RP3) the implants were covered by tartar. In one case, complete bone fill was gained. In the other case, P-B improved slightly.

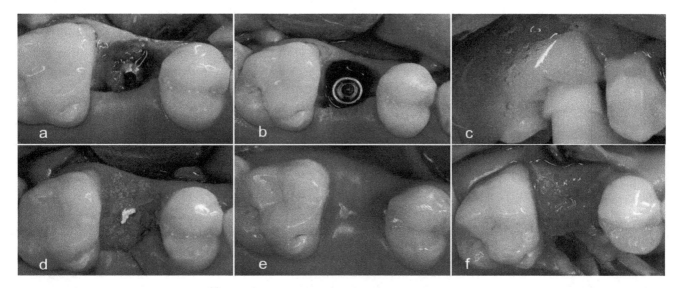

Figure 7. (**a**). A raised flap displays granulation tissue. (**b**). Deep peri-implant RP1 bone defect. (**c**). The spray-head is in place. The film of electrolyte is guided by a sponge. Hydrogen bubbles appear as a result of the process. (**d**). Defect augmented by a mixture of autogenous and natural bone mineral. (**e**). Healed defect after six months. (**f**). Solid bone overgrew the implant.

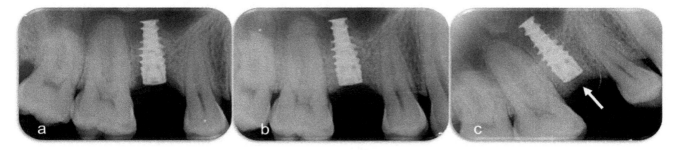

Figure 8. (**a**). The defect at baseline looks much less severe than in clinical reality. (**b**). Augmented defect. (**c**). Six months of healing.

4. Discussion

4.1. Design of Study

The study was designed as a randomized and controlled trial. As none of the current treatment modalities was superior to any other and all of them failed to prove long-term stability and re-osseointegration in a clinical setting [10], they were unsuitable to serve as a control method. None of these methods was considered ethical to use. After lengthy discussion with the ethics committee, we decided to investigate whether additional ablative methods are beneficial to the outcome of the electrolytic approach. For this purpose, we cannot compare the results of this study directly with current treatment modalities. Furthermore, this RCT investigated changes in bone level clinically while most of the published articles focus on the change in clinical parameters. In view of the different endpoints, the data presented in this article cannot be compared directly with existing literature. After six months of healing after second-stage surgery, we will have the chance to assess clinical data (PPD, BoP, secretion) and compare them to existing literature.

The definition of success in the therapy of periimplantitis is a matter of debate. Carcuac et al. approached this question by assessing three outcomes: 1. further marginal bone loss ≤ 0.5 mm, 2. outcome 1 + PD ≤ 5 mm, and 3. outcome 2 + BoP and/or suppuration on probing (SoP) = negative. According to this definition they were able to achieve 69.4%, 55.4% and 33.1% success in an RCT investigating resective surgery [22]. Assuming that elimination of a pocket should resolve the problems, these results are disheartening. In an RCT, after cleaning of the implant surface with plastic curettes and chlorhexidine gel in cases with intrabony defects, Schwarz et al. showed PD changes after four years from 7.1 mm to 4.6 mm when using Bio-Oss and a collagen membrane [23]. BoP reduced from 79 to 28%. Defect configuration seems to have a major effect on PD reduction. Schwarz et al. proved that circumferential intrabony defects exhibit a significantly higher reduction of PD compared to intrabony fenestration defects [24]. Roccuzzo et al. followed 24 patients (two dropouts) with intrabony defects in a case series for seven years. Implants were treated by mechanical debridement and application of EDTA and chlorhexidine gel followed by augmentation with Bio-Oss Collagen. The survival rate was 83.3% for SLA implants and 71.4% for TPS. PD was reduced from 6.6 ± 1.3 to 3.2 ± 0.7 mm in SLA, and 7.2 ± 1.5 to 3.4 ± 0.6 mm in TPS. BoP changed from $75.0 \pm 31.2\%$ to $7.5 \pm 12.1\%$ (SLA), and from $90.0 \pm 12.9\%$ to $30.0 \pm 19.7\%$ (TPS). The authors described successful therapy as PD ≤ 5 mm, negative BoP and no further bone loss. Success was achieved in two of 14 (14.3%) of the TPS and in seven of 12 (58.3%) of the SLA implants [25]. These results are difficult to understand as BoP, according to the definition of peri-implantitis, should have been 100% at baseline. It is not known whether non-infected implants with bone loss were enrolled in the study. This demonstrates the difficulty of using the parameter of BoP as a tool for diagnosing peri-implantitis, as discussed by Coli et al. [26].

4.2. Our Results

The potential of the electrolytic approach has previously been demonstrated in various in vitro tests [15–17,27]. We did not focus on intrabony defects, like the cited studies, but accepted all kinds of defects in our data. Therefore, because of the use of different endpoints, it is not possible to compare our data directly with the studies cited above. Achievement of re-osseointegration can be proved only histologically. In an animal study [27], we proved that complete re-osseointegration could be achieved after the use of EC, whereas with conventional cleaning, the bone filled the defect partially, but was never in direct contact with the implant. Clinically, bone fill cannot be equated with re-osseointegration, although this can happen with high probability after EC. The quality of the gained bone was evaluated by visual inspection, assessment of x-rays, and/or mechanical bone sounding of the most crestal position of the bone at the six predetermined points. Mature and solid bone in direct contact with the implant was detected. This still does not prove re-osseointegration. It may be stated, however, that we achieved complete bone fill (according to this definition) in all intrabony defects (RP1 cases). Complete bone fill was achieved in 50% of all cases – a number which, to the best knowledge of the authors, has not yet been quoted in the literature. In cases with exposure, no flap was raised after six months. The P-B distance could not be assessed under direct visual control. The potential bias seems to be negligible. Former studies demonstrated that even probing with 0.5 N completely lateralizes the peri-implant tissues [28]. In the study bone sounding was performed with high pressure under local anesthesia.

Published clinical studies focus on the change in radio-opalescence in x-rays. We will compare radiologic data in a further follow-up as well as PD and BoP assessments and answer the question of the long-term stability of the EC approach.

The exposure rates (15 sites at suture removal) were much higher than is usual in the hands of the author compared to simultaneous implant placement and augmentation. This happened even though a strict initial phase was applied in order to reduce infection and inflammation. It will be necessary to investigate this issue more closely in future and possibly adapt surgical techniques. Whether the soft tissues could be compromised by the former peri-implant infection is merely a matter of speculation.

Our in vitro data clearly prove the potential of EC for removing bacterial [17]. No data are available regarding whether periimplantitis impacts the healing potential of surrounding soft tissue. The number of exposures exceeds the number of exposures in cases of simultaneous implantation and augmentation according to the author's experience. This requires further studies.

Powder spray has to impact at an angle of 30–60° and a working distance of 3–5 mm according to the manufacturer's manual. Owing to micro- and macrostructure as well as defect anatomy, this prerequisite may not always be met. In our study, we compared EC with a combination of EC and powder spray in order to assess whether additional mechanical debridement enhances outcomes. Our data support previous in vitro results, namely that EC alone is able to clean the implant surface and regain a surface onto which bone grows [17].

Tartar had to be removed in two cases before EC cleaning. It was clearly visible that the surfaces of the implants were damaged by the curettes and the ultrasonic device. Our data prove that regain of bone above the former bone level and clinical reattachment of bone are nevertheless possible.

One implant had to be removed because of various factors (reinfection, malpositioning of the implant, and compliance of the patient). Which of these obstacles was causative for the decision is unclear. This raises the question of which implants should be treated or removed and leads to discussion about the etiology of the individual disease and the regenerative potential of this special defect. It is still a matter of discussion whether the bacterial biofilm is the only causal factor or whether bone loss caused by surgical, mechanical, or patient-related reasons, and bacterial colonization happens secondarily on the exposed surfaces [29]. This debate about etiology is not only an academic question. The success rate of possible treatments correlates with specimen susceptibility and uncorrectable surgical or mechanical obstacles. The number of implants included in the present study was too small to draw statistically significant conclusions about correlations between defect morphology and outcome. Conspicuously, all implants with completely preserved bone walls but intrabony defects (RP1) healed with complete bone fill of the defect. Only two out of nine cases with a vertical component (circumferential bone loss; RP3) achieved complete bone fill. Our data support the results of Schwarz et al. who stated that defect morphology has a major impact on healing [24]. We clearly state that the data from this study are too weak because of the sample size to justify the validity of the suggested RP classification. Initially, we did not plan to discuss the data in this way, but the results showed clear differences without reaching significance. Further studies are necessary to validate the RP classification. We treated all implants with the diagnosis of peri-implantitis. Implants placed with a bad axis, insufficient buccolingual inclination, and inter-implant distance < 3 mm were not excluded. Bone gain was smaller compared to perfectly placed implants according to the clinical impression of the authors. Statistical analysis was not performed because of small sample sizes. Further studies are recommended to clarify this issue. For treatment, planning a classification of bone defects to forecast treatment results would be helpful. Therefore, we herewith introduce a new classification focusing on risk-chance ratio: The Regenerative Potential (RP) Classification. Cup-shaped defects with complete bone walls surrounding the defect have the highest healing potential [24]. If more walls are missing and/or additional risk factors are present, removal of the infected implant may be considered. Further studies are necessary to develop a clear decision tree for determining which implants should be treated or removed and when electrolytic cleaning is helpful for long-term success.

5. Conclusions

Electrolytic cleaning of contaminated implants achieves an implant surface where complete re-osseointegration is possible. This was attained in 50% of the cases. Additional mechanical cleaning by the use of powder spray devices does not improve the results further. The amount of regeneration depends on the regenerative potential of the bone (multiwall craterlike defects perform better than horizontal bone loss). Further confounding factors could not be identified owing to the limited sample size of 24 patients.

Author Contributions: Conceptualization, M.S. and H.Z.; Data curation, M.S. and F.R.; Formal analysis, M.S., F.R., C.R. and H.Z.; Investigation, M.S. and F.R.; Methodology, M.S., U.B. and H.Z.; Project administration, M.S.; Resources, M.S.; Software, C.R.; Supervision, M.S.; Validation, M.S., F.R., C.R., P.W. and H.Z.; Visualization, M.S. and H.Z.; Writing—original draft, M.S. and H.Z.; Writing—review & editing, M.S., F.R., U.B., C.R., P.W. and H.Z.

Acknowledgments: The study was sponsored by GalvoSurge Dental AG; We appreciate Ümniye Balaban, Institute for Biostatistics and Mathematical Modeling Center of Health Sciences, Hospital and Department of Medicine of the Goethe University for her support with the statistics.

References

1. Sendyk, D.I.; Chrcanovic, B.R.; Albrektsson, T.; Wennerberg, A.; Deboni, Z.; Cristina, M. Does Surgical Experience Influence Implant Survival Rate? A Systematic Review and Meta-Analysis. *Int. J. Prosthodont.* **2017**, *30*, 341–347. [CrossRef]
2. Lang, N.P.; Berglundh, T. Periimplant diseases: Where are we now?—Consensus of the Seventh European Workshop on Periodontology. *J. Clin. Periodontol.* **2011**, *38*, 178–181. [CrossRef]
3. Berglundh, T.; Armitage, G.; Araujo, M.G.; Avila-Ortiz, G.; Blanco, J.; Camargo, P.M.; Chen, S.; Cochran, D.; Derks, J.; Figuero, E.; et al. Peri-implant diseases and conditions: Consensus report of workgroup 4 of the 2017 World Workshop on the Classification of Periodontal and Peri-Implant Diseases and Conditions. *J. Periodontol.* **2018**, *89*, S313–S318. [CrossRef]
4. Mombelli, A.; Décaillet, F. The characteristics of biofilms in peri-implant disease. *J. Clin. Periodontol.* **2011**, *38*, 203–213. [CrossRef]
5. Mombelli, A.; Müller, N.; Cionca, N. The epidemiology of peri-implantitis. *Clin. Oral Implant. Res.* **2012**, *23*, 67–76. [CrossRef]
6. Derks, J.; Tomasi, C. Peri-implant health and disease. A systematic review of current epidemiology. *J. Clin. Periodontol.* **2015**, *42*, S158–S171. [CrossRef]
7. Fürst, M.M.; Salvi, G.E.; Lang, N.P.; Persson, G.R. Bacterial colonization immediately after installation on oral titanium implants. *Clin. Oral Implant. Res.* **2007**, *18*, 501–508. [CrossRef]
8. Tastepe, C.S.; van Waas, R.; Liu, Y.; Wismeijer, D. Air powder abrasive treatment as an implant surface cleaning method: A literature review. *Int. J. Oral Maxillofac. Implant.* **2012**, *27*, 1461–1473.
9. Claffey, N.; Clarke, E.; Polyzois, I.; Renvert, S. Surgical treatment of peri-implantitis. *J. Clin. Periodontol.* **2008**, *35*, 316–332. [CrossRef]
10. Esposito, M.; Grusovin, M.G.; Worthington, H.V. Treatment of peri-implantitis: What interventions are effective? A Cochrane systematic review. *Eur. J. Oral Implantol.* **2012**, *5*, S21–S41.
11. de Almeida, J.M.; Matheus, H.R.; Rodrigues Gusman, D.J.; Faleiros, P.L.; Januário de Araújo, N.; Noronha Novaes, V.C. Effectiveness of Mechanical Debridement Combined With Adjunctive Therapies for Nonsurgical Treatment of Periimplantitis: A Systematic Review. *Implant Dent.* **2017**, *26*, 137–144. [CrossRef]
12. del Pozo, J.L.; Rouse, M.S.; Mandrekar, J.N.; Steckelberg, J.M.; Patel, R. The electricidal effect: Reduction of Staphylococcus and pseudomonas biofilms by prolonged exposure to low-intensity electrical current. *Antimicrob. Agents Chemother.* **2009**, *53*, 41–45. [CrossRef]
13. Schwarz, F.; Becker, K.; Sager, M. Efficacy of professionally administered plaque removal with or without adjunctive measures for the treatment of peri-implant mucositis. A systematic review and meta-analysis. *J. Clin. Periodontol.* **2015**, *42*, S202–S213. [CrossRef]
14. Mohn, D.; Zehnder, M.; Stark, W.J.; Imfeld, T. Electrochemical disinfection of dental implants—A proof of concept. *PLoS ONE* **2011**, *6*, e16157. [CrossRef]
15. Zipprich, H.; Ratka, C.; Schlee, M.; Brodbeck, U.; Lauer, H.C.; Seitz, O. Periimplantitistherapie: Durchbruch mit neuer Reinigungsmethode. *Dentalmagazin* **2013**, *31*, 14–17.

16. Schneider, S.; Rudolph, M.; Bause, V.; Terfort, A. Electrochemical removal of biofilms from titanium dental implant surfaces. *Bioelectrochemistry* **2018**, *121*, 84–94. [CrossRef]

17. Ratka, C.; Weigl, P.; Henrich, D.; Koch, F.; Schlee, M.; Zipprich, H. The Effect of In Vitro Electrolytic Cleaning on Biofilm-Contaminated Implant Surfaces. *J. Clin. Med.* **2019**, *8*, 1397. [CrossRef]

18. Schwarz, F.; Herten, M.; Sager, M.; Bieling, K.; Sculean, A.; Becker, J. Comparison of naturally occurring and ligature-induced peri-implantitis bone defects in humans and dogs. *Clin. Oral Implant. Res.* **2007**, *18*, 161–170. [CrossRef]

19. Alomrani, A.N.; Hermann, J.S.; Jones, A.A.; Buser, D.; Schoolfield, J.; Cochran, D.L. The effect of a machined collar on coronal hard tissue around titanium implants: A radiographic study in the canine mandible. *Int. J. Oral Maxillofac. Implant.* **2005**, *20*, 677–686.

20. Laurell, L.; Lundgren, D. Marginal bone level changes at dental implants after 5 years in function: A meta-analysis. *Clin. Implant Dent. Relat. Res.* **2011**, *13*, 19–28. [CrossRef]

21. Albrektsson, T.; Canullo, L.; Cochran, D.; de Bruyn, H. "Peri-Implantitis": A Complication of a Foreign Body or a Man-Made "Disease". Facts and Fiction. *Clin. Implant Dent. Relat. Res.* **2016**, *18*, 840–849. [CrossRef]

22. Carcuac, O.; Derks, J.; Abrahamsson, I.; Wennström, J.L.; Petzold, M.; Berglundh, T. Surgical treatment of peri-implantitis: 3-year results from a randomized controlled clinical trial. *J. Clin. Periodontol.* **2017**, *44*, 1294–1303. [CrossRef]

23. Schwarz, F.; Sahm, N.; Bieling, K.; Becker, J. Surgical regenerative treatment of peri-implantitis lesions using a nanocrystalline hydroxyapatite or a natural bone mineral in combination with a collagen membrane: A four-year clinical follow-up report. *J. Clin. Periodontol.* **2009**, *36*, 807–814. [CrossRef]

24. Schwarz, F.; Sahm, N.; Schwarz, K.; Becker, J. Impact of defect configuration on the clinical outcome following surgical regenerative therapy of peri-implantitis. *J. Clin. Periodontol.* **2010**, *37*, 449–455. [CrossRef]

25. Roccuzzo, M.; Pittoni, D.; Roccuzzo, A.; Charrier, L.; Dalmasso, P. Surgical treatment of peri-implantitis intrabony lesions by means of deproteinized bovine bone mineral with 10% collagen: 7-year-results. *Clin. Oral Implant. Res.* **2017**, *28*, 1577–1583. [CrossRef]

26. Coli, P.; Christiaens, V.; Sennerby, L.; de Bruyn, H. Reliability of periodontal diagnostic tools for monitoring peri-implant health and disease. *Periodontol. 2000* **2017**, *73*, 203–217. [CrossRef]

27. Schlee, M.; Naili, L.; Rathe, F.; Brodbeck, U.; Zipprich, H. Is complete re-osseointegration of an infected dental implant possible—Histological results of a dog study. A short communication. *J. Clin. Med.* **2019**, Submitted.

28. Ericsson, I.; Lindhe, J. Probing depth at implants and teeth. An experimental study in the dog. *J. Clin. Periodontol.* **1993**, *20*, 623–627. [CrossRef]

29. Canullo, L.; Schlee, M.; Wagner, W.; Covani, U. International Brainstorming Meeting on Etiologic and Risk Factors of Peri-implantitis, Montegrotto (Padua, Italy), August 2014. *Int. J. Oral Maxillofac. Implant.* **2015**, *30*, 1093–1104. [CrossRef]

15

Improvement of Quality of Life with Implant-Supported Mandibular Overdentures and the Effect of Implant Type and Surgical Procedure on Bone and Soft Tissue Stability: A Three-Year Prospective Split-Mouth Trial

Ron Doornewaard [1,*], Maarten Glibert [1], Carine Matthys [1], Stijn Vervaeke [1], Ewald Bronkhorst [2] and Hugo de Bruyn [1,2,*]

[1] Department Periodontology & Oral Implantology, Dental School, Faculty Medicine and Health Sciences, Ghent University, De Pintelaan 185, 9000 Ghent, Belgium; maarten.glibert@ugent.be (M.G.); carine.matthys@ugent.be (C.M.); stijn.vervaeke@ugent.be (S.V.)

[2] Section Implantology & Periodontology, Department of Dentistry, Radboudumc, Philips van Leydenlaan 25, 6525 EX Nijmegen, The Netherlands; ewald.bronkhorst@radboudumc.nl

* Correspondence: ron.doornewaard@ugent.be (R.D.); hugo.debruyn@radboudumc.nl (H.d.B.)

Abstract: In fully edentulous patients, the support of a lower dental prosthesis by two implants could improve the chewing ability, retention, and stability of the prosthesis. Despite high success rates of dental implants, complications, such as peri-implantitis, do occur. The latter is a consequence of crestal bone loss and might be related to the implant surface and peri-implant soft tissue thickness. The aim of this paper is to describe the effect of implant surface roughness and soft tissue thickness on crestal bone remodeling, peri-implant health, and patient-centered outcomes. The mandibular overdenture supported by two implants is used as a split-mouth model to scrutinize these aims. The first study compared implants placed equicrestal to implants placed biologically (i.e., dependent on site-specific soft tissue thickness). The second clinical trial compared implants with a minimally to a moderately rough implant neck. Both studies reported an improvement in oral health-related quality of life and a stable peri-implant health after three years follow-up. Only equicrestal implant placement yielded significantly higher implant surface exposure, due to the establishment of the biologic width. Within the limitations of this study, it can be concluded that an implant supported mandibular overdenture significantly improves the quality of life, with limited biologic complications and high survival rates of the implants.

Keywords: bone loss; dental implant; overdenture; implant survival; peri-implantitis; implant surface; soft tissue; split-mouth design; oral health-related quality of life; patient-reported outcome measures

1. Introduction

Edentulousness is widely spread worldwide. According to the WHO the prevalence in the elderly population is 26% in the USA and between 15% and 78% in European countries. Among the edentulous population, a strong negative impact of poor oral conditions on daily life has been described. Edentulism could lead to diet changes where food rich in saturated fats and cholesterol are preferred. Besides diet changes, edentulousness is an independent risk factor for weight loss and could lead to social handicaps related to communication [1].

The support of a dental prosthesis by two implants could improve the chewing ability, retention, and stability of the prosthesis, which could lead to higher satisfaction and health-related quality of life.

Dental implants have been used since the early sixties to replace missing teeth by fixed or removable prostheses. Nowadays, this yields a predictable treatment outcome with success over 95% after 10 years of function [2].

To measure the improvement in health-related quality of life, the Oral Health Impact Profile (OHIP) is a widely used tool to assess currently applied dental procedures. It has also been used for evaluating the quality of life in more invasive surgical interventions in oral surgery [3]. The tool consists of a questionnaire to measure the impact of medical care on functional and social wellbeing [4]. Allen and McMillan reported significant improvement in satisfaction and health-related quality of life for patients who received implant-retained prostheses compared to those who received conventional dentures [5]. A panel of experts published a consensus statement where they described overwhelming evidence for a 2-implant supported overdenture as the first choice of treatment for the edentulous mandible instead of a conventional denture [6].

A recent review focusing on the Patient-Reported Outcome Measures (PROMs) showed compelling evidence to support that the fully edentulous patients experience higher satisfaction with an implant-supported overdenture in the mandible compared to a conventional denture [7]. These findings were confirmed by several other recent systematic reviews and meta-analyses [8–10].

De Bruyn and co-workers also concluded that patient satisfaction is highly individual and satisfaction with an implant-supported overdenture is never guaranteed. Hence, the decision to propose an implant-supported overdenture should be based on proper individual assessment [7].

Despite the improvement of the patient's quality of life and high survival and success rates of dental implants in patients with overdentures, dental implants are not free of complications. The most common complications following implant therapy are peri-implant mucositis (bleeding on probing and inflammation of the peri-implant soft tissues), and peri-implantitis (clinical and radiographic bone loss with or without suppuration). To detect inflammatory changes around the implant, several biologic parameters (plaque, bleeding, and suppuration) must be monitored during the patient's follow-up visits [11].

According to the latest consensus report of the "World Workshop on the Classification of Periodontal and Peri-implant Diseases and Conditions", the main clinical characteristic of peri-implant mucositis is bleeding on gently probing [12]. Erythema, swelling, and/or suppuration may also be present [13]. There is strong evidence from animal and human experimental studies that plaque is the etiological factor for peri-implant mucositis [11,14–18]. Peri-implantitis is described as a plaque-associated pathologic condition occurring in tissues around dental implants, characterized by inflammation in the peri-implant mucosa and subsequent progressive loss of supporting bone. Peri-implantitis sites exhibit clinical signs of inflammation, bleeding on probing, and/or suppuration, increased probing depths and/or recession of the mucosal margin in addition to radiographic bone loss [19]. Peri-implantitis is a consequence of crestal bone loss. Two recent consensus meetings highlighted the influence of implant material, shape and surface characteristics on the occurrence and progression of peri-implantitis. However, evidence for these suggestions is weak and future long-term studies are necessary to analyze these potential risk factors [20,21]. Beside these implant factors also other important factors like surgical, prosthetic, patient-related factors and foreign body reactions may contribute to crestal bone loss [21].

The composition and the topography of the implant surface have been a matter of debate during the last decades. Both composition and topography have their influence on implant surface roughness. The implant surface roughness is expressed in a Sa value. This three-dimensional value expresses an absolute difference in the height of each point compared to the arithmetical mean of the surface [22]. In the early years of implant dentistry two types of implant surfaces were used, the machined/turned surface (Sa = 0.5–1 μm) and the microporous titanium plasma-sprayed surface (Sa > 2 μm). The first one is smooth and the latter could be described as a rough implant surface. Surface modification was done to enlarge the surface, resulting in a greater bone-to-implant contact area. Implant surface modifications were done by sandblasting, acid-etching, anodic oxidation or hydroxyapatite coating.

These techniques resulted in a moderately rough implant surface (Sa = 1–2 μm), which is nowadays the most used surface roughness. Beside the higher bone-to-implant contact [23], a lower clinical failure rate [24] and a higher removal torque was observed compared to the smooth implant surfaces [25]. Hence, the surface modification made it possible to load the implant earlier or even immediately after the surgery. The resulting surface enlargement allowed shorter implants to be used, without jeopardizing the prognosis and with a reduced necessity for bone grafting procedures [2]. Beside the aforementioned benefits, related to faster integration, rough implant systems have been linked to increased bacterial adhesion [26]. The applied model in the latter study does not always mimic the clinical reality. However, A Cochrane systematic review suggested limited evidence that smooth surfaces had a 20% reduced risk of being affected by peri-implantitis over a three-year period [27,28]. This finding led to the commercial production of hybrid dental implants, combining the best of both systems. Hybrid dental implants have a minimally rough coronal part to decrease biofilm formation in the soft tissue crevice and a moderately rough implant body to enhance bone healing and speed up the osseointegration. These hybrid surfaces combine the effect of both surface roughnesses in the same implant. A short-term study indicated that the moderately rough and smooth coronal part showed the same crestal bone remodeling in the initial healing phase [29]. However, long-term studies to describe clinical parameters and peri-implant health are not yet available.

Some patient-related factors, such as certain metabolic syndrome components, medical conditions and/or the use of medication are known to have an effect on implant treatment outcome. Systematic reviews reveal that hyperglycemia has an increased risk for peri-implantitis [30,31], although the risk for more implant failures is comparable with the one observed in healthy patients. [32]. There is inconsistent and controversial evidence about the association with cardiovascular diseases [31]. Another meta-analysis revealed that there was no difference in implant survival rate between patients with and without osteoporosis. However, increased peri-implant bone loss was observed [33]. The intake of bisphosphonates, related to the treatment of osteoporosis, was not associated with an increased implant failure rate [34]. On the other hand, the same systematic review revealed an increased risk for implant failure with the intake of certain selective serotonin reuptake inhibitors and proton pump inhibitors [34]. Patients that are periodontally compromised are at higher risk for implant failure and crestal bone loss when compared with periodontally healthy subjects [35].

Another patient factor related to the failure of integrated implants is smoking. De Bruyn and Collaert described in a large retrospective study significantly higher failure rates of dental implants in smokers compared to non-smokers, both before and after functional loading, especially in the maxilla [36]. These findings are in agreement with a large meta-analysis of 18 studies showing an odds-ratio of 2.17 for implant failures in smokers were compared to non-smokers [37]. Besides implant failure smokers are more prone to peri-implant bone loss [38,39].

Also, biologic variances between patients could influence crestal bone loss around dental implants. Especially, soft tissue dimensions could play an important role in bone remodeling. The effect of peri-implant mucosal tissue thickness on the crestal bone loss was described in an animal study suggesting a certain minimal width of peri-implant mucosa may be required, and that bone resorption may take place allowing a stable soft tissue attachment [40]. The latter was confirmed in a human clinical trial, when there was a soft tissue thickness of 2 mm or less, crestal bone loss up to 1.45 mm may occur [41].

More recently Vervaeke and co-workers concluded that the initial bone remodeling was affected by the thickness of the peri-implant soft tissue [42]. They suggested that bone loss directly after implant placement, due to crestal bone remodeling, precludes the biologic width re-establishment and can be controlled by adapting the vertical depth position of the implant in the bone in relation to the soft tissue thickness at the time of implant placement. Hence, in thin tissues, a deeper subcrestal position in the bone may prevent partial exposure of the crestal part of the implant. Although crestal bone remodeling is a given fact after implant placement, related to the surgical trauma from periosteal elevation, as well as the drilling procedure, it is from a preventive point of view important to have the bone covering the implant as much as possible. Initial crestal bone loss, resulting in the absence of bone contact, can predict a future bone loss in patients prior to the disease. Galindo-Moreno and co-workers concluded that 96% of implants with a marginal bone loss above 2 mm at 18 months had lost 0.44 mm or more at six months post loading [43]. A critical long-term study where implants were placed in the partially edentulous mandible, indicated that bone loss in patients with thin (<2 mm) and a thick mucosa (>2 mm) was identical, when the implants were installed subcrestally to anticipate on the biologic width re-establishment [44].

Another subject of debate is the predictive value of biologic parameters around dental implants. Bleeding on probing, suppuration, plaque formation and probing pocket depth are the most widely used clinical parameters to describe health and/or disease around dental implants. These biologic parameters are most of the times included in the definition of peri-implantitis. However, a largely critical review showed the absence of a correlation between bone loss and the biologic parameters mean probing pocket depth and mean bleeding on probing. The authors also reported inconsistency and incompleteness in reporting on these parameters in the literature, which could affect decision-making in clinical practice [45].

Hence, the aim of this paper is to describe, by means of two prospective clinical split-mouth cohort studies, the effect of implant surface roughness and surgical implant depth positioning on crestal bone remodeling, peri-implant health, and patient-centered outcomes. The mandibular overdenture supported by two dental implants is used as a split-mouth model to scrutinize these aims.

2. Experimental Section

2.1. Patient Population and Surgical/Prosthetic Procedures

This paper includes two prospective split-mouth studies. Both studies included edentulous patients in need of a two-implant supported overdenture in the lower jaw. The same inclusion and exclusion were used for both studies. Inclusion criteria include: (1) Total complete edentulism for at least four months and (2) presence of sufficient residual bone volume to install two implants of 3.5 to 4.0 mm diameter and 8 to 11 mm length. Patients were excluded if they were: (1) Younger than 21, (2) suffered from systemic diseases, (3) current smokers and (4) had general contraindications for oral surgery (full dose head and neck radiation, intravenous administrated bisphosphonates, and ongoing chemotherapy). All patients were treated at the Ghent University Hospital by the same surgeon between January 2013 and September 2014. Twenty-six patients (study 1) received two moderately rough dental implants (Astra Tech Osseospeed TX™, Dentsply implants, York, PA, USA). The control implant was installed equicrestally (group 1), according to the manufacturer's guidelines with the rough implant surface completely surrounded by bone. The vertical position of the test implant (group 2) was adapted to the soft tissue thickness, allowing at least 3 mm space for biologic width establishment [42].

Another 23 patients (study 2) received two dental implants with a difference in implant surface roughness of the coronal part of the implant (Figure 1). All 46 implants were biologically guided taking the soft tissue thickness into account whereby care was taken to ensure a 3 mm soft tissue seal in contact with the abutment. All patients received one moderately rough implant (group 3) (Sa = 1.3 µm) (DCC, Southern implants, Irene, South Africa) and one test implant (group 4). The latter was a hybrid dental implant with a minimally rough coronal neck of 3 mm (Sa = 0.9 µm) combined with a moderately rough body (Sa = 1.3 µm) (MSC, Southern implants, Irene, South Africa).

Although two different brands were used in both studies, all 98 implants installed in the 49 patients were identical at the level of the abutment-implant connection. Implants had the same integrated platform-shift with a smooth implant bevel, the same internal deep conical connection and a similar macro design of the micro-threads on the implant neck.

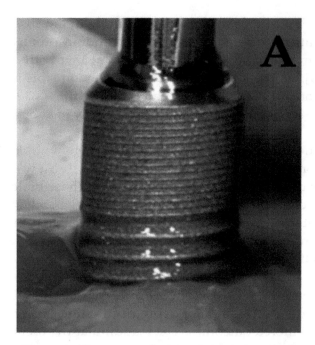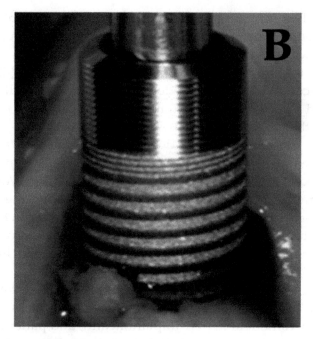

Figure 1. Placement of an implant with a moderately rough surface (**A**) and a hybrid implant with a minimally rough coronal neck (**B**).

Implants were immediately restored if primary stability was achieved (insertion-torque > 25 Ncm). Implants were restored either with locator abutments (study 1) or definitive titanium abutments (Compact Conical Abutments; Southern Implants, Irene, South Africa) and a healing cap with a standard abutment height of 4 mm (study 2).

Before surgery, all patients received new removable dentures in the mandible and maxilla to achieve a correct occlusion, appropriate teeth position, and appropriate smile line. The removable dentures were adapted after surgery to connect with the implants by one experienced prosthodontist. The surgical and prosthetic procedures have been described previously by Vervaeke and co-workers [46] and Glibert and co-workers [29].

The clinical trial has been conducted in full accordance with the Helsinki Decleration (1975) as revised in 2000. All patients were thoroughly informed and signed written informed consent. The study protocol was approved by the ethical committee of the Ghent University Hospital.

2.2. Clinical and Radiographic Examination

Follow-up visits were planned at 1 week, 1, 3, 6, 12, 24, and 36 months after surgery. After soft tissue healing was fully established, three months after surgery, peri-implant health was monitored and probing pocket depths, bleeding on probing and plaque scores were assessed on four implants sites: Midmesial, middistal, midbuccal, and midlingual. The bleeding- and plaque scores were measured on a dichotomous scale (0 = absence of bleeding on probing/absence of plaque; 1 = bleeding on probing/plaque). From the site level scores both for bleeding and plaque mean scores on implant level were calculated.

Digital peri-apical radiographs were taken at baseline (implant placement), at 3, 6, 12, 24, and 36 months using a guiding system in order to obtain the X-rays perpendicular to the film. The radiographic measurements were calibrated using the length of the implant, the distance between the threads or the diameter of the implant. Bone levels were determined as the distance from a reference point, which corresponds with the lower edge of the smooth implant bevel at the implant-abutment interface, to the most crestal bone-to-implant contact point. The baseline bone-to-implant contact levels are assessed from the implant-abutment interface. The baseline from the four experimental groups was logically comparable. Bone loss was determined by the difference of the bone level directly after implant placement and the bone level at the follow-up visit.

If necessary, calculus and plaque were removed and oral hygiene was reinforced during follow-up visits. Instructions with a (electric) toothbrush and interdental brushes were given based on the need, preferences and dexterity or motoric skills of the patient.

To measure the change in oral health-related quality of life the Oral Health Impact Profile-14 questionnaire (OHIP-14) is assessed before surgery, 3, and 12 months after connection of the prosthesis with the implants (Table 1). The questionnaire is based on 14 questions capturing seven domains: Functional limitation, physical pain, psychological discomfort, physical disability, psychological disability, social disability, and handicap. Of these seven domains, two questions need to be answered on a Likert scale. Score 4 is indicating a highly negative answer to the question and 0 means that there is no discomfort at all. The total score of the 14 questions can balance between 56 (maximally negative) to 0 (maximally positive).

Table 1. OHIP-14 questionnaire divided per domain.

Domain 1: Functional Limitation
1   Have you had trouble pronouncing any words because of problems with your teeth, mouth, or denture?
2   Have you felt that your sense of taste has worsened because of problems with your teeth, mouth, or denture?

Domain 2: Physical Pain
3   Have you had painful aching in your mouth?
4   Have you found it uncomfortable to eat any foods because of problems with your teeth, mouth, or denture?

Domain 3: Psychological Discomfort
5   Have you been self-conscious because of your teeth, mouth, or denture?
6   Have you felt tense because of problems with your teeth, mouth, or denture?

Domain 4: Physical Disability
7   Has been your diet been unsatisfactory because of problems with your teeth, mouth, or denture?
8   Have you interrupt meals because of problems with your teeth, mouth, or denture?

Domain 5: Psychological Disability
9   Have you found it difficult to relax because of problems with your teeth, mouth or denture?
10   Have you been a bit embarrassed because of problems with your teeth, mouth, or denture?

Domain 6: Social Disability
11   Have you been a bit irritable with other people because of problems with your teeth, mouth, or denture?
12   Have you had difficulty doing your usual jobs because of problems with your teeth, mouth, or denture?

Domain 7: Handicap
13   Have you felt that life, in general, was less satisfying because of problems with your teeth, mouth, or denture?
14   Have you been totally unable to function because of problems with your teeth, mouth, or denture?

2.3. Statistics

Outcomes are reported with descriptive statistics (mean, SD, median, range, and 95% CI) and boxplots. All analyses concern pair-wise comparisons within patients. For continuous variables paired *t*-tests were applied, for dichotomous variables the McNemar test was used. The 95% confidence intervals are given to show the precision of an estimate of a certain effect.

The sample size for both studies was calculated using SAS Power and Sample size calculator for related samples based on an effect size of 1 mm and a standard deviation of 0.60, with the level of significance set at 0.05 and $\beta = 0.80$. The effect estimation was based on findings Vervaeke et al., 2014 [42].

For the OHIP-14 outcome, the impact of the change was assessed by calculating the "effect size" with the following formula:

((mean-OHIP before surgery) − (mean-OHIP three months after connection))/SD before surgery

As proposed by Cohen 1977 an "effect size" of 0.2 could be interpreted as a small change, 0.6 as a moderate change and > 0.8 as a large change.

3. Results

3.1. Study Population

A sample size of 14 patients for each study was calculated. Hence, minimums of 20 patients (= 40 implants) were consequently included to anticipate future dropouts.

Twenty-six patients in study I were initially treated with one equicrestally (group 1) and one subcrestally (group 2) placed implant. In study II, 23 patients were initially treated with one implant with a moderately rough implant neck (group 3) and one implant with a minimally rough implant neck (group 4). In total four experimental treatment groups were assessed. After a follow-up of at least three years, one patient was excluded, due to anatomical constraints requiring deviation of the surgical protocol. Two patients were excluded after starting smoking and one did not respond to the follow-up invitation. Hence, 45 patients with two implants each were available after a follow-up of three years and none of the implants had failed (survival 100%). A flowchart of the patients' distribution is shown in Figure 2. The study population consisted of 24 men and 21 women with a mean age at implant placement of 64 years (SD = 9.25, range = 43–85).

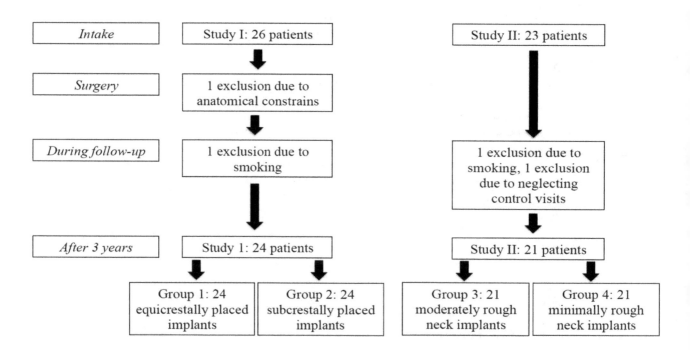

Figure 2. Flowchart of both study populations.

3.2. Mean Bone Level Difference

Table 2 shows the mean bone level and the corresponding changes of the four treatment groups at baseline and after 6, 12, 24, and 36 months. Initially, the bone level of the implants in the four groups is comparable and basically located at the implant crest. In the first six months bone remodeling was 0.7 mm for equicrestally placed implants and ranging from 0–0.3 mm in the other three subcrestally placed groups. Over time no further statistically significant bone level changes occurred in all groups (Figures 3–6). Figures 5 and 6 gives a schematic view of the bone remodeling over time, with the visible implant surface exposure in the equicrestally placed implant group (group 1).

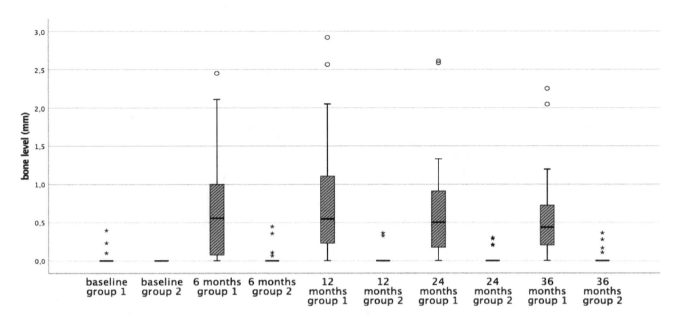

Figure 3. Boxplots representing the bone level at subsequent time points for the equicrestally (group 1) and subcrestally placed implants (group 2). * Outliers (≥3 × IQR above third quartile), ° suspected outliers (between 1.5 × IQR and 3 × IQR above third quartile).

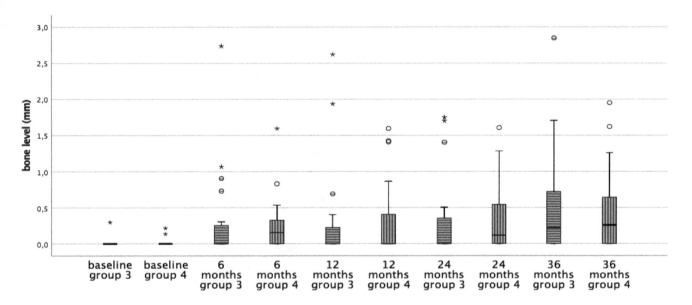

Figure 4. Boxplots representing the bone level at subsequent time points for the implants with a moderately rough neck (group 3) and minimally rough neck (group 4). * Outliers (≥3 × IQR above third quartile), ° suspected outliers (between 1.5 × IQR and 3 × IQR above third quartile).

Between groups the subcrestally placed implants of group 2 lost no bone at all. Groups 3 and 4 showed comparable bone remodeling. Hence, implant surface roughness did not affect initial nor long-term bone remodeling (Figures 4 and 6).

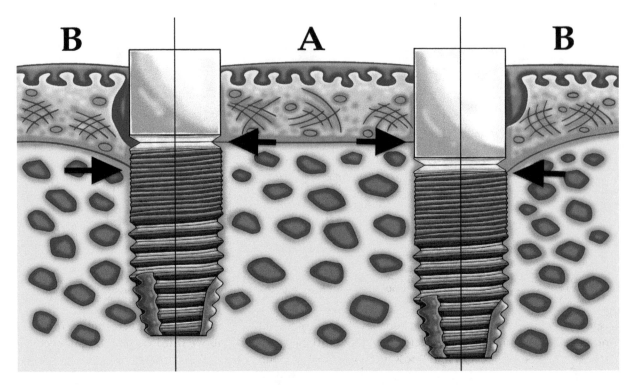

Figure 5. Schematic illustration of study 1, left equicrestally placed implant (group 1) and right subcrestally placed implant (group 2); showing the bone level at baseline (A) and bone level after bone remodeling (B).

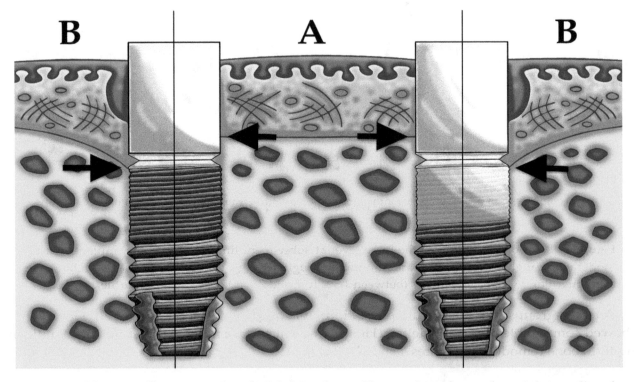

Figure 6. Schematic illustration of study 2, left implant with a moderately rough neck (group 3) and right implant with a minimally rough neck (group 4); showing the bone level at baseline (A) and bone level after bone remodeling (B).

Table 2. Mean bone level for each study group and the bone level difference between respectively equicrestally versus subcrestally placed implants and implants with moderately rough versus minimally rough neck; $p < 0.05$ indicates a statistically significant difference (paired t-test).

	Bone Level										
	Group 1: Equicrestal				Group 2: Subcrestal				Paired Difference		
	Mean (SD)	Median	Min	Max	Mean (SD)	Median	Min	Max	Mean dif	95% CI	p
Baseline	0.03 (0.09)	0.00	0.00	0.40	0.00 (0.00)	0.00	0.00	0.00	0.030	(−0.009,0.070)	0.123
6 months	0.72 (0.74)	0.59	0.00	2.45	0.04 (0.11)	0.00	0.00	0.45	0.678	(0.360,0.996)	<0.001
12 months	0.78 (0.81)	0.54	0.00	2.92	0.03 (0.10)	0.00	0.00	0.36	0.746	(0.397,1.096)	<0.001
24 months	0.69 (0.70)	0.51	0.00	2.61	0.04 (0.10)	0.00	0.00	0.30	0.644	(0.337,0.951)	<0.001
36 months	0.59 (0.59)	0.44	0.00	2.25	0.04 (0.10)	0.00	0.00	0.36	0.549	(0.297,0.802)	<0.001
	Group 3: Moderately Rough Neck				Group 4: Minimally Rough Neck				Paired Difference		
	Mean (SD)	Median	Min	Max	Mean (SD)	Median	Min	Max	Mean dif	95% CI	p
Baseline	0.01 (0.07)	0.00	0.00	0.30	0.02 (0.05)	0.00	0.00	0.22	−0.002	(−0.424,0.037)	0.902
6 months	0.33 (0.64)	0.00	0.00	2.74	0.27 (0.38)	0.18	0.00	1.60	0.064	(−0.118,0.245)	0.474
12 months	0.34 (0.68)	0.00	0.00	2.62	0.34 (0.53)	0.00	0.00	1.61	0.009	(−0.191,0.209)	0.926
24 months	0.36 (0.58)	0.00	0.00	1.75	0.37 (0.49)	0.23	0.00	1.60	−0.014	(−0.170,0.142)	0.853
36 months	0.51 (0.74)	0.22	0.00	2.84	0.45 (0.58)	0.26	0.00	1.95	0.066	(−0.114,0.246)	0.453

3.3. Biologic Parameters

On implant level only a statistically significant difference could be measured for the plaque score at 24 months ($p = 0.042$), with significantly less plaque for the equicrestally placed compared with subcrestally placed implants. However, at all other time points the plaque–and bleeding scores were not statistically significantly different, indicative of peri-implant health (Table 3).

Table 3. Mean plaque and bleeding on probing on implant level at 6, 12, 24 and 36 month for each study group and mean difference between respectively equicrestally versus subcrestally placed implants and implants with moderately rough versus minimally rough neck; $p < 0.05$ indicates a statistically significant difference (paired t-test).

	Plaque				
	Group 1: Equicrestal	Group 2: Subcrestal	Paired Difference		
	Mean (SD)	Mean (SD)	Mean dif	95% CI	p
6 months	0.44 (0.47)	0.52 (0.45)	−0.083	(−0.221,0.055)	0.224
12 months	0.45 (0.39)	0.56 (0.44)	−0.115	(−0.285,0.056)	0.178
24 months	0.42 (0.40)	0.51 (0.40)	−0.091	(−0.178,−0.003)	0.042
36 months	0.39 (0.43)	0.41 (0.42)	−0.022	(−0.148,0.104)	0.724
	Group 3: Moderately Rough Neck	Group 4: Minimally Rough Neck	Paired Difference		
	Mean (SD)	Mean (SD)	Mean dif	95% CI	p
6 months	0.38 (0.33)	0.40 (0.31)	−0.025	(−0.144,0.094)	0.666
12 months	0.37 (0.31)	0.35 (0.31)	0.017	(−0.136,0.169)	0.818
24 months	0.57 (0.36)	0.52 (0.36)	0.054	(−0.030,0.137)	0.189
36 months	0.39 (0.41)	0.43 (0.38)	−0.038	(−0.147,0.072)	0.481
	Bleeding on Probing				
	Group 1: Equicrestal	Group 2: Subcrestal	Paired Difference		
	Mean (SD)	Mean (SD)	Mean dif	95% CI	p
6 months	0.15 (0.22)	0.15 (0.22)	0.000	(−0.093,0.0933)	1.000
12 months	0.19 (0.18)	0.19 (0.18)	0.000	(−0.125,0.125)	1.000
24 months	0.23 (0.30)	0.20 (0.28)	0.023	(−0.090,0.136)	0.680
36 months	0.30 (0.33)	0.23 (0.25)	0.076	(−0.048,0.200)	0.216
	Group 3: Moderately Rough Neck	Group 4: Minimally Rough Neck	Paired Difference		
	Mean (SD)	Mean (SD)	Mean dif	95% CI	p
6 months	0.24 (0.31)	0.23 (0.24)	0.013	(−0.110,0.135)	0.834
12 months	0.20 (0.32)	0.23 (0.24)	−0.033	(−0.189,0.122)	0.653
24 months	0.25 (0.29)	0.30 (0.37)	−0.054	(−0.243,0.136)	0.551
36 months	0.08 (0.14)	0.07 (0.12)	0.013	(−0.084,0.109)	0.789

For the probing pocket depth at implant level only at 24 months a statistically significant difference between equicrestally placed compared to subcrestally placed implants could be observed (Table 4). After three years all groups are comparable indicative of peri-implant health.

Table 4. Mean probing pocket depth on implant level at 6, 12, 24 and 36 months for each study group and the mean difference between respectively equicrestally versus subcrestally placed implants and implants with a moderately rough versus minimally rough neck; $p < 0.05$ indicates a statistically significant difference (paired t-test).

	Probing Pocket Depth								
	Group 1: Equicrestal			Group 2: Subcrestal			Paired Difference		
	Mean (SD)	Min	Max	Mean (SD)	Min	Max	Mean dif	95% CI	p
6 months	1.88 (0.53)	1.00	3.25	2.01 (0.66)	1.00	3.75	−0.135	(−0.311,0.041)	0.125
12 months	1.70 (0.44)	1.00	2.50	1.83 (0.53)	1.00	2.75	−0.130	(−0.312,0.051)	0.149
24 months	2.30 (0.66)	1.50	4.50	2.57 (0.84)	1.25	4.50	−0.261	(−0.473,−0.048)	0.018
36 months	2.42 (0.69)	1.00	4.00	2.59 (0.71)	1.00	3.75	−0.163	(−0.0378,0.052)	0.130
	Group 3: Moderately Rough Neck			Group 4: Minimally Rough Neck			Paired Difference		
	Mean (SD)	Min	Max	Mean (SD)	Min	Max	Mean dif	95% CI	p
6 months	2.93 (0.71)	1.75	5.25	2.88 (0.65)	1.75	4.75	0.050	(−0.142,0.242)	0.592
12 months	2.65 (0.72)	1.75	4.75	2.68 (0.68)	1.75	4.50	−0.033	(−0.221,0.154)	0.709
24 months	2.48 (0.58)	1.25	3.50	2.34 (0.60)	1.00	3,25	0.143	(−0.114,0.401)	0.252
36 months	2.10 (0.68)	1.25	4.25	2.01 (0.58)	1.00	3.00	0.088	(−0.259,0.434)	0.603

3.4. Oral Health-Related Quality of Life

Based on 45 edentulous patients, receiving an implant-supported overdenture, the OHIP-14 index reduced from 13.37/56 (SD 9.97) at baseline to 4.42/56 (SD 4.94) after three months of functional loading. This result in a large effect size of 0.90, suggesting a strong improvement in oral health related quality of life. Between 3 and 12 months, no further changes were observed, resulting in small effect size (0.04), indicative of a very stable result over time (Figure 7). The reduction was statistically significant for all seven domains after three months (Table 5). For functional limitation, physical disability and handicap the effect size was moderate. For the other four domains, a large effect size was observed and most expressed for physical pain with an effect size of 1.04. The latter is logically given the fact that improved denture retention results in less mucosal irritation and consequently fewer complaints related to pain suffering.

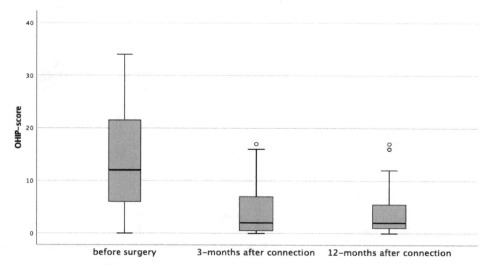

Figure 7. Boxplots representing the Oral Health Impact Profile-14 (OHIP-14) total score before surgery, 3 and 12 months after connection of the prosthesis with the implants. A score of 56 represents a maximal negative appreciation. ° Suspected outliers (between 1.5 × IQR and 3 × IQR above third quartile).

Table 5. Mean OHIP score and the mean difference for each of the seven domains before surgery and three months after connection with the calculated effect-size.

Domain	Mean-OHIP (SD)		Paired Difference			Effect-Size
	Before Surgery	Three Months after Connection	Mean Dif	95% CI	p	
functional limitation	2.30 (1.85)	1.14 (1.42)	1.16	(0.540,1.785)	0.001	0.63
physical pain	3.37 (2.06)	1.21 (1.55)	2.16	(1.440,2.886)	<0.001	1.04
psychological discomfort	2.52 (2.35)	0.65 (1.43)	1.87	(1.034,2.687)	<0.001	0.80
physical disability	2.12 (2.16)	0.44 (0.85)	1.68	(0.971,2.378)	<0.001	0.78
psychological disability	2.21 (1.91)	0.58 (0.93)	1.63	(0.930,2.326)	<0.001	0.85
social disability	1.67 (1.49)	0.16 (0.49)	1.51	(1.007,2.016)	<0.001	1.01
handicap	1.42 (1.48)	0.26 (0.66)	1.16	(0.683,1.642)	<0.001	0.78

4. Discussion

The current paper focuses on implant treatment outcome in patients, which were completely edentulous in both jaws. Retention of the lower denture is a typical problem in this category of patients, especially in the mandible as compared to the maxillary denture. The denture in the mandible is less retentive because of a smaller crestal bone support, a more expressed degree of bone resorption, and unfavorable distribution of occluding forces, as well as additional pressure of the tongue yielding dislocating forces. Often this results in functional discomfort and pain, the latter because of the absence of keratinized mucosa. In the maxilla, the denture is supported on the crest and on the hard structure of the palate, which is covered by keratinized tissue. A vacuum present during mastication, between the palatal coverage of the denture and the underlying tissues, improves the retention. Consequently, fully edentulous patients have more complaints with mandibular dentures and an overdenture retained on two implants has therefore been suggested as of minimal care in order to provide functional comfort [6]. Implant treatment in denture wearing patients can be used for split mouth studies as was the case in the two clinical studies presented in the present paper. The focus was on implant type and surgical procedure, defined as implant survival, crestal bone loss and biologic peri-implant health. The latter is an important aspect because peri-implant diseases may jeopardize treatment outcome in the long run and are often related to aesthetic appreciation. Additionally, the patient-centered outcome was assessed by using a validated Oral Health Related Quality of Life questionnaire.

After three years of follow-up, no implant failures could be recorded in the present study and all remaining patients remained fully functional. This 100% implant survival is in line with current literature on implant overdenture therapy [47].

Initial bone remodeling is a healing phenomenon related to the surgical procedure mainly the exposure of bone and periosteum during implant placement, as well as the depth placement in the bone. Given the fact that implant survival with currently available dental implant systems is successful and quite predictable, the research focuses on implant success. Implant treatment is considered a success when high implant survival is combined with bone stability over time, because the latter reflects the health of the peri-implant tissues. Indeed, worldwide consensus defined that peri implantitis, a disease condition of the implant resulting in pocket formation between the implant and soft tissue, is always preceded by the bone loss [12]. Additionally, soft tissue health also affects the aesthetic outcome, especially in the partially edentulous patient. Although aesthetics was not the key issue in the present paper, the study conditions tested may provide clinical guidelines that do affect aesthetics, as well as peri-implant health outcomes.

In the present paper, minimal initial bone remodeling ranging from 0–0.7 mm was assessed. After the physiological initial bone remodeling, no further bone loss could be observed up to three years of function. The effect of soft tissue thickness and implant surface roughness on the crestal bone loss was evaluated. The applied split-mouth study design corrects for inter-individual variability from the estimates of the treatment effect [48]. The results showed that the initial bone remodeling was affected by the originally present soft tissue thickness, but not by the implant surface roughness. After implant installation, a minimum of 3 mm soft tissue dimensions seems to be necessary for the re-establishment of the so-called "biologic width", indicative of the importance of the biologically guided implant placement. These findings are in accordance with an earlier published systematic review, including meta-analysis. There it is stated that implants placed with an initially thicker peri-implant soft tissue have less radiographic marginal bone loss in the short term [49]. Additionally, an increased early bone remodeling leads to implant surface exposure in patients with thin soft tissues, which increases the risk of on-going bone loss as shown by Vervaeke and colleagues in a nine year follow-up. A greater implant surface exposure increases the bacterial colonization of the implant surface, which could enlarge the chance to induce peri-implantitis [50]. From a clinical point of view, it is highly suggested that the surgeon adapts the surgical position of the implant in relation to the available pre-operative soft-tissue thickness.

It is generally accepted that osseointegration of moderately rough implants is enhanced as compared to minimally rough implants. This resulted in faster treatment protocols and reduced early failures. More recently, it was suggested that a minimally rough implant surface yields less crestal bone loss and less peri-implantitis on the long-term. A recent systematic review, including studies up to 10 years, reported on the survival rate and marginal bone loss of implants with different surface roughness. Implant survival was higher for moderately rough surfaces, but minimally rough surfaces showed the least marginal bone loss [51]. This outcome is in contrast to the outcome presented in another systematic review with meta-analysis. The latter evaluated the influence of the implant collar surface on marginal bone loss and revealed less bone loss for the rougher implant systems. However, 10 out of the 12 included studies showed results with less than five years of function. The only study with 10 years of follow-up showed less bone loss for the implants with a smooth collar compared to the implants with a rough collar. Yet, the authors stated that the results of their systematic review needed to be interpreted cautiously, due to several confounding factors [52]. Another systematic review with meta-analysis, which included only studies with at least, a five-year follow-up showed significantly less bone loss around smooth implant surfaces compared to moderately rough and rough implant surfaces [38]. Recently Donati and co-workers published the results of a 20-year follow-up RCT to evaluate the effect of a modified implant surface. In 51 patients at least one implant with a minimally rough surface and one with a modified surface was installed. The difference in mean bone level change between the two implant-systems was not statistically significant, and the moderate increase of implant surface roughness has no beneficial effect on long-term preservation of the peri-implant marginal bone level. A more detailed analysis of the paper revealed, however, that none of the 32 evaluated smooth implants showed more than 3 mm bone loss, whereas 3 out of the 32 modified implants showed bone loss between 3 and 6 mm. Only two smooth surface implants were diagnosed with peri-implantitis compared with five implants with a modified surface [53].

The findings of our paper are in accordance with the paper of Donati and co-workers, concluding that the surface roughness of the implant neck has no effect on bone level up to three years. The hybrid implant system used in our study combines the benefits of faster osseointegration, due to the moderately rough implant body, and the minimally rough surface around the implant neck suggests it is less prone to develop peri-implantitis [54]. Additionally, several studies conclude the beneficial effect of a smoother surface with a lower incidence of peri-implantitis and less bone loss on the long term. A further long-term follow-up of the current study population will elucidate the latter.

Besides implant survival and bone level stability, also peri-implant health is considered a perquisite for treatment success. Peri-implant health is defined on two levels. Plaque accumulation yields minor inflammation of the soft tissue surrounding the implant- restorative interface, coined as mucositis. It is diagnosed with bleeding of the tissues after probing the crevice between implant and mucosa. In a recent consensus report, the diagnosis of peri-implantitis has been redefined as a combination of probing pocket depths of at least 6 mm in combination with bleeding on probing or a bone level of at least 3 mm apical of the most coronal portion of the intraosseous part of the implant [12]. In our study, no patients showed ongoing bone-loss in combination with bleeding and increasing probing pocket depths. Hence, the incidence of peri-implantitis was 0.0%.

The absence of peri-implantitis was found despite a high plaque level. This could be explained by the elderly, fully edentulous patient population. De Waal and colleagues revealed that edentulous patients restored with implants showed more plaque compared to partially edentulous patients restored with implants. However, the plaque in the fully edentulous patients harbours a potentially less pathogenic peri-implant micro-flora [55,56].

Another explanation for the relatively high plaque scores could be the dexterity problems inducing imperfect cleaning abilities in elderly patients. On the other hand, plaque is screened at a given moment in time during the clinical inspection and this may be several hours after cleaning and not necessarily reflects the overall hygiene of the patient over time.

This is the reason why the bleeding index is considered more useful. It reflects the degree of inflammation as a result of the long-term plaque control and is less momentarily. The current study revealed that high plaque score did not result in high bleeding scores.

The support of a mandibular overdenture by two implants has a significant positive effect on the quality of life. The OHIP-14 score was calculated irrespective of the implant group because it is a patient-related outcome variable. On all the seven domains measured with the OHIP-14 questionnaire a statistically significant difference was measured, all in favor of the support of a mandible overdenture by two implants. These findings are in accordance with a clinical trial reporting a significant improvement in satisfaction and health-related quality of life when subjects who received two implants are compared with subjects requesting a new conventional denture. Besides the improvement in the quality of life, they reported that patients requesting implants reported that tooth loss and denture wearing problems had a much greater impact in their quality of life than patients seeking conventional dentures [5].

5. Conclusions

Within the limitations of this study, it can be concluded that an implant supported mandibular overdenture significantly improves the quality of life, with limited biologic complications and a high survival rate of the implants. All seven domains of the OHIP-14 questionnaire significantly reduced when the mandible overdenture is supported by two implants. No differences were observed in crestal bone remodeling between minimally rough and moderately rough implant surfaces. However, initial bone remodeling was affected by initial soft tissue thickness. Anticipating biologic width re-establishment by adapting the vertical position of the implant in relation to the available soft tissue thickness may avoid peri-implant bone loss. The biologic variance of the patient might be more important compared to the configuration of the implant surface. Long-term follow-up of the study is necessary to determine the influence of early implant surface exposure and implant surface roughness on crestal bone loss, biologic parameters, mechanical complication, and implant survival.

Author Contributions: Conceptualization, R.D. and H.d.B.; methodology, R.D. and E.B.; software, R.D. and E.B.; validation, R.D., H.d.B. and E.B.; formal analysis, R.D., H.d.B. and E.B.; investigation, R.D., M.G., S.V. and C.M.; resources, R.D., H.d.B.; data curation, E.B.; writing—original draft preparation, R.D.; writing—review and editing, H.d.B., M.G. and S.V.; visualization, R.D.; supervision, H.d.B.; project administration, R.D.

Acknowledgments: Special thanks to Mario de Timmerman for the illustrations.

References

1.   Petersen, P.E.; Yamamoto, T. Improving the oral health of older people: the approach of the WHO Global Oral Health Programme. *Community Dent. Oral Epidemiol.* **2005**, *33*, 81–92. [CrossRef] [PubMed]

2.   Buser, D.; Sennerby, L.; De Bruyn, H. Modern implant dentistry based on osseointegration: 50 years of progress, current trends and open questions. *Periodontology 2000* **2017**, *73*, 7–21. [CrossRef] [PubMed]

3. Pelo, S.; Saponaro, G.; Patini, R.; Staderini, E.; Giordano, A.; Gasparini, G.; Garagiola, U.; Azzuni, C.; Cordaro, M.; Foresta, E.; et al. Risks in surgery-first orthognathic approach: complications of segmental osteotomies of the jaws. A systematic review. *Eur. Rev. Med. Pharmacol. Sci.* **2017**, *21*, 4–12.

4. Slade, G.D.; Spencer, A.J. Development and evaluation of the Oral Health Impact Profile. *Community Dent. Health* **1994**, *11*, 3–11.

5. Allen, P.F.; McMillan, A.S. A longitudinal study of quality of life outcomes in older adults requesting implant prostheses and complete removable dentures. *Clin. Oral Implant. Res.* **2003**, *14*, 173–179. [CrossRef]

6. Feine, J.S.; Carlsson, G.E.; Awad, M.A.; Chehade, A.; Duncan, W.J.; Gizani, S.; Head, T.; Lund, J.P.; MacEntee, M.; Mericske-Stern, R.; et al. The McGill consensus statement on overdentures. Mandibular two-implant overdentures as first choice standard of care for edentulous patients. Montreal, Quebec, 24–25 May, 2002. *Int. J. Oral Maxillofac. Implant.* **2002**, *17*, 601–602.

7. De Bruyn, H.; Raes, S.; Matthys, C.; Cosyn, J. The current use of patient-centered/reported outcomes in implant dentistry: a systematic review. *Clin. Oral Implant. Res.* **2015**, *26* (Suppl. 11), 45–56. [CrossRef]

8. Zhang, L.; Lyu, C.; Shang, Z.; Niu, A.; Liang, X. Quality of Life of Implant-Supported Overdenture and Conventional Complete Denture in Restoring the Edentulous Mandible: A Systematic Review. *Implant Dent.* **2017**, *26*, 945–950. [CrossRef]

9. Kutkut, A.; Bertoli, E.; Frazer, R.; Pinto-Sinai, G.; Fuentealba Hidalgo, R.; Studts, J. A systematic review of studies comparing conventional complete denture and implant retained overdenture. *J. Prosthodont. Res.* **2018**, *62*, 1–9. [CrossRef]

10. Sivaramakrishnan, G.; Sridharan, K. Comparison of implant supported mandibular overdentures and conventional dentures on quality of life: A systematic review and meta-analysis of randomized controlled studies. *Aust. Dent. J.* **2016**, *61*, 482–488. [CrossRef]

11. Renvert, S.; Persson, G.R.; Pirih, F.Q.; Camargo, P.M. Peri-implant health, peri-implant mucositis, and peri-implantitis: Case definitions and diagnostic considerations. *J. Periodontol.* **2018**, *89* (Suppl. 1), S304–S312. [CrossRef]

12. Peri-implant diseases and conditions: Consensus report of workgroup 4 of the 2017 World Workshop on the Classification of Periodontal and Peri-Implant Diseases and Conditions. *Br. Dent. J.* **2018**, *225*, 141. [CrossRef]

13. Heitz-Mayfield, L.J.A.; Salvi, G.E. Peri-implant mucositis. *J. Periodontol.* **2018**, *89* (Suppl. 1), S257–S266. [CrossRef]

14. Pontoriero, R.; Tonelli, M.P.; Carnevale, G.; Mombelli, A.; Nyman, S.R.; Lang, N.P. Experimentally induced peri-implant mucositis. A clinical study in humans. *Clin. Oral Implant. Res.* **1994**, *5*, 254–259. [CrossRef]

15. Zitzmann, N.U.; Berglundh, T.; Marinello, C.P.; Lindhe, J. Experimental peri-implant mucositis in man. *J. Clin. Periodontol.* **2001**, *28*, 517–523. [CrossRef] [PubMed]

16. Salvi, G.E.; Aglietta, M.; Eick, S.; Sculean, A.; Lang, N.P.; Ramseier, C.A. Reversibility of experimental peri-implant mucositis compared with experimental gingivitis in humans. *Clin. Oral Implant. Res.* **2012**, *23*, 182–190. [CrossRef] [PubMed]

17. Meyer, S.; Giannopoulou, C.; Courvoisier, D.; Schimmel, M.; Muller, F.; Mombelli, A. Experimental mucositis and experimental gingivitis in persons aged 70 or over. Clinical and biological responses. *Clin. Oral Implant. Res.* **2017**, *28*, 1005–1012. [CrossRef] [PubMed]

18. Araujo, M.G.; Lindhe, J. Peri-implant health. *J. Periodontol.* **2018**, *89* (Suppl. 1), S249–S256. [CrossRef]

19. Schwarz, F.; Derks, J.; Monje, A.; Wang, H.L. Peri-implantitis. *J. Periodontol.* **2018**, *89* (Suppl. 1), S267–S290. [CrossRef]

20. Canullo, L.; Schlee, M.; Wagner, W.; Covani, U.; Montegrotto Group for the Study of Peri-implant Disease. International Brainstorming Meeting on Etiologic and Risk Factors of Peri-implantitis, Montegrotto (Padua, Italy), August 2014. *Int. J. Oral Maxillofac. Implant.* **2015**, *30*, 1093–1104. [CrossRef]

21. Albrektsson, T.; Buser, D.; Chen, S.T.; Cochran, D.; DeBruyn, H.; Jemt, T.; Koka, S.; Nevins, M.; Sennerby, L.; Simion, M.; et al. Statements from the Estepona consensus meeting on peri-implantitis, 2–4 February 2012. *Clin. Implant Dent. Relat. Res.* **2012**, *14*, 781–782. [CrossRef] [PubMed]

22. De Bruyn, H.; Christiaens, V.; Doornewaard, R.; Jacobsson, M.; Cosyn, J.; Jacquet, W.; Vervaeke, S. Implant surface roughness and patient factors on long-term peri-implant bone loss. *Periodontology 2000* **2017**, *73*, 218–227. [CrossRef] [PubMed]

23. Wennerberg, A.; Hallgren, C.; Johansson, C.; Danelli, S. A histomorphometric evaluation of screw-shaped implants each prepared with two surface roughnesses. *Clin. Oral Implant. Res.* **1998**, *9*, 11–19. [CrossRef]

24. Cochran, D.L. A comparison of endosseous dental implant surfaces. *J. Periodontol.* **1999**, *70*, 1523–1539. [CrossRef]

25. Lazzara, R.J.; Testori, T.; Trisi, P.; Porter, S.S.; Weinstein, R.L. A human histologic analysis of osseotite and machined surfaces using implants with 2 opposing surfaces. *Int. J. Periodontics Restor. Dent.* **1999**, *19*, 117–129.

26. Teughels, W.; Van Assche, N.; Sliepen, I.; Quirynen, M. Effect of material characteristics and/or surface topography on biofilm development. *Clin. Oral Implant. Res.* **2006**, *17* (Suppl. 2), 68–81. [CrossRef]

27. Esposito, M.; Coulthard, P.; Thomsen, P.; Worthington, H.V. The role of implant surface modifications, shape and material on the success of osseointegrated dental implants. A Cochrane systematic review. *Eur. J. Prosthodontics Restor. Dent.* **2005**, *13*, 15–31.

28. Esposito, M.; Ardebili, Y.; Worthington, H.V. Interventions for replacing missing teeth: different types of dental implants. *Cochrane Database Syst. Rev.* **2014**, CD003815. [CrossRef]

29. Glibert, M.; Matthys, C.; Maat, R.J.; De Bruyn, H.; Vervaeke, S. A randomized controlled clinical trial assessing initial crestal bone remodeling of implants with a different surface roughness. *Clin. Implant Dent. Relat. Res.* **2018**, *20*, 824–828. [CrossRef]

30. Monje, A.; Catena, A.; Borgnakke, W.S. Association between diabetes mellitus/hyperglycaemia and peri-implant diseases: Systematic review and meta-analysis. *J. Clin. Periodontol.* **2017**, *44*, 636–648. [CrossRef]

31. Papi, P.; Letizia, C.; Pilloni, A.; Petramala, L.; Saracino, V.; Rosella, D.; Pompa, G. Peri-implant diseases and metabolic syndrome components: a systematic review. *Eur. Rev. Med. Pharmacol. Sci.* **2018**, *22*, 866–875. [CrossRef]

32. Moraschini, V.; Barboza, E.S.; Peixoto, G.A. The impact of diabetes on dental implant failure: a systematic review and meta-analysis. *Int. J. Oral Maxillofac. Surg.* **2016**, *45*, 1237–1245. [CrossRef] [PubMed]

33. de Medeiros, F.; Kudo, G.A.H.; Leme, B.G.; Saraiva, P.P.; Verri, F.R.; Honorio, H.M.; Pellizzer, E.P.; Santiago Junior, J.F. Dental implants in patients with osteoporosis: A systematic review with meta-analysis. *Int. J. Oral Maxillofac. Surg.* **2018**, *47*, 480–491. [CrossRef]

34. Jung, R.E.; Al-Nawas, B.; Araujo, M.; Avila-Ortiz, G.; Barter, S.; Brodala, N.; Chappuis, V.; Chen, B.; De Souza, A.; Almeida, R.F.; et al. Group 1 ITI Consensus Report: The influence of implant length and design and medications on clinical and patient-reported outcomes. *Clin. Oral Implant. Res.* **2018**, *29* (Suppl. 16), 69–77. [CrossRef] [PubMed]

35. Safii, S.H.; Palmer, R.M.; Wilson, R.F. Risk of implant failure and marginal bone loss in subjects with a history of periodontitis: a systematic review and meta-analysis. *Clin. Implant Dent. Relat. Res.* **2010**, *12*, 165–174. [CrossRef] [PubMed]

36. De Bruyn, H.; Collaert, B. The effect of smoking on early implant failure. *Clin. Oral Implant. Res.* **1994**, *5*, 260–264. [CrossRef]

37. Hinode, D.; Tanabe, S.; Yokoyama, M.; Fujisawa, K.; Yamauchi, E.; Miyamoto, Y. Influence of smoking on osseointegrated implant failure: a meta-analysis. *Clin. Oral Implant. Res.* **2006**, *17*, 473–478. [CrossRef]

38. Doornewaard, R.; Christiaens, V.; De Bruyn, H.; Jacobsson, M.; Cosyn, J.; Vervaeke, S.; Jacquet, W. Long-Term Effect of Surface Roughness and Patients' Factors on Crestal Bone Loss at Dental Implants. A Systematic Review and Meta-Analysis. *Clin. Implant Dent. Relat. Res.* **2017**, *19*, 372–399. [CrossRef]

39. Vervaeke, S.; Collaert, B.; Cosyn, J.; De Bruyn, H. A 9-Year Prospective Case Series Using Multivariate Analyses to Identify Predictors of Early and Late Peri-Implant Bone Loss. *Clin. Implant Dent. Relat. Res.* **2016**, *18*, 30–39. [CrossRef]

40. Berglundh, T.; Lindhe, J. Dimension of the periimplant mucosa. Biological width revisited. *J. Clin. Periodontol.* **1996**, *23*, 971–973. [CrossRef]

41. Linkevicius, T.; Apse, P.; Grybauskas, S.; Puisys, A. The influence of soft tissue thickness on crestal bone changes around implants: a 1-year prospective controlled clinical trial. *Int. J. Oral Maxillofac. Implant.* **2009**, *24*, 712–719.

42. Vervaeke, S.; Dierens, M.; Besseler, J.; De Bruyn, H. The influence of initial soft tissue thickness on peri-implant bone remodeling. *Clin. Implant Dent. Relat. Res.* **2014**, *16*, 238–247. [CrossRef] [PubMed]

43. Galindo-Moreno, P.; Leon-Cano, A.; Ortega-Oller, I.; Monje, A.; F, O.V.; Catena, A. Marginal bone loss as success criterion in implant dentistry: Beyond 2 mm. *Clin. Oral Implant. Res.* **2015**, *26*, e28–e34. [CrossRef]

44. Canullo, L.; Camacho-Alonso, F.; Tallarico, M.; Meloni, S.M.; Xhanari, E.; Penarrocha-Oltra, D. Mucosa Thickness and Peri-implant Crestal Bone Stability: A Clinical and Histologic Prospective Cohort Trial. *Int. J. Oral Maxillofac. Implant.* **2017**, *32*, 675–681. [CrossRef]

45. Doornewaard, R.; Jacquet, W.; Cosyn, J.; De Bruyn, H. How do peri-implant biologic parameters correspond with implant survival and peri-implantitis? A critical review. *Clin. Oral Implant. Res.* **2018**, *29* (Suppl. 18), 100–123. [CrossRef]

46. Vervaeke, S.; Matthys, C.; Nassar, R.; Christiaens, V.; Cosyn, J.; De Bruyn, H. Adapting the vertical position of implants with a conical connection in relation to soft tissue thickness prevents early implant surface exposure: A 2-year prospective intra-subject comparison. *J. Clin. Periodontol.* **2018**, *45*, 605–612. [CrossRef] [PubMed]

47. Srinivasan, M.; Meyer, S.; Mombelli, A.; Muller, F. Dental implants in the elderly population: A systematic review and meta-analysis. *Clin. Oral Implant. Res.* **2017**, *28*, 920–930. [CrossRef]

48. Lesaffre, E.; Philstrom, B.; Needleman, I.; Worthington, H. The design and analysis of split-mouth studies: what statisticians and clinicians should know. *Stat. Med.* **2009**, *28*, 3470–3482. [CrossRef]

49. Suarez-Lopez Del Amo, F.; Lin, G.H.; Monje, A.; Galindo-Moreno, P.; Wang, H.L. Influence of Soft Tissue Thickness on Peri-Implant Marginal Bone Loss: A Systematic Review and Meta-Analysis. *J. Periodontol.* **2016**, *87*, 690–699. [CrossRef]

50. Quirynen, M.; Abarca, M.; Van Assche, N.; Nevins, M.; van Steenberghe, D. Impact of supportive periodontal therapy and implant surface roughness on implant outcome in patients with a history of periodontitis. *J. Clin. Periodontol.* **2007**, *34*, 805–815. [CrossRef]

51. Wennerberg, A.; Albrektsson, T.; Chrcanovic, B. Long-term clinical outcome of implants with different surface modifications. *Eur. J. Oral Implantol.* **2018**, *11* (Suppl. 1), S123–S136.

52. Koodaryan, R.; Hafezeqoran, A. Evaluation of Implant Collar Surfaces for Marginal Bone Loss: A Systematic Review and Meta-Analysis. *BioMed Res. Int.* **2016**, *2016*, 4987526. [CrossRef] [PubMed]

53. Donati, M.; Ekestubbe, A.; Lindhe, J.; Wennstrom, J.L. Marginal bone loss at implants with different surface characteristics—A 20-year follow-up of a randomized controlled clinical trial. *Clin. Oral Implant. Res.* **2018**, *29*, 480–487. [CrossRef]

54. Raes, M.; D'Hondt, R.; Teughels, W.; Coucke, W.; Quirynen, M. A 5-year randomized clinical trial comparing minimally with moderately rough implants in patients with severe periodontitis. *J. Clin. Periodontol.* **2018**, *45*, 711–720. [CrossRef] [PubMed]

55. De Waal, Y.C.; van Winkelhoff, A.J.; Meijer, H.J.; Raghoebar, G.M.; Winkel, E.G. Differences in peri-implant conditions between fully and partially edentulous subjects: A systematic review. *J. Clin. Periodontol.* **2013**, *40*, 266–286. [CrossRef] [PubMed]

56. De Waal, Y.C.; Winkel, E.G.; Meijer, H.J.; Raghoebar, G.M.; van Winkelhoff, A.J. Differences in peri-implant microflora between fully and partially edentulous patients: A systematic review. *J. Clin. Periodontol.* **2014**, *85*, 68–82. [CrossRef] [PubMed]

16

Cytokine Profile in Patients with Aseptic Loosening of Total Hip Replacements and Its Relation to Metal Release and Metal Allergy

Rune J. Christiansen [1,2,*], Henrik J. Münch [3], Charlotte M. Bonefeld [2], Jacob P. Thyssen [4], Jens J. Sloth [5], Carsten Geisler [2], Kjeld Søballe [3], Morten S. Jellesen [1] and Stig S. Jakobsen [3,*]

[1] Department of Mechanical Engineering, Technical University of Denmark, DK-2800 Kgs. Lyngby, Denmark
[2] Department of Immunology and Microbiology, University of Copenhagen, DK-2200 Copenhagen, Denmark
[3] Institute of Clinical Medicine—Orthopedic Surgery, Aarhus University, DK-8000 Aarhus C, Denmark
[4] Institute of Clinical Medicine, Copenhagen University, Gentofte Hospital, DK-2900 Hellerup, Denmark
[5] National Food Institute, Research Group on Nanobio Science, Technical University of Denmark, DK-2860 Søborg, Denmark
[*] Correspondence: rujuch@mek.dtu.dk (R.J.C.); Stig.Jakobsen@ki.au.dk (S.S.J.)

Abstract: Metal release from total hip replacements (THRs) is associated with aseptic loosening (AL). It has been proposed that the underlying immunological response is caused by a delayed type IV hypersensitivity-like reaction to metals, i.e., metal allergy. The purpose of this study was to investigate the immunological response in patients with AL in relation to metal release and the prevalence of metal allergy. THR patients undergoing revision surgery due to AL or mechanical implant failures were included in the study along with a control group consisting of primary THR patients. Comprehensive cytokine analyses were performed on serum and periimplant tissue samples along with metal analysis using inductive coupled plasma mass spectrometry (ICP-MS). Patient patch testing was done with a series of metals related to orthopedic implant. A distinct cytokine profile was found in the periimplant tissue of patients with AL. Significantly increased levels of the proinflammatory cytokines IL-1β, IL-2, IL-8, IFN-γ and TNF-α, but also the anti-inflammatory IL-10 were detected. A general increase of metal concentrations in the periimplant tissue was observed in both revision groups, while Cr was significantly increased in patient serum with AL. No difference in the prevalence of metal sensitivity was established by patch testing. Increased levels of IL-1β, IL-8, and TNF-α point to an innate immune response. However, the presence of IL-2 and IFN-γ indicates additional involvement of T cell-mediated response in patients with AL, although this could not be detected by patch testing.

Keywords: arthroplasty; replacement; hip; hypersensitivity; contact; allergy and immunology; cytokines; Interleukin-8

1. Introduction

1.1. Background

Aseptic loosening (AL) of implants is the most common reason for revision surgeries in patients with total hip replacements (THRs), representing close to 75% of all cases, with serious consequences for patients and healthcare systems [1,2]. Although the etiology of AL is multifactorial and yet to be fully understood, evidence suggest that the predominant cause of AL is due to a macrophage-driven chronic inflammatory response initiated by implant wear [1,3–5]. This adverse tissue reaction is associated with the innate immune system and can lead to the bone degrading state of osteolysis, subsequently resulting in implant failure by AL.

Cytokines are small messenger molecules that coordinate the immune response by regulating inflammation and modulating cellular activities such as growth, differentiation and survival [6]. Key mediators of osteolysis have been identified as pro-inflammatory cytokines like interleukin (IL)-1β, IL-6, IL-8 and tumor necrosis factor (TNF)-α secreted by activated macrophages. In turn, these cytokines are capable of inducing the differentiation of osteoclast precursor cells into mature, bone resorbing, osteoclasts [1,7–11]. Interferon (IFN)-γ is another important immune regulatory cytokine implicated in bone resorption but also in inflammation progression and cell mediated immunity [12,13].

Macrophages have been established as important mediators of ostolysis, but several other cell types have also been identified in the periimplant tissue of failed implants, including lymphocytic T cells [9,14–16]. T helper (Th) cells, a subtype of T cells, are important regulators of macrophage function and the adaptive immune response, which given rise to the concept of implant-related metal sensitivity. This concept is evolved around a delayed type IV T cell mediated hypersensitivity (DTH), exemplified by allergic contact dermatitis to metal ions (metal allergy). Due to their small size, metal ions are considered to be incomplete antigens, referred to as haptens, and must interact with peptides or proteins to form an antigen able to mount DTH.

In support of the concept above, findings of elevated levels of metal particles and ions have been shown to correlate with an increased prevalence of metal allergy in patients with failing implants [17–21]. Furthermore, some of the most commonly applied alloys for THR like stainless steel (FeCrNiMo), cobalt chromium (CoCrMo) and titanium alloys (Ti6Al4V) contain known sensitizing metals [22].

Immunological studies of AL in THRs, have suggested the involvement of a Th1 cell response, crucial for DTH, due to increased levels of Th1 cell specific cytokines like IFN-γ and IL-2 [4,23]. Previous studies also suggest the involvement of a Th2 and Th17 cell response in AL, which are respectively characterized by the production of IL-4, IL-17 and granulocyte-macrophage colony-stimulating factor (GM-CSF) [24–26]. However, the causal relationship between immune reactions, metal release from implants, and AL is still uncertain.

1.2. Aim

The aim of the present study was to determine and compare levels of THR relevant metals and cytokine profiles from periimplant tissue and blood serum, and to investigate the prevalence of metal allergy in patients undergoing revision surgery due AL, mechanical failure or undergoing primary THR surgery. Periimplant tissue obtained from patients with AL showed a significantly different cytokine profile suggesting the involvement of both innate and adaptive immunity in AL. No prevalence of metal allergy was established in patients with failed implants despite elevated levels of metal ions in the periimplant tissue.

2. Experimental Section

2.1. Patients and Samples

We conducted a prospective case study including three patient groups. This study was approved by the Central Denmark Region Committee on Biomedical Research Ethics (Journal number: 1-10-72-90-13). All patients gave their written informed consent before entering the study.

Criteria for inclusion in the AL (+) group were: revision (entirely or partial) due to aseptic loosening, osteolysis, or unexplainable pain that could not be treated conservatively. The AL (−) group; revision (entirely or partial) due to fracture, dislocation, or component failure. The Control group; patients received a primary THR. Implant components are listed in Table 1.

Table 1. Implant overview. Implant types and materials used for femoral, head, liner and acetabular components are given for patients in the revision groups. In addition to the implant bulk material, model names and surface finish is also listed. cpTi relates to commercially pure titanium and PS to plasma sprayed coatings. FeCrNiMn is also referred to as Orthinox stainless steel.

Patient #	Type	Femoral	Head	Liner	Acetabular
1 AL (+)	MoP	Ti-6Al-4V, ZMR®, uncemented, porous coating	CoCrMo	PE	Ti-6Al-4V, Trilogy®, uncommented, cpTi fiber mesh.
2 AL (+)	MoP	FeCrNiMn, Exeter®, cemented, polished.	CoCrMo	PE	cpTi, Duraloc®, uncemented, porous coating.
3 AL (+)	MoP	CoCrMo, Lubinus®, cemented polished.	CoCrMo	PE	PE, Lubinus®, cemented, all-polycup
4 AL (+)	MoP	FeCrNiM, Exeter®, cemented, polished.	CoCrMo	PE	Ti-6Al-4V, Mallory Head, uncemented, PS.
5 AL (+)	MoP	Ti-6Al-4V, Bi-metric®, uncemented, grit blasted.	CoCrMo	PE	Ti-6Al-4V, Mallory®Head, uncemented, PS.
6 AL (+)	MoM	Ti-6Al-4V, Bi-metric®, uncemented, grit blasted.	CoCrMo	CoCrMo	CoCrMo, ReCap®, uncemented, cpTI PS.
1 AL (−)	MoP	Ti-6Al-7Nb, CLS spotorno®, uncemented, grit blasted.	CoCrMo	PE	Ti-6Al-4V, Trilogy®, uncemented, cpTi fiber mesh.
2 AL (−)	MoP	Ti-6Al-7Nb, CLS spotorno®, uncemented, grit blasted.	CoCrMo	PE	Ti-6Al-4V, Trilogy®, uncemented, cpTi fiber mesh.
3 AL (−)	CoP	Ti-6Al-4V, Biocontact®, uncemented, grit blasted.	Ceramic	PE	Ti-6Al-4V, Plasmacup®, uncemented, plasmapore PS.
4 AL (−)	MoP	FeCrNiMn, Exeter®, cemented, polished.	CoCrMo	PE	cpTi, Pinnacle®, uncemented porocoat, porous coating.
5 AL (−)	MoP	FeCrNiMn, Exeter®, cemented, polished	CoCrMo	PE	Ti-6Al-4V, Trilogy®, uncemented, cpTi fiber mesh.
6 AL (−)	MoP	FeCrNiMn, Exeter®, cemented, polished	CoCrMo	PE	cpTi, Pinnacle®, uncemented porocoat, porous coating.

Criteria for exclusion: infection (positive Kamme-Lindberg biopsies [27]), use of immunomodulating medication, occupational metal exposure, known metal allergies towards implanted metals or secondary osteoarthritis (fracture, inflammation). The mean age for the AL (+) group was 60.8 years with a gender distribution of 4/2 (M/W). For the AL (−) group, the mean age was 73 years, and the distribution was 4/2 (M/W). The control group had a mean age of 62 years and a distribution of 5/3 (M/W). Tissue samples for cytokine and ICP-MS analysis were snap-frozen in liquid nitrogen and stored at −80 °C for later use. Serum obtained from patients blood samples were taken before the operation and stored at −80 °C for later cytokine and ICP-MS analysis.

2.2. Cytokine Profile Analysis

Snap frozen tissue samples from group AL (+), group AL (−) and the control group were mechanically disrupted and homogenized (Precellys®24 and Cryolys®—Bertin Technologies, Bie & Berntsen A/S 2730, Herlev, Denmark) at 4 °C for 4×20 s in lysis buffer containing protease inhibitor cocktail (REF 11836145001, Roche Diagnostics, Indianapolis, IN, USA). Homogenized tissue samples were then spun for 10 min at $10,000 \times G$ at 4 °C (Microcentrifuge 157MP—Ole Dich Instrumentmakers ApS, Hvidovre, Denmark) and the protein concentration in the supernatant was estimated by Bradford protein assay [28] using Coomassie blue (#1610436. Bio-Rad Laboratories, Inc., Hercules, CA, USA). Prior to cytokine analysis, total protein concentrations of the samples were adjusted to 0.5 mg/mL. Cytokine analysis was performed using a validated V-PLEX electrochemiluminescence immunoassays (Meso Scale Discovery, Rockville, MD, USA). A total of 11 cytokines divided on two separate kits were analyzed. Proinflammatory Panel 1 contained; IL-1β, IL-2, IL-4, IL-6, IL-8, IL-10, IFN-γ and TNF-α (catalog # K15049D-1), and cytokine panel 1 kit contained; IL-15, IL-17A, GM-CSF (catalog # K15050D-1). Samples were analyzed in triplicates (MESO QuickPlex SQ 120—Meso Scale Discovery). Calibration curves used to calculate cytokine concentrations were established by fitting to a 4 parameters logistic model with a $1/Y^2$ weighting. Cytokine concentrations were calculated using the Discovery workbench

4.0.12 software (Meso Scale Discovery). Serum samples were analyzed undiluted using the same cytokine kits as used for the tissue.

2.3. Patch Testing

A special patch test series, provided by Smart Practice®(Phoenix, AZ, USA), was used in this study. The patch contained prefabricated panels with metallic compounds associated with orthopedic prostheses on Scanpor tape. Standard metal allergens included; nickel (II) sulphate $NiSO_4$ (1.0 wt.%), potassium dichromate (VI) $K_2Cr_2O_7$ (0.054 wt.%) and cobalt (II) chloride $CoCl_2$ (0.02 wt.%). In addition, a customized panel with the following metals and corresponding titrations were included; vanadium (IV) oxide sulfate hydrate $VOSO_4 \cdot H_2O$ (0.36, 0.18, 0.06, 0.02 wt.%), vanadium (III) chloride VCl_3 (0.24, 0.12, 0.013, 0.04 wt.%), manganese (II) chloride $MnCl_2.4H_2O$ (0.24, 0.08, 0.06, 0.0057 wt.%), aluminum (III) chloride $AlCl_3 \cdot 6H_2O$ (0.72, 0.38, 0.039 wt.%), ammonium molybdate (VI) $(NH_4)_6Mo_7O_{24}$ $4H_2O$ (0.12, 0.013, 0.04 wt.%), titanium (IV) oxalate hydrate $TiC_4O_8 \cdot H_2O$ (0.32, 0.16, 0.08, 0.04 wt.%), titanium (IV) dioxide TiO_2 (0.24 wt.%), potassium titanium (II) oxide oxalate $C_4K_2O_9Ti \cdot 2H_2O$ (2.4, 1.2, 0.6 wt.%), ammonium titanium (II) lactate, solution Ti $[(C_3H_4O_3)_2(NH_4OH)_2]$ (0.16, 0.08, 0.04 wt.%), ammonium titanium (IV) peroxocitrate $(NH_4)_4[Ti_2(C_6H_4O_7)_2(O_2)_2] \cdot 4H_2O$ (0.32, 0.16, 0.08, 0.04 wt.%). methyl methacrylate $C_5H_8O_2$ (2 wt.%), gentamycin sulfate (20 wt.%) and ferrous chloride $FeCl_2$ (2 wt.%) were tested by manually loading of a Finn chamber on Scanpor tape. Patches were applied on the upper back and were occluded for 48 h. Readings were completed 96 h after application [29]. The patients were instructed to remove the panels after 48 h, and not to shower, scratch or expose to sunlight. Reactions were scored using the International Contact Dermatitis Research Group's (ICDRG) criteria [30]. Only definite +1, +2 and +3 reactions were regarded as positive.

2.4. ICP-MS (Serum)

Blood samples were sent to Vejle Hospital, Department of Clinical Biochemistry, Denmark, for determination of chromium and cobalt levels before the surgery. The samples were analyzed by ICP-MS instrument (iCAPq, Thermo Fisher Scientific Inc., Waltham, MA, USA). The samples were diluted with 0.5% HNO_3, gallium was added as an internal standard prior to analysis. The detection limit was 10 nmol/L equivalent to 0.59 ppb (cobalt) and 0.52 ppb (chromium).

2.5. ICP-MS (Tissue and Serum)

Elemental analysis of tissues and titanium (Ti) analysis of blood was performed at the National Food Institute at the Technical University of Denmark.

Elemental analysis in tissues: Tissue samples (0.1–0.5 g) were digested with a mixture of concentrated nitric acid (4 mL; PlasmaPure, SCPScience, Courtaboeuf, France) and hydrogenperoxide (1 mL; Merck, Darmstadt, Germany) in a microwave oven (Multiwave 3000, Anton Paar, Graz, Austria). The concentration of aluminum (Al), vanadium (V), chromium (Cr), cobalt (Co) and nickel (Ni) was determined using ICPMS (iCAPq, Thermo Fisher Scientific, Waltham, MA, USA) using rhodium as an internal standard and external calibration. The ICPMS instrument was run in the kinetic energy discrimination (KED) mode using helium as a collision cell gas. The limit of detection was estimated at 100 µg/kg for all elements.

Determination of Ti in tissue and blood: The acid digests of tissues were also subjected to Ti analysis. Serum subsamples (200 µL) were diluted with 4.8 mL diluent solution consisting of 0.5% Triton X-100, 10% ethanol (both Merck) and 1% nitric acid (SCPScience) prior to the analysis of the concentration of Ti using a triple quadrupole ICPMS (Agilent 8800 ICP-QQQ, Agilent Technologies, Yokogawa, Japan) and using ammonia as a cell gas with determination of Ti after MS/MS mass shift from m/z 48 $\geq$ m/z 150 with scandium (Sc) as internal standard and external calibration. The data quality of Ti analysis was assessed by the analysis of the reference material Seronorm (Sero, Oslo, Norway). The obtained value 7.2 µg/L was in good agreement with the reference value 6.8 µg/L. The limit of detection was estimated at 1 µg/L in serum samples and 20 µg/kg in tissues. All calibration standards and internal standards were produced from certified single-element stock solutions (SCPScience).

2.6. Statistical Analysis

For group comparison the Kruskal-Wallis test was used, and if statistically significant, the Mann-Whitney U test was used to compare between individual groups. By convention, to calculate group medians, metal concentrations below the detection limit were assigned a value of one-half the detection limit. Comparisons were made using the Mann-Whitney test. Contingency tables (patch test) were analyzed using Fisher's exact test. A significance level of $p < 0.05$ was considered statistically significant. Matlab R2014a (8.3.0.532) with statistical toolbox (MathWorks Inc. Natick, MA, USA) was used for statistical analysis. For graphical representation Prism 6.0 (GraphPad Software, San Diego, CA, USA) was used.

3. Results

3.1. Cytokine Profile Analysis

3.1.1. Analysis of Cytokine Levels in Periimplant Tissue

Cytokine levels were measured in periimplant tissue obtained from revision or primary surgery to identify a potential local immune response (Figure 1).

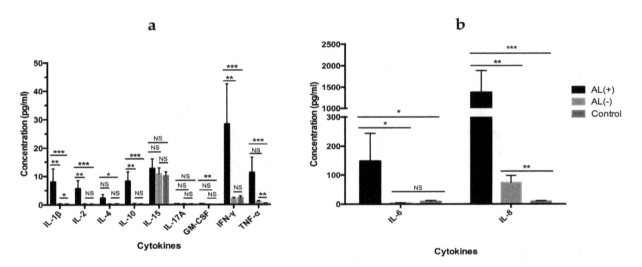

Figure 1. Cytokine profiles of periimplant tissue. Cytokines are shown in graph (**a**) and (**b**) with different concentration scales. Except from IL-15 and IL-17, patients with aseptic loosening AL (+) showed a statistically significant increase in the cytokine levels when compared with the control group. Out of the statistically significant cytokines, IL-4 and TNF-α did not show any statistical significance (NS) when comparing the two revision groups. IL-8 was found to be highly increased in patients with AL. Results are expressed as the mean (±SEM). The Mann-Whitney U test was used for the statistical analysis with a significance level of 0.05. p values are given by $*$ $p < 0.05$, $**$ $p \leq 0.01$, $***$ $p \leq 0.001$.

Altogether, 10 cytokines (IL-1β, IL-2, IL-4, IL-6, IL-8, IL-10, IL-15, IL-17A, IFN-γ and TNF-α) and growth factor GM-CSF were analyzed (Figure 1a/b). We found a highly increased cytokine profile in patients with AL, with a statistical significant increase of IL-1β, IL-2, IL-4, IL-6, IL-8, IL-10, GM-CSF, IFN-γ and TNF-α when compared to the AL (+) and the control group. When compared to the AL (−) group we found a statistically significant increase for all cytokines except from IL-4, IL-15, GM-CSF, and TNF-α. Of note, IL-8 was highly increased and the most strongly associated cytokine with AL.

3.1.2. Analysis of Cytokine Levels in Serum

An identical cytokine profile analysis was performed in serum to investigate a corresponding systemic response (Figure 2). Cytokine levels in serum appeared 10–100 fold lower and although IL-8 and IFN-γ seemed increased in the AL (+) group, no statistical differences could be established. Together these results show a general increase of the investigated cytokine profile, in periimplant tissue obtained from patients with AL, but also that cytokine levels in periimplant tissue are not necessarily reflected in blood serum. Among other increased cytokines, IL-8 was established as the most potent marker of AL.

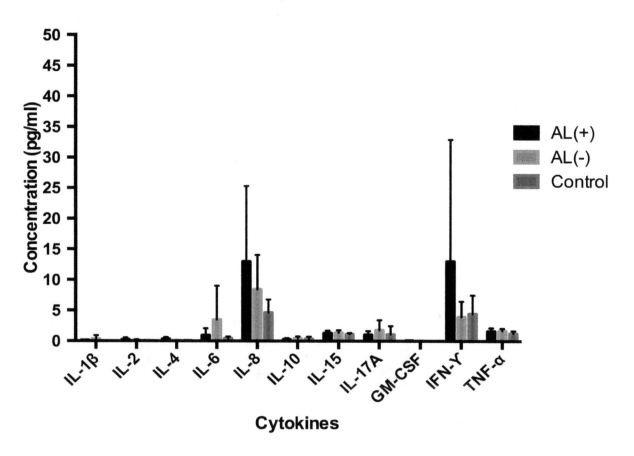

Figure 2. Cytokine profiles in serum. Patients with aseptic loosening are represented as AL (+), patients with dislocations are represented as AL (−) and the controls. Increased IL-8 and IFN-γ levels appeared for the AL (+) group. Results are expressed as the mean concentration (±SEM). No statistically significant differences could be established between the groups using the Mann-Whitney U test with a significance level of 0.05.

3.2. Patch Test

All patient groups were subjected to a comprehensive patch test containing orthopedically relevant metals and methyl methacrylate, the monomer of poly (methyl methacrylate) (PMMA) used as bone cement in THR (Table 2). Positive and doubtful reactions to these metals are summarized in Table 2. No statistical significant differences between either of the groups could be established. Few positive test reaction were observed even for the metals used in the standard series (Cr, Co and Ni), only one reaction to Ni and one to Cr were observed in all three groups. However, three positive reactions for Ti and two positive skin reactions to V were observed in the (AL+) group. In fact, the two positive reactions to V were observed in the same patient who had a positive reaction to Cr (Figure 3).

Table 2. Skin reactions. Positive (+) and doubtful (+?) skin reactions to different metals and methyl methacrylate. Patch test reactions were scored using the International Contact Dermatitis Research Group's (ICDRG) criteria [30]. Only definite +1, +2 and +3 reactions were regarded as positive. No reactions were categorized as +2 and +3 reactions in this study and only compounds with either positive (+1) or doubtful (+?) reactions are listed in the table. Prevalence of positive reactions was tested against the control group using Fisher's exact test with two tailed p values. No statistical significant differences were found.

	AL (+) ($n = 6$)	AL (−) ($n = 6$)	Control ($n = 8$)
	Reactions		
Metal compound (concentration)	+ (+?)	+ (+?)	+ (+?)
Al(III), AlCl$_3$ (0.72%)	0 (0)	0 (0)	0 (1)
Ti(IV), TiC$_4$O$_8$ (0.32%)	0 (0)	1 (0)	2 (0)
Ti(II), C$_4$K$_2$O$_9$Ti (2.4%)	0 (0)	0 (0)	0 (0)
V(III), VCl$_3$ (0.24%)	1 (2)	0 (3)	0 (3)
V(III), VCl$_3$ (0.12%)	1 (0)	0 (1)	0 (3)
V(III), VCl$_3$ (0.013%)	0 (0)	0 (1)	0 (0)
V(III), VCl$_3$ (0.04%)	0 (0)	0 (1)	0 (0)
V(IV), VOSO$_4$ (0.36%)	0 (1)	0 (1)	0 (2)
V(IV), VOSO$_4$ (0.18%)	0 (1)	0 (1)	0 (0)
Cr(VI), K$_2$Cr$_2$O$_7$ (0.054%)	1 (0)	0 (0)	0 (0)
Mn(II), MnCl$_2$ (0.24%)	0 (1)	1 (2)	0 (2)
Ni(II), NiSO$_4$ (5.0%)	0 (0)	0 (0)	1 (1)
Methyl Methacrylate, C$_5$H$_8$O$_2$ (2%)	0 (0)	0 (0)	0 (1)
Total reactions	3 (4)	2 (8)	3 (12)

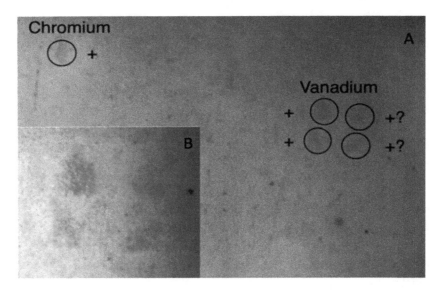

Figure 3. Patch test. (**A**) Example of a positive (+) and a doubtful skin reactions (+?) to vanadium and chromium in a patient from the AL (+) group. (**B**) Enlarged photograph of the skin reaction to vanadium.

3.3. ICP-MS Analysis

3.3.1. Metal Concentrations in Periimplant Tissue

Periimplant tissue was analyzed for Al, Ti, V, Cr, Co and Ni by ICP-MS (Table 3). Raised median concentrations of most metals could be observed in both revision groups, AL (+) and AL (−) as shown in Table 3. Metals found at highest concentrations were, Al, Ti and Cr, although no statistically significant differences could be established between the AL (+) and AL (−) group, however, a difference was observed when compared to the control group. Despite the raised concentrations of Cr observed in the

AL (+) group compared to the control group no statistical significant increase could be determined ($p = 0.074$). These results clearly demonstrate the presence of metal release in the two revision groups.

Table 3. Elemental analysis. Metal concentrations (ppb) measured by ICP-MS in periimplant tissue and blood serum. Titanium, chromium and cobalt were measured in blood serum. Values are shown as group medians with interquartile range below. Statistics are based on medians using the Wilcoxon-Mann-Whitney test with a significance level of 0.05. * Indicate significantly increased values compared to the control group. Elemental analysis for Al, V and Ni was only carried out on tissue samples and are therefore indicated as not available (N/A) for serum samples.

Metal	AL (+) $n = 6$		AL (−) $n = 6$		Control $n = 10$	
	Tissue	Serum	Tissue	Serum	Tissue	Serum
Al	7186 * (1905–29,019)	N/A	3407 * (845–26,709)	N/A	1258 (352–2615)	N/A
Ti	1610 * (891–13,328)	0.65 (0.60–2.95)	12978 * (588–47,078)	1.45 (0.60–3.98)	716.5 (504–1152)	0.60 (0.60–1.00)
V	210 (128–920)	N/A	381 (151–573)	N/A	160 (133–209)	N/A
Cr	3648 (358–21,075)	0.98 * (0.26–3.4)	499 (151–6235)	0.26 (0.26–0.26)	484 (184–1868)	0.26 (0.26–0.26)
Co	210 (128–2724)	0.30 (0.30–1.93)	167 (118–2549)	0.30 (0.30–0.74)	160 (133–209)	0.30 (0.30–0.30)
Ni	772 * (355–2027)	N/A	328 (151–1589)	N/A	212 (162–326)	N/A

3.3.2. Metal Concentrations in Serum

Serum samples were analyzed for Ti, Co and Cr by ICP-MS (Table 3). A statistical significant increase of Cr concentrations in the AL (+) group was found, compared to the control group. No statistical significant increase was observed between the two revision groups ($p = 0.105$). Nevertheless, the highest concentrations of both Co and Cr was found in the AL (+) group. One patient in the control group showed a high concentration of Ti and despite reanalysis, this sample still showed a high Ti concentration, preventing it from being regarded as an outlier. All other Ti concentrations in the control group were at the detection limit of the ICP-MS method. Furthermore, the results show that local metal concentrations in the periimplant tissue can be highly increased compared to serum levels.

4. Discussion

The possibility of metal allergy leading to aseptic loosening has been debated in the literature for many years [21,31–33]. Still, the long-term effect of internally released metals remains unknown and so does the underlining immunological response lead to AL and implant failure [22]. In this study we investigated the correlations between the immunological profile, metal allergy and metal released from implants, in THR patients with AL.

We found that patients with AL had a cytokine profile with statistically significant increased levels of the pro-inflammatory cytokines IL-1β, IL-6, and IL-8, but also Th1 associated cytokines, IL-2 and IFN-γ, and the anti-inflammatory cytokine IL-10, when compared to patients with implant failures due to mechanical causes. Despite a statistically significant and substantial metal exposure both locally and systemically in THR patients, we were not able to prove any systemic effect by cytokine analysis of serum or by positive patch testing. Based on the present study, a systemic effect cannot be ruled out due to the low number of patients enrolled in this study. The findings are, however, in line with the clinical observations, where the adverse effect to implants is predominantly observed locally rather than systemically. A further limitation of this study was the clinical approach, where polyethylene (PE) debris derived from the acetabular liner is most likely contributing the innate part of the cytokine profile observed in the periimplant tissue.

Cytokines play an important role in AL, not only as regulators of osteolysis, but also as important identifiers of the occurring immune response. In our cytokine analysis we included IL-1β IL-2, IL-4, IL-6, IL-8, IL-10, IL-15, IL-17A, GM-CSF, IFN-γ and TNF-α due to their implication in innate and adaptive immunity and their function as osteolytic mediators (Figures 1 and 2). In addition to being involved in the innate immune response, IL-1β, IL-6, IL-8, GM-CSF, and TNF-α have previously been identified as mediators of osteolysis [14,34]. In accordance with these observations, we found elevated levels of these cytokines in the periimplant tissue from the AL (+) group when compared to the control group. When comparing the two revision groups, AL (+) and AL (−), no statistically significant difference was seen for GM-CSF and TNF-α. However, levels of GM-CSF were very low and might be considered without any biological effect. TNF-α is well-known as a strong inducer of osteolysis and is the first proinflammatory cytokine produced in response to many wear particles and stimulates macrophage production of IL-1β and IL-6 [35]. Although no statistically significance is seen for TNF-α between the two revision groups, both IL-1β and IL-6 still showed a statistically significant increase in the AL (+) group. In comparison, other investigators have found low levels of IL-1β and TNF-α in periimplant tissue from patients with failed THRs due to osteolysis [36]. Moreover, they found that IL-6 and IL-8 were consistent with failed implants, suggesting that IL-6 and IL-8 might be the primary drivers of end-stage osteolysis, while IL-1β and TNF-α are critical mediators in the acute phase of inflammation. Interestingly, these observations did indeed correspond well to our findings of IL-6 and notably IL-8, which we found to be the strongest predictor of AL.

The main IL-8 secreting cells are macrophages, osteoblasts and osteoclasts. Studies have shown that IL-8 holds multiple functions in AL and has been found to affect both neutrophils, T cells, monocyte/macrophages and osteoclasts [37,38]. It has been demonstrated that wear particle stimulation of osteoblasts and macrophages promotes IL-8 production, which in turn can lead to both macrophage activation and induce phagocytosis [39]. Interleukin-8 also possess chemotactic properties on neutrophils and T cells and could conceivably play a role in attracting such cells to the periimplant tissue [37,40]. Moreover, IL-8 is shown to promote osteoclastogenesis and the formation of osteoclasts that are capable of secreting IL-8 on their own. Thus, the high levels of IL-8 observed in patients with AL is probably not only caused by an innate immune response but also in part by the osteolytic process taking place in the patients with AL, which could explain the differences in IL-8 observed between the AL (+) and the AL (−) group [40].

As indicators of DTH, IL-2 and IFN-γ levels were statistical significantly increased in the AL (+) group compared to the AL (−), supporting the involvement of a Th1 cell response in AL. This is consistent with other studies, showing lymphocyte reactivity to implant related metals and production of Th1-specific cytokines (IFN-γ and IL-2), and even the generation of metal specific T cells [41,42]. Macrophages are capable of producing IFN-γ but abundant evidence suggests that T cells and natural killer (NK) cells are the major sources of IFN-γ [3,43,44]. Accompanied by the increased levels of IL-2, the increased IFN-γ levels found in patients with AL further support the involvement of a Th1 cell response. Interferon-gamma possess both pro- and anti-inflammatory activities with the functional outcome being dependent on secretion levels, pathogenesis and disease severity [13,44]. Some studies show a protective effect of IFN-γ on osteolysis, possible by inhibiting the early differentiation of osteoclasts, whereas others have shown that IFN-γ promotes osteoclast formation [13]. How IFN-γ affects the progression of AL in this study is difficult to decipher but low levels of IFN-γ does not exert the inhibitory effect on osteoclasts and seems to be limited to the early stage of osteoclast differentiation. Furthermore, IFN-γ can promote osteoclast maturation in the late state of osteoclast formation leading to a shift from the inhibitory effect towards a state of bone resorption [45].

In addition to the Th1 signature cytokines, we also observed an increase of IL-4, along with a statistically significant increase of IL-10 when comparing the two revision groups.

Although the production of these cytokines are related to Th2 cells, IL-10 is also produced by monocytes and regulatory T cells, acting as an anti-inflammatory cytokine, which could regulate cell-mediated reactions involved in AL [46–48]. We were not able to detect any consistent cytokine profile at a systemic level in serum, underlining the difficulty of detecting AL based on the systemic levels of cytokines. In fact, cytokines have a short half-life in serum due to their potent nature as signaling molecules, which makes cytokines very challenging to use as biomarkers in serum [49].

In our analysis of Ti, Co and Cr in serum, we found a statistically significant increase of Cr in the AL (+) group and Ti in the Al (−) group (Table 3). Furthermore, we did detect a correlation between raised Ti concentrations in serum from patients with a stem component made from a Ti containing alloy, which corresponds to the findings of other studies applying the ICP-MS method [50]. Metal release, has previously been shown to increase in patients with poorly functioning implants [17]. From a corrosion point of view, this could be explained by increased micro-motions of the implant leading to fretting corrosion [20,51]. Fretting of the Ti6Al4V and the Orthinox SS alloys could contribute to the statistically significant raise in Al, Ti, and Ni observed in the revision groups (Table 4) [52,53]. Highest concentrations of Co and Cr were detected in the AL (+) group. One patient in this group had a MoM implant but no markedly increased in Co or Cr concentrations were detected in either periimplant tissue or serum from this specific patient. Interestingly, relative low concentrations of Co were found in tissue and blood samples compared to Cr concentrations. This observation has previously been explained by a faster elimination of Co from both the tissue and blood than that of Cr [54]. No upper limits are currently employed to describe critical metal release from implants, but an upper limit of 7 ppb for Co and Cr in blood is often used as an action level for MoM implants [55]. Serum concentrations of this magnitude were not detected in this study. In general, our results confirm previous metal concentrations reported in serum and periimplant tissue from patients with poorly functioning implants [17]. A correlation between the metal content in periimplant tissue but not that of serum has recently been made to a lymphocyte dominated response [56]. This emphasizes the importance of the periimplant environment, in which we found highly raised metal concentrations.

Table 4. Alloy composition. Elemental composition of the different implant alloys found patient groups, based on the ASTM international standard.

Implant Alloy	CoCrMo ASTM-(F75)	Orthinox SS ASTM-(F1586)	cpTi ASTM-(F67)	Ti6Al7Nb ASTM-(F1295)	Ti6Al4V ASTM-(F136)
Element	Composition, wt.%				
Aluminum (Al)	0.10	-	0.03	5.50–6.50	5.5–6.50
Carbon (C)	0.35	0.08	0.08	0.08	0.08
Chromium (Cr)	27–30	19.5–22	-	-	-
Cobalt (Co)	Balance	-	-	-	-
Copper (Cu)	-	0.25	0.10	-	-
Iron (Fe)	0.75	Balance	0.50	0.25	0.25
Manganese (Mn)	1	2–4.25	-	-	-
Molybdenum (Mo)	5–7	2–3	-	-	-
Nickel (Ni)	0.50	9.0–11.0	-	-	-
Niobium (Nb)	-	0.25–0.8	0.015	6.50–7.50	-
Nitrogen (N)	0.25	0.25–0.5	0.15	0.05	0.05
Oxygen (O)	-	-	0.40	0.20	0.13
Tantalum (Ta)	-	-	Balance	0.50	-
Titanium (Ti)	0.10	-	-	Balance	Balance
Tungsten (W)	0.20	-	-	-	-
Vanadium (V)	-	-	-	-	3.5–4.5

In this study implants with different fixation strategies was used i.e. cemented implants and different surface treatments for optimizing stability and osseointegration. Metal release and implant performance is highly dependent on the micro/nano topography of the implant surface [57,58]. Cemented implants have been proved to increased initial stability and minimize micro-motions of cemented parts leading to long survival rates [59]. The downside of this approach is the possible formation of a crevice between the cement and implant, which can provide a highly corrosive environment and lead to accelerated corrosion and subsequently implant failure by AL [60,61]. All uncemented implants in this study had some form of increased roughness applied to their surfaces for optimal osseointegration (Table 1). One of the costs of increasing the surface roughness on implant is an increased functional surface area, which in turn will increase metal release. Especially titanium release has recently become a subject of concern and not only in implants used for THRs [62–65]. Another debated strategy of improving osseointegration is the use of hydroxyapatite (HA) coatings, simulating the bone chemistry and structure. However, recent studies suggest that the long-term effects are not improved compared to other porous coatings or rough sandblasted surfaces [66,67].

Patch testing showed a diverse profile of test reactions across all groups making results difficult to interpret (Table 2). Metals salts are well-known skin irritants and skin reactions may therefore, in reality, be an irritant rather than an allergic reaction. On the other hand, a positive reaction can only occur if the metal reaches the viable layers of the epidermis, and this might be a challenge for some metals [68]. One patient in the AL (+) group had a positive reaction to Cr, which is higher than expected considering that less than 1% of the general population are allergic to Cr [69]. Surprisingly, we found positive reactions to Ti (IV) in the control group, which had not been exposed to Ti containing implants. Although Ti allergy is considered very limited in THRs, in vitro studies of Ti particles suggest that these can initiate innate and adaptive Th2 cell response [68,70]. Within the field of odontology there is a growing concern of the innate immune response associated with Ti, which is believed to cause osteolysis through macrophage secretion of IL1β, IL6, and TNFα [6,71]. A relative high number of skin reactions to V were observed, although most of these were scored as doubtful, true allergy cannot be ruled out. While larger cohort studies have found an increased prevalence of metal allergy in THR patients our study was not powered to examine a possible association [21,72]. Nonetheless, our findings indicate that metal allergy, as tested by patch test, is not likely to be a key driver of AL in most patients.

5. Conclusions

Aseptic loosening of implants is a complex tissue response influenced by various factors. Metal release from implants may generate DTH response capable of accelerating aseptic loosening of implants. In this study, we report a distinct cytokine profile in periimplant tissues between patients with implant failure due to AL, compared to mechanical causes, with statistically significant increased levels of IL-1β, IL-2, IL-4, IL-6, IL-8, IL-10, GM-CSF, IFN-γ and TNF-α. In addition, raised metal concentrations were found in blood and periimplant tissue from patients with failed THRs. Despite these observations, we failed to detect any correlation between the prevalence of metal allergy and failed THRs or AL. This work contributes to a better understanding of the immunologic nature of aseptic loosening and suggests that the immunological events involved in AL are of both innate and adaptive character.

Author Contributions: Composer of manuscript, study design, acquisition of cytokine data, analysis and interpretation of data obtained from ICP-MS and patch test, R.J.C. Research design, acquisition of patch test data, patient recruitment and sample collection from patients and critical revising of manuscript draft, H.J.M. Research design, interpretation of cytokine data, critical revising of manuscript draft and final approval of manuscript, C.M.B. Interpretation of patch test results and critical revising of manuscript draft, J.P.T. Acquisition of ICP-MS data and interpretation of these, J.J.S. Critical revising of manuscript draft, on allergy and cytokine data, C.G. Study design, critical revising and approval of final approval of manuscript, K.S. Interpretation of ICP-MS data and critical revising on corrosion/metal release from implants and final approval of manuscript, M.S.J. Study design, patient recruitment and sample collection from patients and critical revising of manuscript draft and final approval of manuscript, S.S.J.

References

1.   Camuzard, O.; Breuil, V.; Carle, G.F.; Pierrefite-Carle, V. Autophagy Involvement in Aseptic Loosening of Arthroplasty Components. *J. Bone Jt. Surg.* **2019**, *101*, 466–472. [CrossRef] [PubMed]

2.   Ulrich, S.D.; Seyler, T.M.; Bennett, D.; Delanois, R.E.; Saleh, K.J.; Thongtrangan, I.; Kuskowski, M.; Cheng, E.Y.; Sharkey, P.F.; Parvizi, J.; et al. Total Hip Arthroplasties: What Are the Reasons for Revision? *Int. Orthop.* **2008**, *32*, 597–604. [CrossRef] [PubMed]

3.   Cobelli, N.; Scharf, B.; Crisi, G.M.; Hardin, J.; Santambrogio, L. Mediators of the Inflammatory Response to Joint Replacement Devices. *Nat. Rev. Rheumatol.* **2011**, *7*, 600–608. [CrossRef] [PubMed]

4.   Gallo, J.; Goodman, S.B.; Konttinen, Y.T.; Raska, M. Particle Disease: Biologic Mechanisms of Periprosthetic Osteolysis in Total Hip Arthroplasty. *Innate Immun.* **2013**, *19*, 213–224. [CrossRef] [PubMed]

5.   Holt, G.; Murnaghan, C.; Reilly, J.; Meek, R.M.D.; Features, S. The Biology of Aseptic Osteolysis. *Clin. Orthop. Relat. Res.* **2007**, *460*, 240–252. [CrossRef] [PubMed]

6.   Eger, M.; Sterer, N.; Liron, T.; Kohavi, D.; Gabet, Y. Scaling of Titanium Implants Entrains Inflammation-Induced Osteolysis. *Sci. Rep.* **2017**, *7*, 39612. [CrossRef] [PubMed]

7.   Dyskova, T.; Gallo, J.; Kriegova, E. The Role of the Chemokine System in Tissue Response to Prosthetic By-Products Leading to Periprosthetic Osteolysis and Aseptic Loosening. *Front. Immunol.* **2017**, *8*. [CrossRef]

8.   Hallab, N.J.; Jacobs, J.J. Chemokines Associated with Pathologic Responses to Orthopedic Implant Debris. *Front. Endocrinol.* **2017**, *8*, 5. [CrossRef]

9.   Nich, C.; Takakubo, Y.; Pajarinen, J.; Ainola, M.; Salem, A.; Sillat, T.; Rao, A.J.; Raska, M.; Tamaki, Y.; Takagi, M.; et al. Macrophages-Key Cells in the Response to Wear Debris from Joint Replacements. *J. Biomed. Mater. Res. A* **2013**, *101*, 3033–3045. [CrossRef]

10. Stea, S.; Visentin, M.; Granchi, D.; Ciapetti, G.; Donati, M.; Sudanese, A.; Zanotti, C.; Toni, A. Cytokines and Osteolysis Around Total Hip Prostheses. *Cytokine* **2000**, *12*, 1575–1579. [CrossRef]

11. Wolfe, J.; Goldberg, J.; Harris, H. Production of Cytokines around Loosened Cemented Acetabular Components. *J. Bone Jt. Surg.* **1993**, *75*, 663–879.

12. Fiorillo, L.; Cervino, G.; Herford, A.; Lauritano, F.; D'Amico, C.; Lo Giudice, R.; Laino, L.; Troiano, G.; Crimi, S.; Cicciù, M. Interferon Crevicular Fluid Profile and Correlation with Periodontal Disease and Wound Healing: A Systemic Review of Recent Data. *Int. J. Mol. Sci.* **2018**, *19*, 1908. [CrossRef] [PubMed]

13. Tang, M.; Tian, L.; Luo, G.; Yu, X. Interferon-Gamma-Mediated Osteoimmunology. *Front. Immunol.* **2018**, *9*. [CrossRef] [PubMed]

14. Goodman, S.B.; Huie, P.; Song, Y.; Schurman, D.; Maloney, W.; Woolson, S.; Sibley, R. Cellular Profile and Cytokine Production at Prosthetic Interfaces. Study of Tissues Retrieved from Revised Hip and Knee Replacements. *J. Bone Joint Surg. Br.* **1998**, *80*, 531–539. [CrossRef] [PubMed]

15. Kadoya, Y.; Revell, P.A.; Al-Saffar, N.; Kobayashi, A.; Scott, G.; Freeman, M.A.R. Bone Formation and Bone Resorption in Failed Total Joint Arthroplasties: Histomorphometric Analysis with Histochemical and Immunohistochemical Technique. *J. Orthop. Res.* **1996**, *14*, 473–482. [CrossRef] [PubMed]

16. Büdinger, L.; Hertl, M. Immunologic Mechanisms in Hypersensitivity Reactions to Metal Ions: An Overview. *Allergy* **2000**, *55*, 108–115. [CrossRef]

17. Hallab, N.J.; Mikecz, K.; Vermes, C.; Skipor, A.; Jacobs, J.J. Orthopaedic Implant Related Metal Toxicity in Terms of Human Lymphocyte Reactivity to Metal-Protein Complexes Produced from Cobalt-Base and Titanium-Base Implant Alloy Degradation. *Mol. Cell. Biochem.* **2001**, *222*, 127–136. [CrossRef] [PubMed]

18. Sundfeldt, M.; Carlsson, L.V.; Johansson, C.B.; Thomsen, P.; Gretzer, C. Aseptic Loosening, Not Only a Question of Wear: A Review of Different Theories. *Acta Orthop.* **2006**, *77*, 177–197. [CrossRef]

19. Grosse, S.; Haugland, H.K.; Lilleng, P.; Ellison, P.; Hallan, G.; Høl, P.J. Wear Particles and Ions from Cemented and Uncemented Titanium-Based Hip Prostheses-A Histological and Chemical Analysis of Retrieval Material. *J. Biomed. Mater. Res. Part B Appl. Biomater.* **2015**, *103*, 709–717. [CrossRef]

20. McGrath, L.R.; Shardlow, D.L.; Ingham, E.; Andrews, M.; Ivory, J.; Stone, M.H.; Fisher, J. A Retrieval Study of Capital Hip Prostheses with Titanium Alloy Femoral Stems. *J. Bone Jt. Surg. Ser. B* **2001**, *83*, 1195–1201. [CrossRef]

21. Frigerio, E.; Pigatto, P.D.; Guzzi, G.; Altomare, G. Metal Sensitivity in Patients with Orthopaedic Implants: A Prospective Study. *Contact Dermat.* **2011**, *64*, 273–279. [CrossRef]

22. Hallab, N. Metal Sensitivity in Patients with Orthopedic Implants. *J. Clin. Rheumatol.* **2001**, *7*, 215–218. [CrossRef]

23. Schmidt, M.; Goebeler, M. Immunology of Metal Allergies. *JDDG J. Der Dtsch. Dermatol. Ges.* **2015**, *13*, 653–659. [CrossRef]

24. Summer, B.; Paul, C.; Mazoochian, F.; Rau, C.; Thomsen, M.; Banke, I.; Gollwitzer, H.; Dietrich, K.; Mayer-Wagner, S.; Ruzicka, T.; et al. Nickel (Ni) Allergic Patients with Complications to Ni Containing Joint Replacement Show Preferential IL-17 Type Reactivity to Ni. *Contact Dermat.* **2010**, *63*, 15–22. [CrossRef] [PubMed]

25. Arora, A.; Song, Y.; Chun, L.; Huie, P.; Trindade, M.; Smith, R.L.; Goodman, S. The Role of the TH1 and TH2 Immune Responses in Loosening and Osteolysis of Cemented Total Hip Replacements. *J. Biomed. Mater. Res. A* **2003**, *64*, 693–697. [CrossRef]

26. Looney, R.J.; Schwarz, E.M.; Boyd, A.; O'Keefe, R.J. Periprosthetic Osteolysis: An Immunologist's Update. *Curr. Opin. Rheumatol.* **2006**, *18*, 80–87. [CrossRef] [PubMed]

27. Kamme, C.L.L. Aerobic and Anaerobic Bacteria in Deep Infections after Total Hip Arthroplasty: Differential Diagnosis between Infectious and Non-Infectious Loosening. *Clin. Orthop. Relat. Res.* **1981**, *154*, 201–207. [CrossRef]

28. Bradford, M.M. A Rapid and Sensitive Method for the Quantitation of Microgram Quantities of Protein Utilizing the Principle of Protein-Dye Binding. *Anal. Biochem.* **1976**, *72*, 248–254. [CrossRef]

29. Todd, D.J.; Hasdlev, J.; Metwali, M.; Allen, G.E.; Burrows, D. Day 4 Is Better than Day 3 for a Single Patch Test Reading. *Contact Dermat.* **1996**, *34*, 402–404. [CrossRef]

30. Wilkinson, D.S.; Fregert, S.; Magnusson, B.; Bandmann, H.J.; Calnan, C.D.; Cronin, E.; Hjort, N.; Maibach, H.J.; Malten, K.E.; Meneghini, C.L.; et al. Terminology of Contact Dermatitis. *Acta Derm. Venereol.* **1970**, *50*, 287–292.

31. Krecisz, B.; Kieć-Swierczyńska, M.; Bakowicz-Mitura, K. Allergy to Metals as a Cause of Orthopedic Implant Failure. *Int. J. Occup. Med. Environ. Health* **2006**, *19*, 178–180. [CrossRef]

32. Thyssen, J.P.; Jakobsen, S.S.; Engkilde, K.; Johansen, J.D.; Søballe, K.; Menné, T. The Association between Metal Allergy, Total Knee Arthroplasty, and Revision. *Acta Orthop.* **2015**, *86*, 378–383. [CrossRef]

33. Granchi, D.; Cenni, E.; Giunti, A.; Baldini, N. Metal Hypersensitivity Testing in Patients Undergoing Joint Replacement. *J. Bone Jt. Surg. Br.* **2012**, *94-B*, 1126–1134. [CrossRef]

34. Konttinen, Y.; Xu, J.W.; Pätiälä, H.; Imai, S.; Waris, V.; Li, T.F.; Goodman, S.; Nordsletten, L.; Santavirta, S. Cytokines in Aseptic Loosening of Total Hip Replacement. *Curr. Orthop.* **1997**, *11*, 40–47. [CrossRef]

35. Hirayama, T.; Tamaki, Y.; Takakubo, Y.; Iwazaki, K.; Sasaki, K.; Ogino, T.; Goodman, S.B.; Konttinen, Y.T.; Takagi, M. Toll-like Receptors and Their Adaptors Are Regulated in Macrophages after Phagocytosis of Lipopolysaccharide-Coated Titanium Particles. *J. Orthop. Res.* **2011**, *29*, 984–992. [CrossRef]

36. Shanbhag, A.S.; Kaufman, A.M.; Hayata, K.; Rubash, H.E. Assessing Osteolysis with Use of High-Throughput Protein Chips. *J. Bone Jt. Surg. Am.* **2007**, *89*, 1081–1089. [CrossRef]

37. Baggiolini, M.; Loetscher, P.; Moser, B. Interleukin-8 and the Chemokine Family. *Int. J. Immunopharmacol.* **1995**, *17*, 103–108. [CrossRef]

38. Bendre, M.S.; Montague, D.C.; Peery, T.; Akel, N.S.; Gaddy, D.; Suva, L.J. Interleukin-8 Stimulation of Osteoclastogenesis and Bone Resorption Is a Mechanism for the Increased Osteolysis of Metastatic Bone Disease. *Bone* **2003**, *33*, 28–37. [CrossRef]

39. Fritz, E.A.; Jacobs, J.J.; Roebuck, A. Chemokine IL-8 Induction by Particulate Wear Debris in Osteoblasts Is Mediated by NF-KB. *J. Orthop. Res.* **2005**, *23*, 1249–1257. [CrossRef]

40. Qin, S.; Larosa, G.; Campbell, J.J.; Smith-heath, H.; Kassam, N.; Zeng, L.; Butcher, E.C.; Mackay, C.R. Expression of Monocyte Chemoattractant Protein-1 and Interleukin-8 Receptors on Subsets of T Cells: Correlation with Transendothelial Chemotactic Potential. *Eur. J. Immunol.* **1996**, *26*, 640–647. [CrossRef]

41. Chan, E.; Cadosch, D.; Gautschi, O.P.; Sprengel, K.; Filgueira, L. Influence of Metal Ions on Human Lymphocytes and the Generation of Titanium-Specific T-Lymphocytes. *J. Appl. Biomater. Biomech.* **2011**, *9*, 137–143. [CrossRef]

42. Hallab, N.J.; Anderson, S.; Stafford, T.; Glant, T.; Jacobs, J.J. Lymphocyte Responses in Patients with Total Hip Arthroplasty. *J. Orthop. Res.* **2005**, *23*, 384–391. [CrossRef]

43. Valladares, R.D.; Nich, C.; Zwingenberger, S.; Li, C.; Swank, K.R.; Gibon, E.; Rao, A.J.; Yao, Z.; Goodman, S.B. Toll-like Receptors-2 and 4 Are Overexpressed in an Experimental Model of Particle-Induced Osteolysis. *J. Biomed. Mater. Res. Part A* **2014**, *102*, 3004–3011. [CrossRef]

44. Lees, J.R. Interferon Gamma in Autoimmunity: A Complicated Player on a Complex Stage. *Cytokine* **2015**, *74*, 18–26. [CrossRef]

45. Kim, J.W.; Lee, M.S.; Lee, C.H.; Kim, H.Y.; Chae, S.U.; Kwak, H.B.; Oh, J. Effect of Interferon-γ on the Fusion of Mononuclear Osteoclasts into Bone-Resorbing Osteoclasts. *BMB Rep.* **2012**, *45*, 281–286. [CrossRef]

46. Couper, K.; Blount, D.; Riley, E. IL-10: The Master Regulator of Immunity to Infection. *J. Immunol.* **2008**, *180*, 5771–5777. [CrossRef]

47. Van Roon, J.A.G.; Van Roy, J.L.A.M.; Gmelig-Meyling, F.H.J.; Lafeber, F.P.J.G.; Bijlsma, J.W.J. Prevention and Reversal of Cartilage Degradation in Rheumatoid Arthritis by Interleukin-10 and Interleukin-4. *Arthritis Rheum.* **1996**, *39*, 829–835. [CrossRef]

48. Perretti, M.; Szabó, C.; Thiemermann, C. Effect of Interleukin-4 and Interleukin-10 on Leucocyte Migration and Nitric Oxide Production in the Mouse. *Br. J. Pharmacol.* **1995**, *116*, 2251–2257. [CrossRef]

49. Tarrant, J.M. Blood Cytokines as Biomarkers of In Vivo Toxicity in Preclinical Safety Assessment: Considerations for Their Use. *Toxicol. Sci.* **2010**, *117*, 4–16. [CrossRef]

50. Sarmiento-González, A.; Marchante-Gayón, J.M.; Tejerina-Lobo, J.M.; Paz-Jiménez, J.; Sanz-Medel, A. High-Resolution ICP–MS Determination of Ti, V, Cr, Co, Ni and Mo in Human Blood and Urine of Patients Implanted with a Hip or Knee Prosthesis. *Anal. Bioanal. Chem.* **2008**, *391*, 2583–2589. [CrossRef]

51. Revell, P.A. The Combined Role of Wear Particles, Macrophages and Lymphocytes in the Loosening of Total Joint Prostheses. *J. R. Soc. Interface* **2008**, *5*, 1263–1278. [CrossRef]

52. Pound, B.G. Corrosion Behavior of Metallic Materials in Biomedical Applications. I. Ti and Its Alloys. *Corros. Rev.* **2014**, *32*, 1–20. [CrossRef]

53. Pellier, J.; Geringer, J.; Forest, B. Fretting-Corrosion between 316L SS and PMMA: Influence of Ionic Strength, Protein and Electrochemical Conditions on Material Wear. Application to Orthopaedic Implants. *Wear* **2011**, *271*, 1563–1571. [CrossRef]

54. Merritt, K.; Brown, S.A. Distribution of Cobalt Chromium Wear and Corrosion Products and Biologic Reactions. *Clin. Orthop. Relat. Res.* **1996**, *329*, 233–243. [CrossRef]

55. Hart, A.J.; Sabah, S.A.; Bandi, A.S.; Maggiore, P.; Tarassoli, P.; Sampson, B.; Skinner, J.A. Sensitivity and Specificity of Blood Cobalt and Chromium Metal Ions for Predicting Failure of Metal-on-Metal Hip Replacement. *J. Bone Jt. Surg. Br. Vol.* **2011**, *93-B*, 1308–1313. [CrossRef]

56. Lohmann, C.H.; Meyer, H.; Nuechtern, J.V.; Singh, G.; Schmotzer, H.; Morlock, M.M. Periprosthetic Tissue Metal Content but Not Serum Metal Content Predicts the Type of Tissue Response in Failed Small-Diameter Metal-on-Metal Total Hip Arthroplasties. *J. Bone Jt. Surg.* **2013**, *95*, 1561–1568. [CrossRef]

57. Cicciù, M.; Fiorillo, L.; Herford, A.S.; Crimi, S.; Bianchi, A.; D'Amico, C.; Laino, L.; Cervino, G. Bioactive Titanium Surfaces: Interactions of Eukaryotic and Prokaryotic Cells of Nano Devices Applied to Dental Practice. *Biomedicines* **2019**, *7*, 12. [CrossRef]

58. Cervino, G.; Fiorillo, L.; Iannello, G.; Santonocito, D.; Risitano, G.; Cicciù, M. Sandblasted and Acid Etched Titanium Dental Implant Surfaces Systematic Review and Confocal Microscopy Evaluation. *Materials (Basel)* **2019**, *12*, 1763. [CrossRef]

59. Howell, J.R. Cemented Hip Arthroplasty: Why I Do It. *Orthop. Trauma* **2018**, *32*, 13–19. [CrossRef]

60. Thomas, S.R.; Shukla, D.; Latham, P.D. Corrosion of Cemented Titanium Femoral Stems. *J. Bone Jt. Surg. Br.* **2004**, *86-B*, 974–978. [CrossRef]

61. Cohen, J. Current Concepts Review. Corrosion of Metal Orthopaedic Implants. *J. Bone Jt. Surg. Am.* **1998**, *80*, 1554. [CrossRef]

62. Cadosch, D.; Sutanto, M.; Chan, E.; Mhawi, A.; Gautschi, O.P.; von Katterfeld, B.; Simmen, H.P.; Filgueira, L. Titanium Uptake, Induction of RANK-L Expression, and Enhanced Proliferation of Human T-Lymphocytes. *J. Orthop. Res.* **2010**, *28*, 341–347. [CrossRef]

63. Dmd, R.T.; Albrektsson, T.; Dds, S.G.; Prgomet, Z.; Tengvall, P.; Dds, A.W. Osseointegration and Foreign Body Reaction: Titanium Implants Activate the Immune System and Suppress Bone Resorption during the First 4 Weeks after Implantation. *Clin. Implant Dent. Relat. Res.* **2018**, *2017*, 82–91. [CrossRef]

64. Cadosch, D.; Chan, E.; Gautschi, O.P.; Meagher, J.; Zellweger, R.; Filgueira, L. Titanium IV Ions Induced Human Osteoclast Differentiation and Enhanced Bone Resorption in Vitro. *J. Biomed. Mater. Res. A* **2009**, *91*, 29–36. [CrossRef]

65. Nuevo-Ordóñez, Y.; Montes-Bayón, M.; Blanco-González, E.; Paz-Aparicio, J.; Raimundez, J.D.; Tejerina, J.M.; Peña, M.A.; Sanz-Medel, A. Titanium Release in Serum of Patients with Different Bone Fixation Implants and Its Interaction with Serum Biomolecules at Physiological Levels. *Anal. Bioanal. Chem.* **2011**, *401*, 2747–2754. [CrossRef]

66. Lazarinis, S.; Mäkelä, K.T.; Eskelinen, A.; Havelin, L.; Hallan, G.; Overgaard, S.; Pedersen, A.B.; Kärrholm, J.; Hailer, N.P. Does Hydroxyapatite Coating of Uncemented Cups Improve Long-Term Survival? An Analysis of 28,605 Primary Total Hip Arthroplasty Procedures from the Nordic Arthroplasty Register Association (NARA). *Osteoarthr. Cartil.* **2017**, *25*, 1980–1987. [CrossRef]

67. Hailer, N.P.; Lazarinis, S.; Mäkelä, K.T.; Eskelinen, A.; Fenstad, A.M.; Hallan, G.; Havelin, L.; Overgaard, S.; Pedersen, A.B.; Mehnert, F.; et al. Hydroxyapatite Coating Does Not Improve Uncemented Stem Survival after Total Hip Arthroplasty! *Acta Orthop.* **2015**, *86*, 18–25. [CrossRef]

68. Fage, S.W.; Muris, J.; Jakobsen, S.S.; Thyssen, J.P. Titanium: A Review on Exposure, Release, Penetration, Allergy, Epidemiology, and Clinical Reactivity. *Contact Dermat.* **2016** *74*, 323–345. [CrossRef]

69. Thyssen, J.P.; Jensen, P.; Carlsen, B.C.; Engkilde, K.; Menné, T.; Johansen, J.D. The Prevalence of Chromium Allergy in Denmark Is Currently Increasing as a Result of Leather Exposure. *Br. J. Dermatol.* **2009**, *161*, 1288–1293. [CrossRef]

70. Mishra, P.K.; Wu, W.; Rozo, C.; Hallab, N.J.; Benevenia, J.; Gause, W.C. Micrometer-Sized Titanium Particles Can Induce Potent Th2-Type Responses through TLR4-Independent Pathways. *J. Immunol.* **2011**, *187*, 6491–6498. [CrossRef]

71. Eger, M.; Hiram-Bab, S.; Liron, T.; Sterer, N.; Carmi, Y.; Kohavi, D.; Gabet, Y. Mechanism and Prevention of Titanium Particle-Induced Inflammation and Osteolysis. *Front. Immunol.* **2018**, *9*. [CrossRef]

72. Thomas, P.; Braathen, L.R.; Dörig, M.; Aubock, J.; Nestle, F.; Werfel, T.; Willert, H.G. Increased Metal Allergy in Patients with Failed Metal-on-Metal Hip Arthroplasty and Peri-Implant T-Lymphocytic Inflammation. *Allergy Eur. J. Allergy Clin. Immunol.* **2009**, *64*, 1157–1165. [CrossRef]

17

The Effect of Tapered Abutments on Marginal Bone Level: A Retrospective Cohort Study

Simone Marconcini [1,*], **Enrica Giammarinaro** [2], **Ugo Covani** [1], **Eitan Mijiritsky** [3], **Xavier Vela** [4] **and Xavier Rodríguez** [5]

1   Department of Surgical, Medical, Molecular and Critical Area Pathology, University of Pisa, 56124 Pisa, Italy
2   Tuscan Dental Institute, Versilia General Hospital, 55041 Lido di Camaiore, Italy
3   Department of Otolaryngology Head and Neck Surgery and Maxillofacial Surgery, Tel-Aviv Sourasky Medical Center, Sackler School of Medicine, 61503 Tel Aviv, Israel
4   Department of Maxillofacial Surgery and Implantology, International University of Catalunya, 08001 Barcelona, Spain
5   Department of Oral Implantology, European University of Madrid, 28001 Madrid, Spain
*   Correspondence: simosurg@gmail.com

Abstract: Background: Early peri-implant bone loss has been associated to long-term implant-prosthetic failure. Different technical, surgical, and prosthetic techniques have been introduced to enhance the clinical outcome of dental implants in terms of crestal bone preservation. The aim of the present cohort study was to observe the mean marginal bone level around two-part implants with gingivally tapered abutments one year after loading. Methods: Mean marginal bone levels and change were computed following radiological calibration and linear measurement on standardized radiographs. Results: Twenty patients who met the inclusion criterion of having at least one implant with the tapered prosthetic connection were included in the study. The cumulative implant success rate was 100%, the average bone loss was -0.18 ± 0.72 mm, with the final bone level sitting above the implant platform most of the time ($+1.16 \pm 0.91$ mm). Conclusion: The results of this cohort study suggested that implants with tapered abutments perform successfully one year after loading and that they are associated with excellent marginal bone preservation, thus suggesting that implant-connection macro-geometry might have a crucial role in dictating peri-implant bone levels.

Keywords: bone loss; convergence; clinical study

1. Introduction

Long-term dental implant survival has been extensively documented under different conditions, so that contemporary clinical dentistry has been focusing on means to achieve predictable implant success. Most of the authors agree on the fact that minimal marginal bone loss should be observed one year within the implant loading, as this quantity is a predictor of the long-term implant survival and success [1]. The extent of post-loading bone remodeling has been mainly related to two different phenomena: (1) The microbial infiltration at the implant-abutment (IA) micro-gap—with consequent inflammation and bone demineralization [2]; (2) the implant-abutment (IA) design [3].

The most accounted risk factor for marginal bone loss has been long considered the inflammatory infiltrate at the IA gap [4]. The understanding of the complex biological events impacting the cervical bone surrounding submerged implants begun with the fundamental animal histometric study by Ericsson [5] who typified the inflammatory infiltrate as a consistent finding in matching IA interfaces. This circumscribed inflammation resulted in a round connective demarcation wall that ultimately leads to bone demineralization and resorption [2,6,7]. Different studies indicated less marginal bone resorption around mis-matching implants (implants with a platform switching connection—PS)—when compared to matching implants—as well as a different organization of the connective tissue fibers [8]. Several theories have been proposed to explain this clinical manifestation, such as the shifting of the inflammatory infiltrate away from the bone, the additional room for protective connective tissue proliferation, or, best, the creation of a geometrical stop for biological width apical establishment. In fact, in matching implants, the fixture first thread is also the first topographic point where the rehabilitation turns from a smaller to a wider diameter, creating a mechanical retention for connective tissues. In short, marginal bone loss should be inevitable, at least to this extent [9]. In PS implants, the implant-abutment discrepancy acts equally, but at a more coronal level—at the platform level—where the connective fibers are retained. It could be hypothesized that the rehabilitation macro-geometry dictates soft and hard tissue position, independent of the effect of the inflammatory infiltrate produced by the gap [10,11].

The gingivally convergent abutment was developed with the idea of maximizing the available space for soft tissues, which is occupied by the bulky metal shoulder in divergent abutments [12]. The sloping profile of gingival convergent abutments would allow tissue to slide coronally in the early phases of healing, creating a thick connective seal above the IA gap.

What is really bearing the brunt of preserving marginal bone levels? Is it either the relative location of the implant-abutment (IA) junction or is it the connection macro-geometry?

The specific aim of this cohort study was to investigate the clinical and radiological outcome of implants with a convergent implant-abutment connection one year after loading.

2. Materials and Methods

This study was a retrospective, non-interventional analysis of consecutive patients treated with dental implants with a gingivally convergent abutment connection (Shelta XA, Sweden & Martina, Via Veneto 19, 35020, Due Carrare, Padova, Italy). This study was based on patients consecutively treated on a routine basis at one specialistic center (BORG, Carrer de la Mare de Déu de Sales, 67 08840 Viladecans, Barcelona, Spain) during the period from 2016 to 2018.

2.1. Inclusion and Exclusion Criteria

The medical records of patients who had at least one two-part implant rehabilitated with a convergent abutment with a one-year follow-up were reviewed. Patients were included if presenting a complete set of follow-up radiographs and intra-oral digital photographs. All implants were placed at a slightly sub-crestal level. Patient records were excluded if they did not present for bi-annual follow-up visits, if they had been rehabilitated with overdentures or full-arch prosthesis or if the implants had been placed with simultaneous guided bone regeneration.

2.2. Data Collection and Analysis

Data were directly entered into an Excel spreadsheet and then converted to a .csv file format in order to be read by the software for statistical analysis. The following population describing the variables were collected: Age, gender, implant characteristics (diameter, length), implant location (tooth number and anterior/posterior, maxillary/ mandibular), type of implant-supported prosthetic restoration (single crown or partial bridge), and follow-up time.

2.3. Radiologic Marginal Bone Level Evaluation

Routine peri-apical radiographs obtained via the long-cone paralleling technique with a loop film holder (Rinn, Dentsply Australia Pty Ltd, Pacific Hwy, St Leonards NSW 2065, Australia) were used to measure the marginal bone levels. Radiographs were standardized by means of individual resin bites. The distance between the implant–abutment connection and the first bone-to-implant contact (fBIC) on mesial and distal surfaces was recorded. The scale was calibrated by the width of the dental implant achieving a unique pixel/mm ratio (Figure 1). Radiographic bone levels were calculated at the moment of prosthetic transfer connection (impression taking), at loading, and every six months after loading.

The mean marginal bone level for each implant was computed merging mesial and distal variations. The marginal bone change was defined as the difference between the last follow-up and the baseline MBL value, with negative values denoting a loss in bone height.

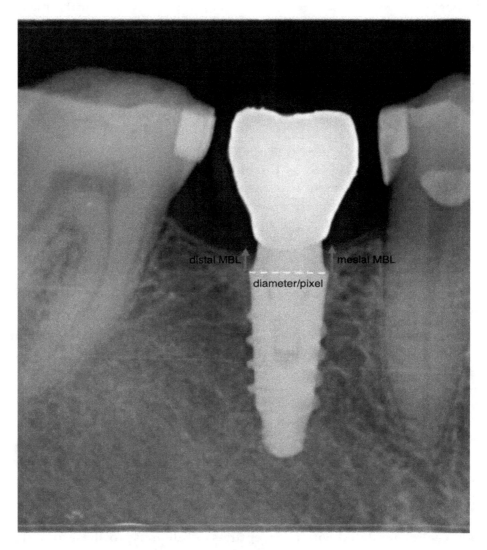

Figure 1. The picture is a schematic representation of the calibration performed on the software to achieve bone level linear measurements. The scale was set and calibrated by the width of the dental implant.

All measurements were performed by a single examiner (SM). The intra-examiner reproducibility was evaluated using the intraclass correlation analysis from the measurements in 10 patients, which revealed a strong correlation coefficient of 0.982 for MBL radiological measurements. Measurements were performed via the OsirisX software (Pixmeo SARL, 266 Rue de Bernex, CH-1233 Bernex, Switzerland).

2.4. Dichotomous Outcomes

- Implant failure was identified with eventual implant mobility or persistent infection, and whenever the implant presented signs and symptoms that led to the implant removal.
- Survival and success rates (SRs and CSRs, respectively) for implants, were calculated according to the criteria defined by Buser et al. in 1997 [13]. Successful implants were those showing a mean radiological peri-implant bone resorption within 1.5 mm during the first year of loading, and less than 0.2 mm/year during the following years.

2.5. Statistical Analysis

Descriptive and longitudinal statistics was performed on the R free software version 3.5.1 (02-07-2018). The longitudinal nonparametric analysis on marginal bone levels was implemented on the ld.f1 function within the package nparLD. This non-parametric method exhibits a competitive performance for small sample sizes and outliers. In the per-implant analysis, the ANOVA-type statistic (ATS) was calculated for the global alternatives with 'time' as the fixed su-plot factor. A p value < 0.05 has been used as a cut-off for significance and a robust analysis of variance and a Spearman's correlation coefficient has been performed. A further mixed effect model (function lmer within package lme4) was used to control for crossed random effects posed by patients contributing with more than one implant. This formula expects that there is going to be multiple responses per patient, and these responses will depend on each subject's baseline level. This effectively resolved the non-independence that stemmed from having multiple responses by the same subject.

3. Results

3.1. Study Population

In total, 20 patients received 36 implants. The mean age at the implant insertion was 56.2 ± 10.2 years (Table 1). Of the 20 patients, 65.0% were female and 35.0% were male. Of the 36 implants, 24 (66.6%) were placed in the maxilla and 12 (33.3%) were placed in the mandible. Implant diameters ranged from 3.8 mm to 5.0 mm—the mode being 4.2 mm diameter (70%)—and implant lengths ranged from 8.5 mm to 15 mm. Sixteen implants (44.4%) were splinted. Implants were more frequently placed in upper premolar positions (60%). Abutment heights ranged from 4 mm to 6 mm.

Table 1. Demographic data and clinical characteristics.

	Male	Female	Total
Number of Patients	7	13	20
Number of Implants	9	27	36
Mean Age			56.2 ± 10.2
Age Range			39–76

3.2. Survival and Adverse Events

At the last follow up, all 36 implants were healthy, stable and there were no reported failures; thus, the implant had a cumulative survival rate of 100%. No failure, defined as signs and symptoms that led to the implant removal, could be recorded. Therefore, the cumulative success rate was 100%. The average follow-up period was 1.5 years after loading.

3.3. Bone Levels

All the implants were radiographically examined by one author alien to the treatment procedure (SM) with the OsiriX DICOM viewer (Pixmeo SARL, 266 Rue de Bernex, CH-1233 Bernex, Switzerland).

The mean marginal bone level was +1.39 ± 0.91 mm at the moment of the prosthetic-transfer connection for definitive impression-taking (considered as the study baseline, Figure 2). One year after loading, the mean marginal bone level reached +1.16 ± 0.911 mm (Figure 2) with an average overall change of −0.18 ± 0.72 mm, occurring above the platform level at large (Figure 3). The change over time was significant (p value = 0.01) when the implant was modeled as the first cluster of analysis and the time was set as the only sub-plot factor (Table 2). The fitness of the model has been confirmed also with the mixed-effects model considering the random effect posed by patients contributing with more than one implant. The mean amount of bone resorption to be expected one year after loading was normally distributed (Figure 4).

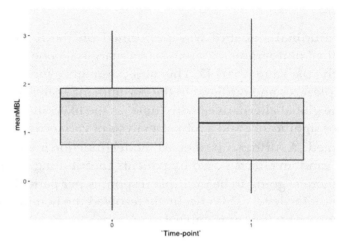

Figure 2. Box-plot of the mean marginal bone levels at the baseline and one year after loading.

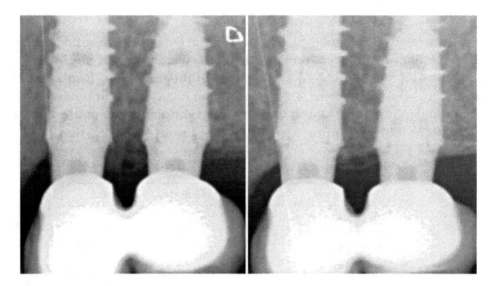

Figure 3. Radiographic appearance of the marginal bone levels at adjacent implants loaded with tapered abutment at loading (left) and one year after (right).

Table 2. Mean marginal bone level (MBL) in function by year, mm (per implant analysis) and statistical significance of time-effect according to the Behrens-Fisher test and the ANOVA results for implant-related factors.

Time-point	Mesial MBL	Distal MBL	Mean MBL	Delta MBL	*p*-value
Mean MBL in function by year, mm (per implant analysis) and statistical significance of time-effect.					
Overall					
Baseline	1.47 ± 0.87	1.30 ± 1.01	1.39 ± 0.91		
1-year	1.28 ± 0.98	1.04 ± 0.92	1.16 ± 0.91	−0.18 ± 0.72	0.01
Mandible					
Baseline	0.90 ± 0.76	0.55 ± 0.87	0.72 ± 0.77		
1-year	0.76 ± 0.67	0.47 ± 0.61	0.61 ± 0.60	−0.10 ± 0.29	0.19
Sub-plot factor analysis for "*Mandible* vs. *Maxilla* relative *treatment effect*" <MBL ~ jaw p-value 6.58×10^{-7}					
Maxilla					
Baseline	1.72 ± 0.81	1.63 ± 0.89	1.68 ± 0.72		
1-year	1.51 ± 1.02	1.29 ± 0.92	1.40 ± 0.93	−0.22 ± 0.84	0.06

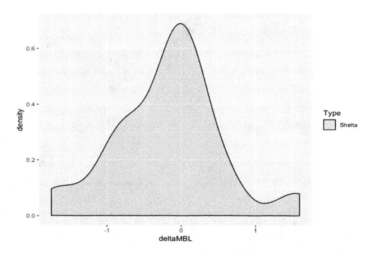

Figure 4. Density plot of the mean marginal bone change frequency distribution one year after loading in the entire cohort. The plot exquisitely shows a bell-shaped curve denoting a predictable amount of marginal bone resorption for the implant-abutment studied: most of the observations converged around zero.

The categorical data describing the implant-related factors and position (diameter, length, abutment height, jaw) were modeled on the multiway test. The implant diameter and length did not appear to affect the marginal bone, however, there was a relative significant effect given by the abutment height (p value < 0.05) in the mixed model: Longer abutments showed better marginal bone preservation at a one-year evaluation (Table 3). To investigate the question about which of the three abutment height categories differed, multiple comparisons with the Bonferroni adjustment were applied. The relationship held only for abutments longer than 5 mm; still, the linearity could not be confirmed.

Implants placed in the mandible and in the maxilla did not differ in terms of 1-year marginal bone loss, however, the first bone-to-implant contact at implants placed in the mandible was significantly lower than that of the maxilla most of the times (p value < 0.001).

Table 3. Mean marginal bone level (MBL) by implant abutment-height by year.

Sub-plot factor analysis for *"Abutment Height treatment effect"* <MBL ~ abutment height p-value 0.05					
Time-point	**mesial MBL**	**distal MBL**	**mean MBL**	**delta MBL**	***p*-value**
4 mm					
Baseline	1.31 ± 0.96	0.97 ± 0.98	1.15 ± 0.94		
1-year	1.08 ± 0.91	0.77 ± 1.03	0.93 ± 0.93	-0.20 ± 0.83	0.36
5 mm					
Baseline	1.54 ± 0.86	1.52 ± 1.03	1.53 ± 0.92		
1-year	1.34 ± 1.08	1.16 ± 0.86	1.25 ± 0.94	-0.20 ± 0.70	0.17
6 mm					
Baseline	1.80 ± 0.69	1.43 ± 0.80	1.62 ± 0.70		
1-year	1.87 ± 0.35	1.53 ± 0.56	1.70 ± 0.43	0.08 ± 0.34	0.05

3.4. Secondary Outcomes: Soft Tissues

Peri-implant soft tissues appeared healthy and thick at each visit after loading (Figure 5). At the provisional prosthesis loading, 96% and 95% of the 36 implants had a papilla index >2 for the mesial and distal side, respectively. At the last follow up, 97% and 94% of the implants had a papilla index >2 for the mesial and distal side, respectively.

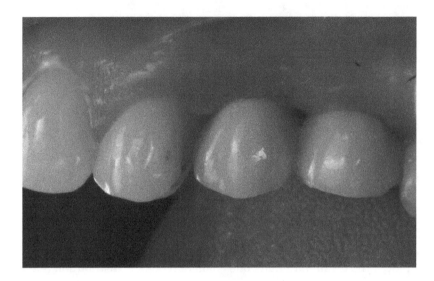

Figure 5. Clinical appearance of vestibular and inter-proximal soft tissues around adjacent implants loaded with tapered abutment.

4. Discussion

In the present study, the one-year healing around two-part implants with a gingival convergent abutment profile was evaluated. In 90% of the implants analyzed, the radiological bone level extended coronal to the IA border, at the abutment level. It is suggested that bone preservation may occur coronal to the IA connection of two-part implants loaded with convergent abutment profile as a consequence of advantageous macro-geometry, independent of the effect of the inflammatory infiltrate at the gap, and of the establishment of biologic width after prosthesis connection.

Results derived from animal studies showed that marginal bone resorption of about 2 mm occurred around two-part implants [14,15]. However, Welander et al. [16] suggested that osseointegration could occur coronal to the IA junction of two-part implants when the fixture was placed 2 mm sub-crestally.

A number of factors, according to prevalent literature, might influence the first-year marginal bone loss, such as neck configuration, surgical trauma, occlusal overload, mucositis, micro-gap colonization, biologic width formation, and flapless or flapped procedures [17–19]. The stability of the marginal bone levels might be determined by other factors, different from those acting during the healing phase. One of these factors is represented by the apico-coronal location of the implant head in respect to the bone crest [20]. In a recent systematic review, it was assessed that the effect of the sub-crestal implant positioning compared with equi-crestal position on the bone and soft tissues around dental implants with platform switching design: The authors reported that platform switch implants placed in a sub-crestal position had shown less marginal bone resorption when compared to implants placed with their head at the crest level [21].

The radiographic observation of post-loading bone remodeling generally coincided with the level of the first thread, and some authors suggested that this would be a consequence of the soft tissue's attempt to sit on top of the dental implant creating a mechanical protective seal [22].

Davarpanah [23] also observed that bone resorption around the implants placed at the supra-crestal level was less than that of the implants placed at the crestal level. However, it is true that when the thread is moved in a coronal direction, the implant platform is moved upward as well. For this reason, it would be impossible to demonstrate the relative influence of each contributing factor on bone resorption. Flores-Guillen et al. [24] compared submerged and trans mucosal platform switch implants and found that there were no differences at a five-year evaluation in terms of marginal bone loss achieving a mean value of −0.73 ± 0.81 mm. Therefore, the cumulative screening literature suggested that platform switching or, more in general, connection macro-geometry is more critical than the relative position of the platform crest module in determining early bone remodeling.

The recent systematic review by Messias et al. suggested that reporting the marginal bone change is insufficient for the correct evaluation of the implant performance: The authors recommended to report the crestal bone levels, in particular where no data is provided relative to the healing period [25]. Furthermore, reporting at which level the crestal bone is in an intimate contact with the implant seemed reasonable and more convenient for describing the effect of the IA macro-geometry on the marginal bone. In the present study, the overall bone change was -0.18 ± 0.72 mm one year after loading, occurring above the platform level, in any case. In fact, the one-year mean bone level was $+1.16 \pm 0.91$ mm with a significant difference between the lower and upper jaw. The mean bone gain from the baseline to the last follow-up occurred in 33.0% of the implants analyzed, which is twice the frequency observed by Flores-Guillen et al. in the platform switch implants in the same given period [24].

Few studies evaluated the tissue response around the tapered convergent abutments [26]. The use of the tapered abutments, not only could improve the peri-implant bone level, but also diminish the sulcus length. In fact, it has been suggested that the biological phenomenon of the peri-implant bone preservation would be related with the circular connective tissue fibers stabilization around the abutment and the presence of a shallow sulcus [27]. In the present study, the cumulative implant success rate was 100%, with no implant showing any sign or symptom of mucositis or prosthetic complication. Peri-implant mucosa appeared healthy-pink, thick, and firm at each visit after loading. The plausible biologic explanation should be sought in the wound healing process that starts after the abutment connection: The convergent abutment would create a housing effect that protects the surrounding biological structures maintaining tissue stability over time.

The multiway analysis conducted on this study displayed a significant relative effect of the abutment height on the marginal bone loss: Implants with longer abutments (>5 mm) appeared to have minimal bone resorption. It has been hypothesized that an abutment with a height <2 mm does not provide sufficient soft tissue for establishing the peri-implant biologic width [28]. The establishment of the peri-implant biologic width follows the implant placement and connective tissue attachment to the abutment. Long abutments might be associated with a thicker gingival biotype, which in turn would be more effective at preventing inflammatory infiltration.

The present cohort study has different limitations that should be taken into account. First, the study design was retrospective, and a single-cohort, thus reducing the meaningfulness and external validity of the results. The implant was chosen as the first cluster of analysis which does not guarantee independence between implants, however the mixed effect model applied took the random effect posed by patients into account, not revealing any significant discrepancy with the fixed effect model. It must be remarked that the radiographic artifact of a stable first bone-to-implant contact does not necessarily imply histologic osseo-integration. However, the imaging accuracy of digital radiography is high with a precision of 0.1 mm or less. Still, the clinical relevance of such small entities is questionable and difficult to repeat among different operators [29]. Furthermore, the present study is a single cohort study without an internal control group.

5. Conclusions

Overall, the present study showed that implants rehabilitated with tapered abutments yielded excellent hard- and soft-tissue outcomes. In particular, after one year of loading, marginal bone levels consistently appeared above the implant platform, at the abutment level, with minimal bone change. It was suggested that the implant-connection macro-geometry might dictate peri-implant bone levels. Therefore, further prospective randomized trials are strongly recommended to support the present findings.

Author Contributions: All of the authors contributed with the investigation, supervision, writing, review, and editing of the study. The study conceptualization must be acknowledged to S.M., U.C., E.M., X.V., and X.R. Data curation, data visualization, and analysis must be acknowledged to S.M., E.G., X.V., and X.R.

References

1. Oh, T.J.; Yoon, J.; Misch, C.E.; Wang, H.L. The causes of early implant bone loss: Myth or science? *J. Periodontol.* **2002**, *73*, 322–333. [CrossRef] [PubMed]

2. Piattelli, A.; Vrespa, G.; Petrone, G.; Iezzi, G.; Annibali, S.; Scarano, A. Role of the micro-gap between implant and abutment: A retrospective histologic evaluation in monkeys. *J. Periodontol.* **2003**, *74*, 346–352. [CrossRef] [PubMed]

3. Jung, Y.C.; Han, C.H.; Lee, K.W. A 1-year radiographic evaluation of marginal bone around dental implants. *Int. J. Oral Maxillofac. Implants* **1996**, *11*, 811–818. [PubMed]

4. Astrand, P.; Engquist, B.; Dahlgren, S.; Gröndahl, K.; Engquist, E.; Feldmann, H. Astra Tech and Brånemark system implants: A 5-year prospective study of marginal bone reactions. *Clin. Oral Implant. Res.* **2004**, *15*, 413–420. [CrossRef] [PubMed]

5. Ericsson, I.; Persson, L.G.; Berglundh, T.; Marinello, C.P.; Lindhe, J.; Klinge, B. Different types of inflammatory reactions in peri-implant soft tissues. *J. Clin. Periodontol.* **1995**, *22*, 255–261. [CrossRef] [PubMed]

6. Canullo, L.; Quaranta, A.; Teles, R.P. The microbiota associated with implants restored with platform switching: A preliminary report. *J. Periodontol.* **2010**, *81*, 403–411. [CrossRef] [PubMed]

7. Canullo, L.; Pellegrini, G.; Allievi, C.; Trombelli, L.; Annibali, S.; Dellavia, C. Soft tissues around long-term platform switching implant restorations: A histological human evaluation. Preliminary results. *J. Clin. Periodontol.* **2011**, *38*, 86–94. [CrossRef]

8. Buser, D.; Wittneben, J.; Bornstein, M.M.; Grütter, L.; Chappuis, V.; Belser, U.C. Stability of contour augmentation and esthetic outcomes of implant-supported single crowns in the esthetic zone: 3-year results of a prospective study with early implant placement postextraction. *J. Periodontol.* **2011**, *82*, 342–349. [CrossRef]

9. Östman, P.O.; Hellman, M.; Sennerby, L. Ten years later. Results from a prospective single-centre clinical study on 121 oxidized (TiUnite™) Brånemark implants in 46 patients. *Clin. Implant Dent. Relat. Res.* **2012**, *14*, 852–860. [CrossRef]

10. Finelle, G.; Papadimitriou, D.E.V.; Souza, A.B.; Katebi, N.; Gallucci, G.O.; Araújo, M.G. Peri-implant soft tissue and marginal bone adaptation on implant with non-matching healing abutments: Micro-CT analysis. *Clin. Oral Implant. Res.* **2015**, *26*, e42–e46. [CrossRef]

11. Rodríguez, X.; Navajas, A.; Vela, X.; Fortuño, A.; Jimenez, J.; Nevins, M. Arrangement of Peri-implant Connective Tissue Fibers Around Platform-Switching Implants with Conical Abutments and Its Relationship to the Underlying Bone: A Human Histologic Study. *Int. J. Periodontics Restor. Dent.* **2016**, *36*, 533–540.

12. Canullo, L.; Tallarico, M.; Pradies, G.; Marinotti, F.; Loi, I.; Cocchetto, R. Soft and hard tissue response to an implant with a convergent collar in the esthetic area: Preliminary report at 18 months. *Int. J. Esthet. Dent.* **2017**, *12*, 306–323. [PubMed]

13. Buser, D.; Mericske-Stern, R.; Bernard, J.P.; Behneke, A.; Behneke, N.; Hirt, H.P.; Belser, U.C.; Lang, N.P. Long-term evaluation of non-submerged ITI implants. Part 1: 8-year life table analysis of a prospective multi-center study with 2359 implants. *Clin. Oral Implant. Res.* **1997**, *8*, 161–172. [CrossRef]

14. Hermann, J.S.; Cochran, D.L.; Nummikoski, P.V.; Buser, D. Crestal bone changes around titanium implants. A radiographic evaluation of unloaded nonsubmerged and submerged implants in the canine mandible. *J. Periodontol.* **1997**, *68*, 1117–1130. [CrossRef] [PubMed]

15. Hermann, J.S.; Schoolfield, J.D.; Schenk, R.K.; Buser, D.; Cochran, D.L. Influence of the size of the microgap on crestal bone changes around titanium implants. A histometric evaluation of unloaded non-submerged implants in the canine mandible. *J. Periodontol.* **2001**, *72*, 1372–1383. [CrossRef] [PubMed]

16. Welander, M.; Abrahamsson, I.; Berglundh, T. The mucosal barrier at implant abutments of different materials. *Clin. Oral Implant. Res.* **2008**, *19*, 635–641.

17. Qian, J.; Wennerberg, A.; Albrektsson, T. Reasons for marginal bone loss around oral implants. *Clin. Implant. Dent. Relat. Res.* **2012**, *14*, 792–807. [CrossRef]

18. Sanz-Sánchez, I.; Sanz-Martín, I.; Carrillo de Albornoz, A.; Figuero, E.; Sanz, M. Biological effect of the abutment material on the stability of peri-implant marginal bone levels: A systematic review and meta-analysis. *Clin. Oral Implant. Res.* **2018**, *29* (Suppl. 18), 124–144. [CrossRef]

19. Albrektsson, T.; Buser, D.; Sennerby, L. Crestal bone loss and oral implants. *Clin. Implant. Dent. Relat. Res.* **2012**, *14*, 783–791. [CrossRef]

20. Schwarz, F.; Hegewald, A.; Becker, J. Impact of implant-abutment connection and positioning of the machined collar/microgap on crestal bone level changes: A systematic review. *Clin. Oral Implant. Res.* **2014**, *225*, 417–425. [CrossRef]

21. Valles, C.; Rodríguez-Ciurana, X.; Clementini, M.; Baglivo, M.; Paniagua, B.; Nart, J. Influence of subcrestal implant placement compared with equicrestal position on the peri-implant hard and soft tissues around platform-switched implants: A systematic review and meta-analysis. *Clin. Oral Investig.* **2018**, *22*, 555–570. [CrossRef] [PubMed]

22. Khayat, P.G.; Hallage, P.G.; Toledo, R.A. An investigation of 131 consecutively placed wide screw-vent implants. *Int. J. Oral Maxillofac. Implant.* **2001**, *16*, 827–832.

23. Davarpanah, M.; Martinez, H.; Tecucianu, J.F. Apical-coronal implant position: Recent surgical proposals. Technical note. *Int. J. Oral Maxillofac. Implant.* **2000**, *15*, 865–872.

24. Flores-Guillen, J.; Álvarez-Novoa, C.; Barbieri, G.; Martín, C.; Sanz, M. Five-year outcomes of a randomized clinical trial comparing bone-level implants with either submerged or transmucosal healing. *J. Clin. Periodontol.* **2018**, *45*, 125–135. [CrossRef] [PubMed]

25. Messias, A.; Nicolau, P.; Guerra, F. Titanium dental implants with different collar design and surface modifications: A systematic review on survival rates and marginal bone levels. *Clin. Oral Implant. Res.* **2019**, *30*, 20–48. [CrossRef] [PubMed]

26. Cocchetto, R.; Canullo, L. The "hybrid abutment": A new design for implant cemented restorations in the esthetic zones. *Int. J. Esthet. Dent.* **2015**, *10*, 186–208. [PubMed]

27. Rodríguez-Ciurana, X.; Vela-Nebot, X.; Segalà-Torres, M.; Calvo-Guirado, J.L.; Cambra, J.; Méndez-Blanco, V.; Tarnow, D.P. The effect of interimplant distance on the height of the interimplant bone crest when using platform-switched implants. *Int. J. Periodontics Restor. Dent.* **2008**, *29*, 141–151.

28. Galindo-Moreno, P.; León-Cano, A.; Ortega-Oller, I.; Monje, A.; Suárez, F.; ÓValle, F.; Spinato, S.; Catena, A. Prosthetic Abutment Height is a Key Factor in Peri-implant Marginal Bone Loss. *J. Dent. Res.* **2014**, *93*, 80S–85S. [CrossRef]

29. De Bruyn, H.; Vandeweghe, S.; Ruyffelaert, C.; Cosyn, J.; Sennerby, L. Radiographic evaluation of modern oral implants with emphasis on crestal bone level and relevance to peri-implant health. *Periodontol 2000*, **2000**, *62*, 256–270. [CrossRef]

Permissions

All chapters in this book were first published by MDPI; hereby published with permission under the Creative Commons Attribution License or equivalent. Every chapter published in this book has been scrutinized by our experts. Their significance has been extensively debated. The topics covered herein carry significant findings which will fuel the growth of the discipline. They may even be implemented as practical applications or may be referred to as a beginning point for another development.

The contributors of this book come from diverse backgrounds, making this book a truly international effort. This book will bring forth new frontiers with its revolutionizing research information and detailed analysis of the nascent developments around the world.

We would like to thank all the contributing authors for lending their expertise to make the book truly unique. They have played a crucial role in the development of this book. Without their invaluable contributions this book wouldn't have been possible. They have made vital efforts to compile up to date information on the varied aspects of this subject to make this book a valuable addition to the collection of many professionals and students.

This book was conceptualized with the vision of imparting up-to-date information and advanced data in this field. To ensure the same, a matchless editorial board was set up. Every individual on the board went through rigorous rounds of assessment to prove their worth. After which they invested a large part of their time researching and compiling the most relevant data for our readers.

The editorial board has been involved in producing this book since its inception. They have spent rigorous hours researching and exploring the diverse topics which have resulted in the successful publishing of this book. They have passed on their knowledge of decades through this book. To expedite this challenging task, the publisher supported the team at every step. A small team of assistant editors was also appointed to further simplify the editing procedure and attain best results for the readers.

Apart from the editorial board, the designing team has also invested a significant amount of their time in understanding the subject and creating the most relevant covers. They scrutinized every image to scout for the most suitable representation of the subject and create an appropriate cover for the book.

The publishing team has been an ardent support to the editorial, designing and production team. Their endless efforts to recruit the best for this project, has resulted in the accomplishment of this book. They are a veteran in the field of academics and their pool of knowledge is as vast as their experience in printing. Their expertise and guidance has proved useful at every step. Their uncompromising quality standards have made this book an exceptional effort. Their encouragement from time to time has been an inspiration for everyone.

The publisher and the editorial board hope that this book will prove to be a valuable piece of knowledge for researchers, students, practitioners and scholars across the globe.

List of Contributors

Sergio Alexandre Gehrke
Biotecnos Research Center, Montevideo 11100, Uruguay
Department of Biotechnology, Catholic University of Murcia, 30107 Murcia, Spain

Raphaél Bettach
Department of Cariology and Comprehensive Care, New York University, New York, NY 10010, USA
77220 Gretz-Armainvilliers, France

Benoit Cayron
37000 Tours, France

Gilles Boukhris
75012 Paris, France

Berenice Anina Dedavid
Department of Materials Engineering, Pontificial Catholic University of Rio Grande do Sul, Porto Alegre 90619-900, Brazil

Juan Carlos Prados Frutos
Department of Medicine and Surgery, Faculty of Health Sciences, Rey Juan Carlos University, 28933 Madrid, Spain

Diego Lops, Alessandro Rossi, Antonino Palazzolo and Eugenio Romeo
Department of Prosthodontics, School of Dentistry, University of Milan, 20142 Milan, Italy

Riccardo Guazzo and Luca Sbricoli
Department of Neurosciences, University of Padua, 35121 Padua, Italy

Vittorio Favero
Section of Dentistry and Maxillofacial Surgery, Department of Surgery, University of Verona, 37134 Verona, Italy

Mattia Manfredini
Department of Oral Surgery, Fondazione Policlinico Ca' Granda, 20141 Milan, Italy

Lyly Sam and Pathawee Khongkhunthian
Center of Excellence for Dental Implantology, Faculty of Dentistry, Chiang Mai University, Chiang Mai 50200, Thailand

Siriporn Chattipakorn
Department of Oral Biology and Diagnostic Sciences, Faculty of Dentistry, Chiang Mai University, Chiang Mai 50200, Thailand

Iulia Roatesi
Department of Histology and Cytology, Dental Medicine Faculty, Carol Davila University of Medicine and Pharmacy, 050474 Bucharest, Romania

Simona Roatesi
Department of Applied Informatics, Ferdinand I Military Technical Academy, 050141 Bucharest, Romania

Thaiz Carrera-Arrabal, Fabricio Passador-Santos, Carlos Eduardo Sorgi da Costa, Frank Róger Teles Costa, Antonio Carlos Aloise, Marcelo Henrique Napimoga and André Antonio Pelegrine
Faculdade São Leopoldo Mandic, Instituto de Pesquisas São Leopoldo Mandic, Campinas 13045-755, Brazil

José Luis Calvo-Guirado
Department of Oral and Implant Surgery, Faculty of Health Sciences, Universidad Católica San Antonio de Murcia (UCAM), 30002 Murcia, Spain

Juan Manuel Aragoneses
Department of Dental Research in Universidad Federico Henríquez y Carvajal (UFHEC), Santo Domingo 10107, Dominican Republic

Pietro Montemezzi, Francesco Ferrini, Enrico Gherlone and Paolo Capparè
Dental School, Vita-Salute San Raffaele University, 20132 Milan, Italy
Department of Dentistry, IRCCS San Raffaele Hospital, 20132 Milan, Italy

Giuseppe Pantaleo
UniSR-Social.Lab (Research Methods), Faculty of Psychology, Vita-Salute San Raffaele University, 20132 Milan, Italy

Nak-Hyun Choi and Eun-Jin Park
Department of Prosthodontics, School of Medicine, Ewha Womans University, Seoul 07985, Korea

Hyung-In Yoon
Department of Prosthodontics, School of Dentistry and Dental Research Institute, Seoul National University, Seoul 03080, Korea

Tae-Hyung Kim
Kim and Lee Dental Clinic, Seoul 06626, Korea

Annalena Bethke and Manja von Stein-Lausnitz
Department of Prosthodontics, Geriatric Dentistry and Craniomandibular Disorders, Charité—Universitätsmedizin Berlin, corporate member of Freie Universität Berlin, Humboldt-Universität zu Berlin, and Berlin Institute of Health, Aßmannshauser Str. 4-6, 14197 Berlin, Germany

Stefano Pieralli, Felix Burkhardt and Benedikt Christopher Spies
Department of Prosthodontics, Geriatric Dentistry and Craniomandibular Disorders, Charité—Universitätsmedizin Berlin, corporate member of Freie Universität Berlin, Humboldt-Universität zu Berlin, and Berlin Institute of Health, Aßmannshauser Str. 4-6, 14197 Berlin, Germany
Department of Prosthetic Dentistry, Faculty of Medicine, Center for Dental Medicine, Medical Center—University of Freiburg, Hugstetter Str. 55, 79106 Freiburg, Germany

Ralf-Joachim Kohal
Department of Prosthetic Dentistry, Faculty of Medicine, Center for Dental Medicine, Medical Center—University of Freiburg, Hugstetter Str. 55, 79106 Freiburg, Germany

Kirstin Vach
Institute of Medical Biometry and Statistics, Faculty of Medicine, Medical Center—University of Freiburg, University of Freiburg, Stefan-Meier-Str. 26, 79104 Freiburg, Germany

Jun-Beom Lee, Yang-Jo Seol, Yong-Moo Lee, Young Ku and In-Chul Rhyu
Department of Periodontology, Seoul National University School of Dentistry, Seoul 03080, Korea

Ye-Hyeon Jo and In-Sung Luke Yeo
Department of Prosthodontics, School of Dentistry and Dental Research Institute, Seoul National University, Seoul 03080, Korea

Jung-Yoo Choi
Dental Research Institute, Seoul National University, Seoul 03080, Korea

Adrien Naveau
Department of Prosthodontics, Dental Science Faculty, University of Bordeaux, 33000 Bordeaux, France
Dental and Periodontal Rehabilitation Unit, Saint Andre Hospital, Bordeaux University Hospital, 33000 Bordeaux, France

Kouhei Shinmyouzu
Department of Oral Implants, Kyushu Dental University, Kitakyushu, Fukuoka 803-8580, Japan

Tanpopo Dental Clinic, Nerima ward, Tokyo 178-0062, Japan

Colman Moore
Department of Nano Engineering, University of California San Diego, La Jolla, CA 92093, USA

Limor Avivi-Arber
Faculty of Dentistry, University of Toronto, Toronto M5G1G6, ON M5G 1G6, Canada

Jesse Jokerst
Department of Nano Engineering, University of California San Diego, La Jolla, CA 92093, USA
Materials Science Program, University of California San Diego, La Jolla, CA 92093, USA
Department of Radiology, University of California San Diego, La Jolla, CA 92093, USA

Sreenivas Koka
Private practice, Koka Dental Clinic, San Diego, CA 92111, USA
Advanced Prosthodontics, Loma Linda University School of Dentistry, Loma Linda, CA 92350, USA
Advanced Prosthodontics, University of California Los Angeles School of Dentistry, Los Angeles, CA 90095, USA

Teresa Lombardi
Private Practice, 87011 Cassano allo Ionio, Italy

Federico Berton, Antonio Rapani, Francesca Piovesana, Giulia Barbati, Roberto Di Lenarda and Claudio Stacchi
Department of Medical, Surgical and Health Sciences, University of Trieste, 34129 Trieste, Italy

Stefano Salgarello
Department of Medical and Surgical Specialties, Radiological Sciences and Public Health, University of Brescia, 25123 Brescia, Italy

Erika Barbalonga
Private Practice, 6600 Locarno, Switzerland

Caterina Gregorio
Department of Statistics, University of Padova, 35121 Padova, Italy

Pierluigi Coli
Edinburgh Dental Specialists, Edinburgh EH2 4BA, UK

Lars Sennerby
Edinburgh Dental Specialists, Edinburgh EH2 4BA, UK
Department of Maxillofacial Surgery, University of Gothenburg, 413 90 Gothenburg, Sweden

Xingting Han, Sebastian Spintzyk, Lutz Scheideler, Ping Li, Jürgen Geis-Gerstorfer and Frank Rupp
Section Medical Materials Science and Technology, University Hospital Tübingen, Osianderstr. 2–8, D-72076 Tübingen, Germany

Dong Yang, Chuncheng Yang and Dichen Li
State Key Laboratory for Manufacturing System Engineering, School of Mechanical Engineering, Xi'an Jiaotong University, Xi'an 710054, China

Markus Schlee
Department of Maxillofacial Surgery, Goethe University, 60590 Frankfurt am Main, Germany

Florian Rathe
Department of Prosthodontics, Danube University, 3500 Krems, Austria

Urs Brodbeck
Private Practice, 8051 Zürich, Switzerland

Christoph Ratka, Paul Weigl and Holger Zipprich
Department of Prosthodontics, Goethe University, 60590 Frankfurt am Main, Germany

Ron Doornewaard, Maarten Glibert, Carine Matthys and Stijn Vervaeke
Department Periodontology & Oral Implantology, Dental School, Faculty Medicine and Health Sciences, Ghent University, De Pintelaan 185, 9000 Ghent, Belgium

Ewald Bronkhorst
Section Implantology & Periodontology, Department of Dentistry, Radboudumc, Philips van Leydenlaan 25, 6525 EX Nijmegen, The Netherlands

Hugo de Bruyn
Department Periodontology & Oral Implantology, Dental School, Faculty Medicine and Health Sciences, Ghent University, De Pintelaan 185, 9000 Ghent, Belgium
Section Implantology & Periodontology, Department of Dentistry, Radboudumc, Philips van Leydenlaan 25, 6525 EX Nijmegen, The Netherlands

Rune J. Christiansen
Department of Mechanical Engineering, Technical University of Denmark, DK-2800 Kgs. Lyngby, Denmark

Department of Immunology and Microbiology, University of Copenhagen, DK-2200 Copenhagen, Denmark

Henrik J. Münch, Kjeld Søballe and Stig S. Jakobsen
Institute of Clinical Medicine—Orthopedic Surgery, Aarhus University, DK-8000 Aarhus C, Denmark

Charlotte M. Bonefeld and Carsten Geisler
Department of Immunology and Microbiology, University of Copenhagen, DK-2200 Copenhagen, Denmark

Jacob P. Thyssen
Institute of Clinical Medicine, Copenhagen University, Gentofte Hospital, DK-2900 Hellerup, Denmark

Jens J. Sloth
National Food Institute, Research Group on Nanobio Science, Technical University of Denmark, DK-2860 Søborg, Denmark

Morten S. Jellesen
Department of Mechanical Engineering, Technical University of Denmark, DK-2800 Kgs. Lyngby, Denmark

Simone Marconcini and Ugo Covani
Department of Surgical, Medical, Molecular and Critical Area Pathology, University of Pisa, 56124 Pisa, Italy

Enrica Giammarinaro
Tuscan Dental Institute, Versilia General Hospital, 55041 Lido di Camaiore, Italy

Eitan Mijiritsky
Department of Otolaryngology Head and Neck Surgery and Maxillofacial Surgery, Tel-Aviv Sourasky Medical Center, Sackler School of Medicine, 61503 Tel Aviv, Israel

Xavier Vela
Department of Maxillofacial Surgery and Implantology, International University of Catalunya, 08001 Barcelona, Spain

Xavier Rodríguez
Department of Oral Implantology, European University of Madrid, 28001 Madrid, Spain

Index

Printed in the USA
CPSIA information can be obtained
at www.ICGtesting.com
JSHW051400091023
49903JS00006B/222